Quality Improvement

Editors

HEATHER C. KAPLAN
MUNISH GUPTA

CLINICS IN PERINATOLOGY

www.perinatology.theclinics.com

Consulting Editor
LUCKY JAIN

June 2023 • Volume 50 • Number 2

ELSEVIER

1600 John F. Kennedy Boulevard • Suite 1800 • Philadelphia, Pennsylvania, 19103-2899

http://www.theclinics.com

CLINICS IN PERINATOLOGY Volume 50, Number 2
June 2023 ISSN 0095-5108, ISBN-13: 978-0-323-96050-2

Editor: Kerry Holland
Developmental Editor: Karen Justine S. Dino

Clinics in Perinatology (ISSN 0095-5108) is published quarterly by Elsevier Inc., 360 Park Avenue South, New York, NY 10010-1710. Months of issue are March, June, September, and December. Business and Editorial Offices: 1600 John F. Kennedy Blvd., Ste. 1800, Philadelphia, PA 19103-2899. Customer Service Office: 3251 Riverport Lane, Maryland Heights, MO 63043. Periodicals postage paid at New York, NY and additional mailing offices. Subscription prices are $341.00 per year (US individuals), $713.00 per year (US institutions), $387.00 per year (Canadian individuals), $872.00 per year (Canadian institutions), $461.00 per year (international individuals), $872.00 per year (international institutions), $100.00 per year (US and Canadian students), and $195.00 per year (International students). International air speed delivery is included in all Clinics subscription prices. All prices are subject to change without notice. **POSTMASTER:** Send address changes to *Clinics in Perinatology*, Elsevier Health Sciences Division, Subscription Customer Service, 3251 Riverport Lane, Maryland Heights, MO 63043. **Customer Service: Telephone: 1-800-654-2452** (U.S. and Canada); **1-314-447-8871** (outside U.S. and Canada). **Fax: 1-314-447-8029. E-mail: journalscustomerservice-usa@elsevier.com** (for print support); **journalsonlinesupport-usa@elsevier.com** (for online support).

Reprints. For copies of 100 or more, of articles in this publication, please contact the Commercial Reprints Department, Elsevier Inc., 360 Park Avenue South, New York, NY 10010-1710. Tel. 212-633-3874; Fax: 212-633-3820; E-mail: reprints@elsevier.com.

Clinics in Perinatology is also published in Spanish by McGraw-Hill Interamericana Editores S.A., P.O. Box 5-237, 06500 Mexico D.F., Mexico.

Clinics in Perinatology is covered in *MEDLINE/PubMed (Index Medicus) Current Contents, Excepta Medica, BIOSIS* and *ISI/BIOMED.*

Contributors

CONSULTING EDITOR

LUCKY JAIN, MD, MBA
George W. Brumley Jr Professor and Chairman, Emory University School of Medicine, Department of Pediatrics; Chief Academic Officer, Children's Healthcare of Atlanta; Executive Director, Emory + Children's Pediatric Institute, Atlanta, Georgia, USA

EDITORS

HEATHER C. KAPLAN, MD, MSCE
Associate Professor, Department of Pediatrics, University of Cincinnati College of Medicine, Perinatal Institute, James M. Anderson Center for Health Systems Excellence, Cincinnati Children's Hospital Medical Center, Cincinnati, Ohio, USA

MUNISH GUPTA, MD, MMSc
Assistant Professor in Pediatrics, Harvard Medical School, Beth Israel Deaconess Medical Center, Boston, Massachusetts, USA

AUTHORS

ANNA AXELIN, RN, PhD
Associate Professor, Department of Nursing Science, University of Turku, Turku, Finland

FABIANA BACCHINI, MSc, BJ
Executive Director, Canadian Premature Babies Foundation, Etobicoke, Ontario, Canada

CHAIM M. BELL, MD, PhD
Professor, University of Toronto, Physician in Chief, Sinai Health System, Toronto, Ontario, Canada

SANDHYA S. BRACHIO, MD
Assistant Professor of Pediatrics, Division of Neonatology, Department of Pediatrics, Columbia University Vagelos College of Physicians and Surgeons, New York, New York, USA

JENNIFER CALLAGHAN-KORU, PhD, MHS
Associate Professor, Department of Internal Medicine, University of Arkansas for Medical Sciences, Fayetteville, Arkansas, USA

LEAH H. CARR, MD
Assistant Professor Pediatrics, Division of Neonatology, Department of Pediatrics, Department of Biomedical and Health Informatics, Children's Hospital of Philadelphia, Children's Hospital of Philadelphia Newborn Care at the Hospital of the University of Pennsylvania, Department of Pediatrics, University of Pennsylvania Perelman School of Medicine, Philadelphia, Pennsylvania, USA

LORI CHRIST, MD
Associate Professor of Pediatrics, Division of Neonatology, Department of Pediatrics, Children's Hospital of Philadelphia, Children's Hospital of Philadelphia Newborn Care at the Hospital of the University of Pennsylvania, Department of Pediatrics, University of Pennsylvania Perelman School of Medicine, Philadelphia, Pennsylvania, USA

KATHERINE COUGHLIN, MD
Sharp Mary Birch Hospital for Women and Newborns, San Diego, California, USA

BYRON CROWE, MD
Department of Medicine, Beth Israel Deaconess Medical Center, Boston, Massachusetts, USA

GEOFFREY CURRAN, PhD
Professor, Department of Pharmacy Practice, University of Arkansas for Medical Sciences, Little Rock, Arkansas, USA

ERIKA EDWARDS, PhD, MPH
Vermont Oxford Network, Department of Pediatrics, Robert Larner, MD, College of Medicine, University of Vermont, Department of Mathematics and Statistics, College of Engineering and Mathematical Sciences, University of Vermont, Burlington, Vermont, USA

DANIELLE EHRET, MD, MPH
Associate Professor, Pediatrics, Asfaw Yemiru Green and Gold Professor, Global Health, University of Vermont, Larner College of Medicine, Chief Medical Officer and Director of Global Health, Vermont Oxford Network, Burlington, Vermont, USA

AZADEH FARZIN, MD, MHS
Attending Neonatologist, Pediatrix of Maryland/Adventist Healthcare, Rockville, Maryland, USA

DARIA F. FERRO, MD
Assistant Professor, Department of Pediatrics, University of Pennsylvania Perelman School of Medicine, Division of General Pediatrics, Department of Pediatrics, Department of Biomedical and Health Informatics, Children's Hospital of Philadelphia, Center for Pediatric Research, Philadelphia, Pennsylvania, USA

LINDA S. FRANCK, RN, PhD, FRCPCH, FAAN
Professor and Chair in Pediatric Nursing, Department of Family Health Care Nursing, University of California San Francisco, San Francisco, California, USA

JESSICA GAULTON, MD, MPH
Department of Neonatology, Beth Israel Deaconess Medical Center, Boston, Massachusetts, USA

WENDI GU, MD
Postdoctoral Fellow, Division of Neonatology, Department of Pediatrics, Columbia University Vagelos College of Physicians and Surgeons, New York, New York, USA

MUNISH GUPTA, MD, MMSc
Assistant Professor in Pediatrics, Harvard Medical School, Beth Israel Deaconess Medical Center, Boston, Massachusetts, USA

LOUIS P. HALAMEK, MD
Professor, Division of Neonatal and Developmental Medicine, Department of Pediatrics, Stanford University, Palo Alto, California, USA

LEON DUPREE HATCH III, MD, MPH
Associate Professor, Department of Pediatrics, Division of Neonatology, Faculty, Center for Child Health Policy, Critical Illness, Brain Dysfunction, and Survivorship Center, Vanderbilt University Medical Center, Nashville, Tennessee, USA

BEENA D. KAMATH-RAYNE, MD, MPH
Vice President, Global Newborn and Child Health, American Academy of Pediatrics, Itasca, Illinois, USA

HEATHER C. KAPLAN, MD, MSCE
Associate Professor, Department of Pediatrics, University of Cincinnati College of Medicine, Perinatal Institute, James M. Anderson Center for Health Systems Excellence, Cincinnati Children's Hospital Medical Center, Cincinnati, Ohio, USA

ASHISH KC, MBBS, MHCM, PhD
Associate Professor, Global Health, Sahlgrenska Academy, School of Public Health and Community Medicine, Gothenburg University, Gothenburg, Sweden; Department of Women's and Children Health, Uppsala University, Uppsala, Sweden

BRIAN KING, MD
Assistant Professor, Newborn Medicine, Department of Pediatrics, University of Pittsburgh School of Medicine, Pittsburgh, Pennsylvania, USA

KATELIN P. KRAMER, MS, MD
Department of Pediatrics, University of California, San Francisco, Benioff Children's Hospital, San Francisco, California, USA

MELISSA LIEBOWITZ, MD
Envision Physician Services, St. Francis Hospital, Colorado Springs, Colorado, USA

NINA MENDA, MD, MHQS
Department of Pediatrics, University of Wisconsin-Madison, Madison, Wisconsin, USA

RAVI M. PATEL, MD, MSc
Associate Professor of Pediatrics, Emory University School of Medicine, Children's Healthcare of Atlanta, Atlanta, Georgia, USA

MICHAEL A. POSENCHEG, MD
Chief Medical Officer and Vice President, Penn Presbyterian Medical Center, Professor of Clinical Pediatrics, Perelman School of Medicine at the University of Pennsylvania, Neonatologist, The Children's Hospital of Philadelphia, Philadelphia, Pennsylvania, USA

LLOYD P. PROVOST, MS
Associates in Process Improvement, Austin, Texas, USA

ROHIT RAMASWAMY, PhD, MPH
Professor of Pediatrics, Cincinnati Children's Medical Center Hospital, Cincinnati, Ohio, USA

ERICK RIDOUT, MD
Fellow, American Academy of Pediatrics, St George, Utah, USA

ELIZABETH E. ROGERS, MD
Department of Pediatrics, University of California, San Francisco, Benioff Children's Hospital, San Francisco, California, USA

ASAPH ROLNITSKY, MSc HQ, MD
DAN Women and Babies Program, Associate Director, Newborn and Developmental Paediatrics, Assistant Professor, University of Toronto, Sunnybrook Health Sciences Centre, Toronto, Ontario, Canada

LISA SAIMAN, MD, MPH
Professor of Pediatrics, Division of Pediatric Infectious Diseases, Department of Pediatrics, Columbia University Vagelos College of Physicians and Surgeons, Department of Infection Prevention and Control, NewYork-Presbyterian Hospital, New York, New York, USA

LAUREN A. SANLORENZO, MD, MPH
Assistant Professor, Department of Pediatrics, Division of Neonatology, Columbia University Irving Medical Center, New York, New York, USA

JULES SHERMAN, MFA
Director, Biodesign Program, Children's National Hospital, Washington, DC, USA

NICOLE R. VAN VEENENDAAL, MD, MPH
Neonatologist, Department of Pediatrics, Emma Children's Hospital, The Amsterdam UMC Location University of Amsterdam, Amsterdam, the Netherlands

BOGALE WORKU, MD
Professor of Pediatrics and Child Health, Addis Ababa University, Ethiopian Pediatric Society, Addis Ababa Chapter Office, Addis Ababa, Ethiopia

NICOLE K. YAMADA, MD, MS
Clinical Associate Professor, Division of Neonatal and Developmental Medicine, Department of Pediatrics, Stanford University, Palo Alto, California, USA

Contents

> This article reviews several common quality improvement methodologies, including the Model for Improvement, Lean, and Six Sigma. We demonstrate how these methods are based on a similar improvement science foundation. We describe the tools used to understand problems in the context of systems and the mechanisms to learn and build knowledge, using specific examples from the neonatology and pediatric literature. We conclude with a discussion on the importance of the human side of change in quality improvement, including team formation and culture.

> Like many implemented organizational changes, quality improvement (QI) projects demonstrate frequent decline after implementation. Factors associated with successfully sustained change are leadership, change characteristics, system capacity for changes and the resources required, and processes to maintain, evaluate, and communicate results. This review uses lessons from change theory and behavioral sciences to discuss change and sustainment of improvement efforts, to list models to support maintenance, and to provide evidence-based practical suggestions to enable the sustainability of QI interventions.

> Effective quality improvement (QI) depends on rigorous analysis of time-series data through methods such as statistical process control (SPC). As use of SPC has become more prevalent in health care, QI practitioners must also be aware of situations that warrant special attention and potential modifications to common SPC charts, which include skewed continuous data, autocorrelation, small persistent changes in performance, confounders, and workload or productivity measures. This article reviews these situations and provides examples of SPC approaches for each.

Implementation science is an interdisciplinary field that seeks to contribute
generalizable knowledge that can improve the translation of clinical evidence in routine care. To promote the integration of implementation science approaches with health care quality improvement, the authors offer
a framework that links the Model for Improvement with implementation
strategies and methods. Perinatal quality improvement teams can
leverage the robust frameworks of implementation science to diagnose
implementation barriers, select implementation strategies, and assess
the strategies' contribution to improving care. Partnerships between implementation scientists and quality improvement teams could accelerate
efforts by both groups to achieve measurable improvements in care.

Improvements in respiratory care have resulted in improved outcomes for
preterm infants over the past three decades. To target the multifactorial
nature of neonatal lung diseases, neonatal intensive care units (NICUs)
should consider developing comprehensive respiratory quality improvement programs that address all drivers of neonatal respiratory disease.
This article presents a potential framework for developing a quality
improvement program to prevent bronchopulmonary dysplasia in the
NICU. Drawing on available research and quality improvement reports,
the authors discuss key components, measures, drivers, and interventions
that should be considered when building a respiratory quality improvement
program devoted to preventing and treating bronchopulmonary dysplasia.

We discuss the burden of health care-associated infections (HAIs) in the
neonatal ICU and the role of quality improvement (QI) in infection prevention and control. We examine specific QI opportunities and approaches to
prevent HAIs caused by Staphylococcus aureus , multidrug-resistant
gram-negative pathogens, Candida species, and respiratory viruses, and
to prevent central line-associated bloodstream infections (CLABSIs) and
surgical site infections. We explore the emerging recognition that many
hospital-onset bacteremia episodes are not CLABSIs. Finally, we describe
the core tenets of QI, including engagement with multidisciplinary teams
and families, data transparency, accountability, and the impact of larger
collaborative efforts to reduce HAIs.

Neonates requiring intensive care are in a critical period of brain development that coincides with the neonatal intensive care unit (NICU) hospitalization, placing these infants at high risk of brain injury and long-term

neurodevelopmental impairment. Care in the NICU has the potential to be both harmful and protective to the developing brain. Neuro-focused quality improvement efforts address 3 main pillars of neuroprotective care: prevention of acquired injury, protection of normal maturation, and promotion of a positive environment. Despite challenges in measurement, many centers have shown success with consistent implementation of best and potentially better practices that may improve markers of brain health and neurodevelopment.

Human factors science teaches us that patient safety is achieved not by disciplining individual health care professionals for mistakes, but rather by designing systems that acknowledge human limitations and optimize the work environment for them. Incorporating human factors principles into simulation, debriefing, and quality improvement initiatives will strengthen the quality and resilience of the process improvements and systems changes that are developed. The future of patient safety in neonatology will require continued efforts to engineer and re-engineer systems that support the humans who are at the interface of delivering safe patient care.

Both quality improvement (QI) and design thinking (DT) methodologies have their unique strengths and weaknesses. Although QI sees problems through a process-centered lens, DT leverages a human-centered approach to understand how people think, behave, and act when encountering a problem. By integrating these 2 frameworks, clinicians have a unique opportunity to rethink how to solve problems in health care by elevating the human experience and putting empathy back at the center of medicine.

There is strong evidence that family-centered care (FCC) improves the health and safety of infants and families in neonatal settings. In this review, we highlight the importance of common, evidence-based quality improvement (QI) methodology applied to FCC and the imperative to engage in partnership with neonatal intensive care unit (NICU) families. To further optimize NICU care, families should be included as essential team members in all NICU QI activities, not only FCC QI activities. Recommendations are provided for building inclusive FCC QI teams, assessing FCC, creating culture change, supporting health-care practitioners and working with parent-led organizations.

The electronic health record (EHR) offers an exciting opportunity for quality improvement efforts. An understanding of the nuances of a site's EHR landscape including the best practices in clinical decision support design, basics of data capture, and acknowledgment of the potential unintended consequences of technology change is essential to ensuring effective usage of this powerful tool.

Value is defined as health outcomes achieved per dollar spent. Addressing value in quality improvement (QI) efforts can help optimize patient outcomes while reducing unnecessary spending. In this article, we discuss how QI focused on reducing morbidities frequently reduces costs, and how proper cost accounting can help demonstrate improvements in value. We provide examples of high-yield opportunities for value improvement in neonatology and review the literature associated with these topics. Opportunities include reducing neonatal intensive care admissions for low-acuity infants, sepsis evaluations in low-risk infants, unnecessary total parental nutrition use, and utilization of laboratory and imaging.

Quality improvement methodologies, coupled with basic neonatal resuscitation and essential newborn care training, have been shown to be critical ingredients in improving neonatal mortality. Innovative methodologies, such as virtual training and telementoring, can enable the mentorship and supportive supervision that are essential to the continued work of improvement and health systems strengthening that must be done after a single training event. Empowering local champions, building effective data collection systems, and developing frameworks for audits and debriefs are among the strategies that will create effective and high-quality health care systems.

Applying an equity lens to quality improvement (QI) by collecting, reviewing, and using data that measure health disparities helps identify whether QI interventions improve outcomes evenly and equally across the population or have a greater impact in an advantaged or disadvantaged group. Methodological issues inherent in measuring disparities include appropriately selecting data sources; ensuring reliability and validity of equity data; choosing a suitable comparison group; and understanding between-group variation. The integration and utilization of QI techniques to promote equity is dependent on meaningful measurement to develop targeted interventions and provide a means of ongoing real-time assessment.

PROGRAM OBJECTIVE
The goal of *Clinics in Perinatology* is to keep practicing perinatologists, neonatologists, obstetricians, practicing physicians and residents up to date with current clinical practice in perinatology by providing timely articles reviewing the state of the art in patient care.

TARGET AUDIENCE
Perinatologists, neonatologists, obstetricians, practicing physicians, residents and healthcare professionals who provide patient care utilizing findings from *Clinics in Perinatology*.

LEARNING OBJECTIVES
Upon completion of this activity, participants will be able to:
1. Recognize how quality improvement initiatives can positively impact the evolution of care.
2. Discuss quality improvement approaches to reduce and/or eliminate HAIs in the neonatal intensive care.
3. Review quality improvement initiatives to improve value and reduce waste.

ACCREDITATION
The Elsevier Office of Continuing Medical Education (EOCME) is accredited by the Accreditation Council for Continuing Medical Education (ACCME) to provide continuing medical education for physicians.

The EOCME designates this journal-based CME activity for a maximum of 14 *AMA PRA Category 1 Credit*(s)™. Physicians should claim only the credit commensurate with the extent of their participation in the activity.

All other health care professionals requesting continuing education credit for this enduring material will be issued a certificate of participation.

DISCLOSURE OF CONFLICTS OF INTEREST
The EOCME assesses conflict of interest with its instructors, faculty, planners, and other individuals who are in a position to control the content of CME activities. All relevant conflicts of interest that are identified are thoroughly vetted by EOCME for fair balance, scientific objectivity, and patient care recommendations. EOCME is committed to providing its learners with CME activities that promote improvements or quality in healthcare and not a specific proprietary business or a commercial interest.

The planning committee, staff, authors, and editors listed below have identified no financial relationships or relationships to products or devices they or their spouse/life partner have with commercial interest related to the content of this CME activity:
Anna Axelin, RN, PhD; Fabiana Bacchini, MSc, BJ; Chaim M. Bell, MD, PhD; Sandhya S. Brachio, MD; Jennifer Callaghan-Koru, PhD, MHS; Leah H. Carr, MD; Lori Christ, MD; Katherine Coughlin, MD; Byron Crowe, MD; Geoffrey Curran, PhD; Erika Edwards, PhD, MPH; Danielle Ehret, MD, MPH; Azadeh Farzin, MD, MHS; Daria F. Ferro, MD; Linda Franck, RN, PhD, FRCPCH, FAAN; Jessica Gaulton, MD, MPH; Wendi Gu, MD; Munish Gupta, MD, MMSc; Louis P. Halamek, MD; L. Dupree Hatch, III, MD, MPH; Lucky Jain, MD, MBA; Lynette Jones, MSN, RN-BC; Beena Kamath-Rayne, MD, MPH; Heather C. Kaplan, MD, MSCE; Ashish KC, MBBS, MHCM, PhD; Brian King, MD; Katelin P. Kramer, MS, MD; Melissa Liebowitz, MD; Nina Menda, MD, MHQS; Michael A. Posencheg, MD; Lloyd P. Provost, MS; Rohit Ramaswamy, PhD, MPH; Erick Ridout, MD; Elizabeth E. Rogers, MD; Asaph Rolnitsky, MSc HQ, MD; Lisa Saiman, MD, MPH; Lauren A. Sanlorenzo, MD, MPH; Jules Sherman, MFA; Jeyanthi Surendrakumar; Nicole R. Van Veenendaal, MD, MPH; Bogale Worku, MD; Nicole K. Yamada, MD, MS

The planning committee, staff, authors, and editors listed below have identified financial relationships or relationships to products or devices they or their spouse/life partner have with commercial interest related to the content of this CME activity:
Ravi M. Patel MD, MSc: Consultant: Noveome Biotherapeutics, Inc.; Advisor: Infant Bacterial Therapeutics AB

UNAPPROVED/OFF-LABEL USE DISCLOSURE
The EOCME requires CME faculty to disclose to the participants:
1. When products or procedures being discussed are off-label, unlabelled, experimental, and/or investigational (not US Food and Drug Administration [FDA] approved); and
2. Any limitations on the information presented, such as data that are preliminary or that represent ongoing research, interim analyses, and/or unsupported opinions. Faculty may discuss information about

pharmaceutical agents that is outside of FDA-approved labelling. This information is intended solely for CME and is not intended to promote off-label use of these medications. If you have any questions, contact the medical affairs department of the manufacturer for the most recent prescribing information.

TO ENROLL
To enroll in the *Clinics in Perinatology* Continuing Medical Education program, call customer service at 1-800-654-2452 or sign up online at http://www.theclinics.com/home/cme. The CME program is available to subscribers for an additional annual fee of USD 254.00.

METHOD OF PARTICIPATION
In order to claim credit, participants must complete the following:
1. Complete enrolment as indicated above.
2. Read the activity.
3. Complete the CME Test and Evaluation. Participants must achieve a score of 70% on the test. All CME Tests and Evaluations must be completed online.

CME INQUIRIES/SPECIAL NEEDS
For all CME inquiries or special needs, please contact elsevierCME@elsevier.com.

CLINICS IN PERINATOLOGY

SERIES OF RELATED INTEREST

Obstetrics and Gynecology Clinics of North America
https://www.obgyn.theclinics.com

THE CLINICS ARE AVAILABLE ONLINE!
Access your subscription at:
www.theclinics.com

Foreword

When It Comes to Quality of Care, One Is Not Zero

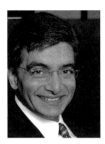

Lucky Jain, MD, MBA
Consulting Editor

Nothing matters more than the quality of care we provide to our patients. Indeed, one unintended death or case of serious harm is not zero. Every clinician strives to get to perfection, but is zero truly achievable?

Nearly every health care system keeps track of and reports serious safety events. The highest level of harm in such trackers is generally reserved for death or permanent harm. As will be evident from articles in this issue of the *Clinics in Perinatology*, we have come a long way in improving patient safety and reducing preventable harm. When accidents do occur, systems spend considerable time and effort pinpointing the cause and finding ways to deliver safer care. However, the overarching conclusion hasn't changed over time: our systems are not built to be fail-safe. They rely too heavily on individual human effort to operate safely. No surprise that errors occur easily when there is lapse in such heroic effort or attention.

How then can we achieve higher reliability? For such discussions, attention often turns to the airline industry, which operates 100,000 flights every day without a single failure! In fact, data show that the risk of a fatal airplane crash is 1 in 16 million.[1] That is

Clin Perinatol 50 (2023) xv–xvii
https://doi.org/10.1016/j.clp.2023.03.003
0095-5108/23/© 2023 Published by Elsevier Inc.

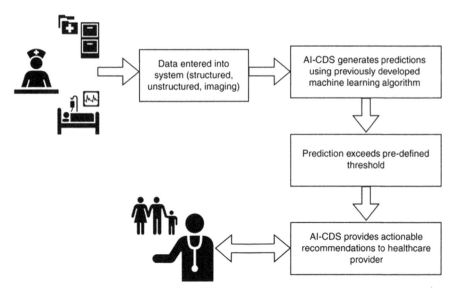

Fig. 1. Functioning of an artificial intelligence clinical decision support (AI-CDS) tool. Electronic health data exist in a variety of formats, including structured (in discrete fields) or unstructured (such as in narrative notes). The machine learning algorithm may then be applied to these test data. When a desired threshold of disease probability is reached, a best practice alert may be provided to the treatment team. (*From* Ramgopal S, Sanchez-Pinto LN, Horvat CM, Carroll MS, Luo Y, Florin TA. Artificial intelligence-based clinical decision support in pediatrics. Pediatr Res. 2023;93(2):334–341.)

well below the six-sigma target of 3.4 defects in a million. This is a shining example of engineering excellence and a *system approach* to quality improvement in an entire industry. It uses a consistent approach to address errors without focusing on heroism or blame.

So where do we go from here? As we discussed in the last issue of the *Clinics in Perinatology* devoted to quality, the *Science of Improvement* is becoming firmly embedded in our culture, but it has only brought incremental change.[2] Attention is now turning to advanced methods of tapping into giant sets of health data and harnessing them to provide computerized clinical decision support (CDS). Coupled with machine learning (which employs algorithms to derive clinically useful patterns from data), CDS can provide real-time interventions to standardize care and improve quality (**Fig. 1**).[3] As one set of authors recently wrote, a diverse group of stakeholders will need to come together to refine the task of developing validated tools from high-resolution data sets.[3] Availability of models with high predictive accuracy will ease the burden of the busy clinician who is constantly bombarded with high volumes of complex data and reduce the chances of errors.

Our 2017 issue of the *Clinics in Perinatology* devoted to Quality Improvement garnered much attention and praise.[2] This current issue not only has expanded the scope and purpose of the discipline but also provides hope that focus on quality and patient safety will ultimately lead to better outcomes. Drs Gupta and Kaplan are to be congratulated for engaging top experts in the field to assemble a true state-of-the-art offering. As always, I am grateful to the authors for their valuable contributions and to my publishing partners at Elsevier (Kerry Holland and Karen Dino) for their help in bringing this valuable resource to you.

Lucky Jain, MD, MBA
Department of Pediatrics
Emory University School of Medicine
Children's Healthcare of Atlanta
2015 Uppergate Drive Northeast
Atlanta, GA 30322, USA

REFERENCES

1. Anne Sophie A, van Dalen HM, Strandbygaard J, et al. Six sigma in surgery: how to create a safer culture in the operating theatre using innovative technology. Br J Anesth 2021;127:817–20.
2. Jain L. Quality improvement: the journey continues. Clin Perinatol 2017;44:xv–xvi.
3. Ramgopal S, Sanchez-Pinto NL, Horvat CM, et al. Artificial intelligence-based clinical decision support in pediatrics. Pediatr Res 2023;93:334–41.

Preface

A Tipping Point for Quality Improvement in Neonatal Intensive Care

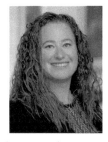
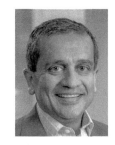

Heather C. Kaplan, MD, MSCE   Munish Gupta, MD, MMSc
Editors

It has now been more than 20 years since the Institute of Medicine's landmark reports "To Err is Human" and "Crossing the Quality Chasm," often considered the unofficial launch of the modern movement in health care safety and quality. It has been 5 years since *Clinics in Perinatology* last devoted an issue to Quality Improvement (QI) in neonatology. Are we making progress?

By many indicators, yes. The neonatology QI community has steadily grown. Quality and safety are now core components of education for all medical disciplines, and advanced training programs are spreading. Neonatal intensive care units (NICUs) are dedicating more time and resources to building QI infrastructure, and it would be a challenge to find a unit that is not a member of a state or national perinatal quality collaborative. National networks have shown significant and sustained improvements in outcomes for preterm infants across thousands of NICUs.[1,2] Review studies attribute broad improvements in neonatal outcomes to QI efforts.[3–5]

One measure of the growth of this community is the dramatic increase in the number of publications focused on neonatal QI. Searching PubMed using the terms "neonatal" and "quality improvement" shows a steady increase in publications over the past two decades, with over 500 publications per year from 2018 to 2021 (**Fig. 1**). At the least, this shows widespread and growing belief that QI can impact neonatal care. Perhaps this also shows that we have reached a "tipping point" where QI has become "the way we do things around here."

We should embrace this growth and this success, but we should also recognize the gaps and challenges that persist. And these are not trivial. The maternal health crisis in the United States is worsening, and preterm birth rates are increasing. As we see progress in survival of extremely preterm infants, rates of certain morbidities remain

Clin Perinatol 50 (2023) xix–xxi
https://doi.org/10.1016/j.clp.2023.03.001
0095-5108/23/© 2023 Published by Elsevier Inc.

perinatology.theclinics.com

Publications by Year
Pubmed: "Neonatal" and "Quality Improvement"

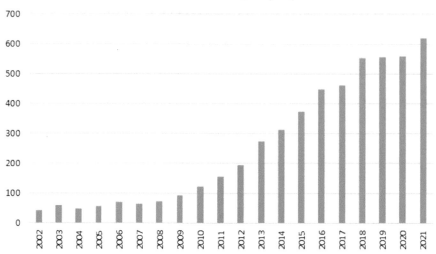

Fig. 1. Neonatal QI publications by year.

stubbornly high. We are becoming more aware of disparities in care and the impact of racism, but interventions that have improved equity remain few and far between.

For those of us engaged in neonatal QI, our challenges include ensuring the robustness of our QI efforts. Systematic reviews reveal inconsistent and even poor use of appropriate methods in QI publications.[6,7] In addition, questions have been raised regarding the scientific rigor of QI methods.[8] Unfortunately, neonatology is not spared from concerns regarding QI quality.[9]

We hope this issue of *Clinics in Perinatology* can help our growing community try to address some of these challenges. We sought to include articles that highlight how QI in neonatology has advanced over the past 5 years, and articles that show us what we can be doing now as well as what we should be doing in the future.

We are thankful for the outstanding group of authors that contributed to this issue. We begin with a series of articles that offer new insights into the QI methods we are using to improve processes and outcomes of care, including a review of common improvement frameworks, an exploration of strategies for sustaining improvement, examples of challenging cases in statistical process control, and approaches for augmenting our traditional QI methods with lessons from implementation science. We then turn to specific clinical improvement topics, with reviews of current and future improvement efforts targeting bronchopulmonary dysplasia, neonatal infection, neurodevelopment, and patient safety. We explore new and emerging topics with reviews of human-centered design thinking, innovations in family-centered care, use of the electronic health record more effectively in improvement, and approaches to addressing value and waste. We conclude the issue targeting equity with a review of QI initiatives in global health and a discussion of measuring equity for improvement efforts.

Now that QI has become part of the daily work for so many of us, we hope we can take our efforts one step further by incorporating tools and ideas from these articles. By using more sophisticated and robust methods, by pushing hard on outcomes that have been difficult to move, by continuing to focus not only on current but also on future problems, and by committing to equity, we expect to reach a true tipping point where the quality of our care and outcomes will exponentially improve.

Heather C. Kaplan, MD, MSCE
Department of Pediatrics
University of Cincinnati College of Medicine
Perinatal Institute, Cincinnati Children's Hospital Medical Center
3333 Burnet Avenue
Cincinnati, OH 45229, USA

Munish Gupta, MD, MMSc
Harvard Medical School
Beth Israel Deaconess Medical Center
330 Brookline Avenue
Boston, MA 02215, USA

E-mail addresses:
heather.kaplan@cchmc.org (H.C. Kaplan)
mgupta@bidmc.harvard.edu (M. Gupta)

REFERENCES

1. Horbar JD, Edwards EM, Greenberg LT, et al. Variation in performance of neonatal intensive care units in the United States. JAMA Pediatr 2017;171(3):e164396.
2. Ellsbury DL, Clark RH, Ursprung R, et al. A multifaceted approach to improving outcomes in the NICU: the Pediatrix 100 000 Babies Campaign. Pediatrics 2016;137(4):e20150389.
3. Spitzer AR. Has quality improvement really improved outcomes for babies in the neonatal intensive care unit? Clin Perinatol 2017;44(3):469–83.
4. Pearlman SA. Advancements in neonatology through quality improvement. J Perinatol 2022;42(10):1277–82.
5. Ellsbury DL, Clark RH. Does quality improvement work in neonatology improve clinical outcomes? Curr Opin Pediatr 2017;29(2):129–34.
6. Knudsen SV, Laursen HVB, Johnsen SP, et al. Can quality improvement improve the quality of care? A systematic review of reported effects and methodological rigor in plan-do-study-act projects. BMC Health Serv Res 2019;19(1):683.
7. Taylor MJ, McNicholas C, Nicolay C, et al. Systematic review of the application of the plan-do-study-act method to improve quality in healthcare. BMJ Qual Saf 2014; 23(4):290–8.
8. Grady D, Redberg RF, O'Malley PG. Quality improvement for quality improvement studies. JAMA Intern Med 2018;178(2):187.
9. Hu ZJ, Fusch G, Hu C, et al. Completeness of reporting of quality improvement studies in neonatology is inadequate: a systematic literature survey. BMJ Open Qual 2021;10(2):1–8.

Common Quality Improvement Methodologies Including the Model for Improvement, Lean, and Six Sigma

Katherine Coughlin, MD[a], Michael A. Posencheg, MD[b],*

KEYWORDS

- System of Profound Knowledge • Model for Improvement • Lean • Six Sigma
- Psychology of change

KEY POINTS

- The System of Profound Knowledge, described by W. Edwards Deming, is the basis for many of the quality improvement methodologies used today.
- A successful quality improvement initiative requires understanding a system, defining the problem, applying tools to create change, and tracking data longitudinally to assess the impact of changes made.
- The Model for improvement, Lean methodology, Six Sigma, and the other methods discussed utilize different structures and tools, but also have overlapping characteristics. Choosing a methodology depends on local expertise and the type of problem to be solved.
- Success in quality improvement requires a structured approach, but equally important is an understanding of the human side of change, as described in the Psychology of Change.

INTRODUCTION

From the 1980s to the present day, we have moved from an emphasis on quality assurance to one of quality improvement in health care. In this article, we will review the foundation of modern-day quality improvement methodologies used in health care. We will describe the most common methodologies with specific examples of their practical applications in neonatology or pediatrics. Lastly, special attention will be paid to the development of teams that do quality improvement (QI) work as well as the importance of engaging people in the effectiveness and sustainability of our efforts.

[a] Sharp Mary Birch Hospital for Women and Newborns, 8555 Aero Drive #340, San Diego CA 92123, USA; [b] Division of Neonatology, Hospital of the University of Pennsylvania, 3400 Spruce Street, Ravdin Building, 8th floor, Philadelphia, PA 19104, USA
* Corresponding author.
E-mail address: michael.posencheg@pennmedicine.upenn.edu

Clin Perinatol 50 (2023) 285–306
https://doi.org/10.1016/j.clp.2023.02.002   perinatology.theclinics.com
0095-5108/23/© 2023 Elsevier Inc. All rights reserved.

The System of Profound Knowledge

Quality improvement originated in the manufacturing sector and was adapted for use in health care. The foundation of current methodologies is based on the original work of Joseph Juran, Walter Shewhart, and W. Edwards Deming. Juran was an engineer and management consultant who is best known for his work on the cost of poor quality. He introduced the concept of the Juran Trilogy, combining quality planning, quality control, and quality improvement into an interrelated continuum to drive improvement and outcomes. Shewhart was an engineer and statistician who is best known for his work on the modern-day Plan-Do-Study-Act (PDSA) cycle with Deming as well as introducing the importance of time-series data in the form of control charts or "Shewhart charts". Deming was an engineer and management consultant best known for his improvement work in Japan after World War II. He is the author of several books, highlighted by Out of the Crisis, in which he introduced us to the System of Profound Knowledge.[1] He stated that to improve our organizations or problem, we sought to solve it was imperative to view them through a lens of four inter-related domains. He defined these domains as

- Appreciation of a system: Our outcomes are created by the systems that produce them, including people, process, and tools or equipment.
- Theory of knowledge: This describes how we learn to gain the necessary knowledge to make change.
- Understanding variation: The notion that everything in life has inherent variation and we must understand and differentiate meaningful from non-meaningful differences.
- Psychology or the human side of change: Understanding how people respond to change and human nature.

The system thinking introduced to us by Deming in this model is at the foundation of all of our quality improvement methodologies. Paul Batalden is often credited with the quote, "Every system is perfectly designed to get the results it gets". To address the problem you are trying to solve, you must change the system that creates it. Each of the QI methods outlined below gives us tools to make changes in our systems to get different results. Upon close inspection, one can see evidence for each of the domains of the System of Profound Knowledge, in addition to system thinking, in the descriptions below.

The Model for Improvement

History

The Model for Improvement is the most frequently used QI methodology in neonatology and is widely used in health care in general. It was developed by the Associates in Process Improvement (API), a group of improvers who worked with W. Edwards Deming from the 1980s to early 1990s. They recognized that the ideas set forth by Deming were revolutionary and could have dramatic impact if applied to health care. They appreciated that frequent, small tests of change were critical in successful process improvement projects, and they aimed to make Deming's concepts applicable to all settings. The initial model built around the core concept of the PDSA cycle, by adding three foundational questions, to create the Model for Improvement.[2,3]

The Model for Improvement was first published in 1996 by the API authors with the Improvement Guide.[3] This book remains a comprehensive resource for anyone pursuing quality improvement in health care. The API has subsequently worked very closely with the Institute for Healthcare Improvement (IHI) in an effort to adapt process improvement methods successfully to the health care industry. The IHI website (IHI.

org) is an excellent place to seek education, tools, and a multitude of other resources for the successful use of the Model for Improvement.

The Methodology
The Model for Improvement is shown in **Fig. 1**. It begins by asking three questions.

1. What are we trying to accomplish?
2. How will we know that a change is an improvement?
3. What changes can we make that will result in improvement?

To expand on these core questions, a quality improvement initiative should therefore include

- A clear aim statement focusing on the problem to be solved.
- A family of measures that describe the system that produces the problem in the aim statement.
- A description of the theory behind the problem and ideas (otherwise known as a driver diagram) that may then affect the desired outcome.
- The use of PDSA cycles for rapid tests of change and learning.
- A plan for moving from testing to implementation and sustainability.[3]

Project Design and Execution
What are we trying to accomplish? The first step is creating an aim, which answers the question, "What are we trying to accomplish?" A SMART aim is recommended as it forces attention to detail and accountability. SMART stands for Specific,

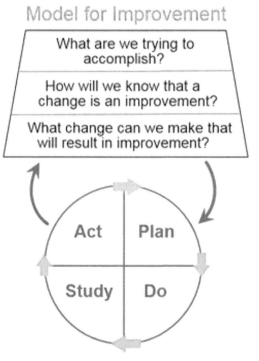

Fig. 1. The Model for Improvement. (*From* Langley GJ, Moen RD, Nolan KM, Nolan TW, Norman CL, Provost LP. The Improvement Guide: A Practical Approach to Enhancing Organizational Performance, 2nd Edition. New Jersey: John Wiley & Sons, Inc.; 2009. p. 24 and 97; with permission.)

Measurable, Actionable, Realistic, and Time-bound. A clear aim statement also ensures the entire team is aligned with the project goal and scope.

Example: *We aim to reduce the number of days to first skin-to-skin in infants born less than 29 weeks' GA at Sharp Mary Birch Hospital from a baseline of 14 days to a goal of 7 days by January 2022.*

Another important aspect of this first question is understanding the team's theory of what "drives" the project goal. Or, conversely one could ask, what contributes to the current problem? A high-yield tool used to answer these questions is the driver diagram. It organizes the teams' thought process, helps outline possible change ideas, and is a great way to help those outside of the team understand the big picture. After the aim statement, primary and secondary drivers impacting the system or problem can be defined. From the secondary drivers will come inspiration for specific change ideas. The driver diagram is also a working document, so one should edit and refine as the team learns along the way. **Fig. 2** provides an example of a driver diagram using the skin-to-skin aim above.

How will we know that a change is an improvement?. To answer this question, one needs to establish a family of measures. Setting and tracking the appropriate measures will allow a team to understand whether the changes they are making actually lead to improvement (vs improvement being due to some other, unexpected, but concurrent change in the system). It is important to remember that measurement in the Model for Improvement is not the same as measurement in research. Measures are meant to stabilize biases (rather than control for them), bring knowledge to local practice, and gather "just enough" data.[4]

A project should include three types of measures when utilizing the Model for Improvement: outcome measures, process measures, and balancing measures.

Outcome Measures: Include the primary goal of the project, or the higher-level problem one is attempting to solve.

For Example: Day of first skin-to-skin in infants born less than 29 weeks' GA.

Process Measures: These measures attempt to identify if the changes implanted are actually affecting your outcome. A project should have at least two process measures, typically two to four.

For Example: After creating eligibility criteria for skin-to-skin, what percentage of eligible infants are actually being held in the first week of life? How often are nurses using the appointment cards or beside checklists we created?

Balancing Measures: These measures ask whether changes meant to improve one part of a system inadvertently cause problems in another area or if there is an alternative explanation for changes in the outcome measure. Each project should have at least one balancing measure.

For Example: The rate of unplanned extubation, safety events, or equipment malfunction during skin-to-skin.

It is important to pick measures that can be realistically tracked over time by the team. In other words, data that are not overly difficult to find or extract on a regular basis.

What change can we make that will result in improvement? Fundamental changes to systems and processes are key to creating meaningful improvement in outcomes. Change ideas can come from many tools, and the driver diagram (mentioned above) provides a logical way to describe a theory of improvement for a QI project. An alternate way to generate change ideas is through the use of change concepts. A change concept is a category or theme for improvement ideas that have previously proven to

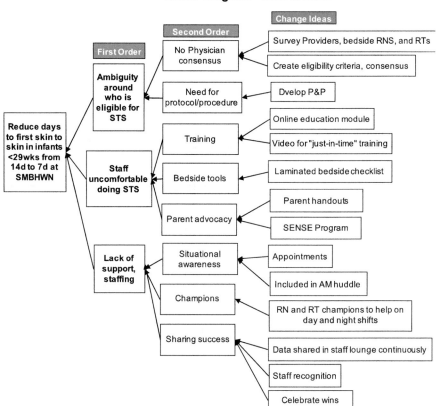

Fig. 2. Example of a driver diagram using a project improving skin-to-skin care.

be successful across many types of QI projects. Therefore, using them can help guide or inspire specific change ideas. There are many change concepts, in fact, the Improvement Guide defines 72 of them.[3] **Box 1** notes some higher-level examples, but the list is not exhaustive. Lastly, change ideas can come from the utilization of lateral thinking or creativity techniques. Edward deBono has described certain provocations that allow us to exit our usual ruts of thinking, allowing us to generate novel solutions to problems. One of his best-known provocation techniques is the Six Thinking Hats.[5]

Using plan-do-study-act cycles. Testing and implementing change ideas is at the core of the Model for Improvement. After identifying an idea for change on a driver diagram or other tool, the team should proceed to use the PDSA cycle to test the change before implementation. See **Fig. 3** for a depiction of the PDSA cycle. Systems in health care are complex, and testing our change ideas using the PDSA cycle allows us to both see the impact of our change idea as well as learn more about our system as we alter it. Thus, the PDSA cycle is a process for both improvement and for learning. The improvement team can then adjust their change ideas during testing to arrive at a better solution before implementation. The following are some details for each phase of the PDSA cycle.

Box 1
A selection of different change concepts

Examples of change concepts
  Eliminate waste
  Improve workflow
  Optimize inventory
  Producer/customer interface
  Manage time
  Focus on variation
  Error proofing
  Focus on product or service

- Plan: Plan in detail how the change will be tested. Each PDSA cycle should have specific questions the cycle is expected to answer with predictions of what the answers to those questions will be.
- Do: Carry out the plan you have designed, testing the change in a subgroup of people or patients (ie, one pod in the unit, one nursing team, or a narrowed gestational age range).
- Study: Examine how the change is working in real time; get feedback from staff, track your measures. Starting small will make this feasible and efficient. Comparing findings to the questions/predictions outlined in the Plan section will lead to learning about your system.
- Act: Adopt, adapt, or abandon. Is the intervention working? Then begin to scale up. Often there are aspects that are working, and aspects that need adjustment. Is the intervention not making a difference or too difficult to implement? Then, pivot early and start on the next PDSA cycle with a new change idea.

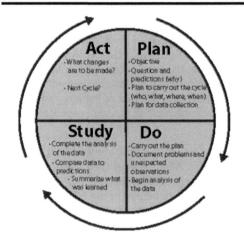

Fig. 3. A more detailed look at the PDSA cycle. (*From* Langley GJ, Moen RD, Nolan KM, Nolan TW, Norman CL, Provost LP. The Improvement Guide: A Practical Approach to Enhancing Organizational Performance, 2nd Edition. New Jersey: John Wiley & Sons, Inc.; 2009. p. 24 and 97; with permission.)

Finally, much attention has been paid to how large of a scale or scope a PDSA cycle should have. The PDSA cycle was designed to be used iteratively, starting at a small scale, to fine-tune change ideas as the team learns about the system and processes they are changing. Three factors should be taken into consideration when determining the size of a PDSA cycle: the confidence the team has that the change idea will lead to improvement, the cost of failure, and the amount of resistance noted in the staff involved. The lower the confidence, higher the cost, and more resistant the staff is, the smaller the size of your initial cycles should be.

Time-series data for improvement. To demonstrate whether or not a change resulted in meaningful improvement, it is important to track the data over time. In the Model for Improvement (and other methodologies), the preferred way to do this is by using run charts or control charts. The chart should tell the story of a project over time and will ideally include baseline data, a goal, and annotation of changes in the system (which could be intentional or unintentional) including the PDSA cycles. They should be updated regularly to provide real-time feedback for the team.[3] **Fig. 4** provides an example of a control chart from the skin-to-skin project. Numerous references provide guidance for creating run charts and control charts.[6,7]

Selected examples from the literature. There are many excellent examples in pediatrics and neonatology utilizing the Model for Improvement. Despite not being classic research projects, many of them have truly advanced the field in areas ranging from reducing central line associated blood stream infections (CLABSIs), to implementing evidenced-based care, to the execution of state-wide collaborative projects.[8]

A common issue that plagues neonatologists is how to manage documentation and discharge surrounding apnea of prematurity. Coughlin and colleagues used the Model for Improvement with the goal of reducing variation surrounding the management of apnea of prematurity.[9] In this project, with a lack of clear evidence-based guidelines, the group chose creating a protocol, operational

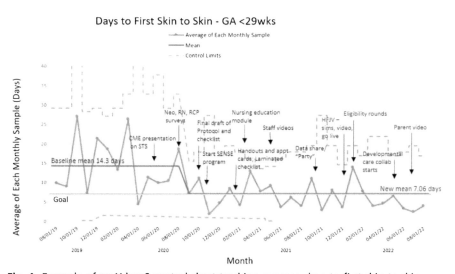

Fig. 4. Example of an X-bar S control chart tracking average days to first skin-to-skin.

definitions, and group consensus to improve the quality of care. They used a pareto chart, shown in **Fig. 5**, as a tool to answer the help answer the question, "what is the problem?" which helped identify gaps in the baseline process that needed to be addressed.

A pareto chart is a type of bar chart that helps a team identify the "vital few" issues that contribute most to the problem they are trying to solve. In this case, it was the most frequent issues with documentation, which was created from a 2-week chart audit. A pareto chart is not specific to the Model for Improvement and could be used in concert with any methodology. It is appropriate for any scenario where you are attempting to understand the different factors contributing to a problem and how much weight each one carries. PDSA cycles included documentation changes for nurses, reminder cards at bedside, revising management of events occurring with oral feeding attempts, spreading over time from one bay to the entire unit, and clinical consensus on a 5-day "event watch." They significantly reduced variation in practice without increasing their balancing measure of the length of stay, as shown in **Fig. 6**.

Safe, effective transport is another common issue in neonatology. Glenn and colleagues used the Model for Improvement to increase the percentage of preterm or low birth weight infants who were admitted with normothermia.[10] Some of their PDSA cycles included standardizing the use of polyethylene wraps and gel packs, standardizing incubator temperature, improved continuous temperature monitoring, and a checklist for referring hospitals. The thought process and theory behind the interventions are evident in their driver diagram, depicted in **Fig. 7**. They demonstrated significant improvement over time in infants admitted with normothermia on their well-annotated control chart, shown in **Fig. 8**.

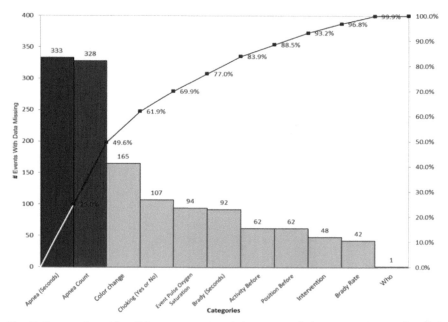

Fig. 5. Pareto chart identifying commonly missing parts of documentation in the EMR apneic event flowsheet. EMR, electronic medical record. (Reproduced with permission from Journal Pediatrics, Vol. 145(2), Page(s) e20190861, © 2020 by the AAP.)

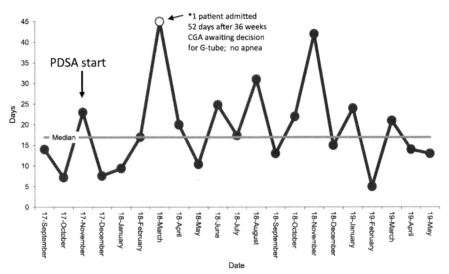

Fig. 6. Run chart tracking a balancing measure of length of stay beyond 36 weeks' CGA in a project standardizing discharge management of apnea events. CGA, corrected gestational age. (Reproduced with permission from Journal Pediatrics, Vol. 145(2), Page(s) e20190861. © 2020 by the AAP.)

Lean Methodology

History
We likely owe the existence of Lean in part to Henry Ford and his creation of the assembly line. However, lean methodology itself originated in Japan, specifically, the Toyota Corporation, which was actually initially the Toyoda Cotton Spinning and Weaving Company founded in 1918. For that reason, much of the terminology used

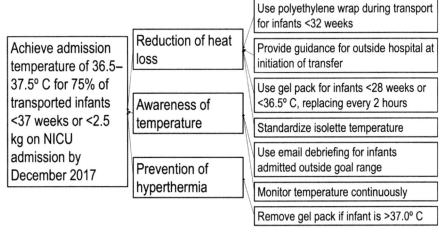

Fig. 7. Driver diagram for a project aimed at improving thermoregulation on transport. (*From* Glenn T, Price R, Culbertson L, Yalcinkaya G. Improving thermoregulation in transported preterm infants: a quality improvement initiative. J Perinatol. 2021;41(2):339 to 345.)

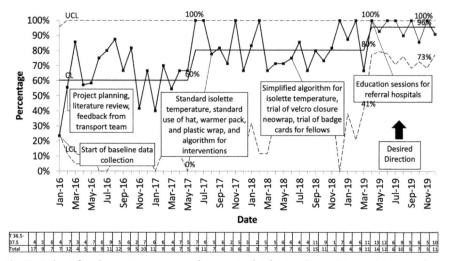

Fig. 8. P-chart for the main outcome of percent of infants admitted in goal temperature range. From Glenn T, Price R, Culbertson L, Yalcinkaya G. Improving thermoregulation in transported preterm infants: a quality improvement initiative. J Perinatol. 2021;41(2):339 to 345.

in Lean is Japanese with origins from textile operations. For example, "*jidoka*" means a loom that stops automatically if a thread breaks, much like the phrase "stop the line" used in Lean today.

The Toyota Motor Company was established as a separate entity in 1937 and continued to carry forward and expand on measures to improve efficiency in manufacturing, building on what Ford started. After World War II, Toyota re-committed to quality improvement using Lean and saw a large increase in productivity; the Toyota Production System was born and refined. Deming, along with Joseph Juran, actually visited and taught the Japanese Union of Scientists and Engineers (JUSE) in the 1950s and this collaboration led to the methods known as "Total Quality Control," which we will revisit later in this article.[2,11]

Lean spread and continued to gain popularity in the manufacturing and service contexts over the next several decades with a focus on removing waste (*muda*) and focusing on value-added workflows. In the early 2000s, Lean began being used in health care. Although health care differs from manufacturing, there are many aspects of health care that are amenable to Lean approaches. Examples include reducing wait times, standardizing procedures, complex care coordination, and improving the supply chain.[12] The literature suggests that Lean can improve health care operational effectiveness; however, implementation is often very localized.[13] Several health care organizations have adopted Lean management, but its use in pediatrics remains somewhat sporadic.[14]

The Methodology

Lean philosophy is made up of lean principles that ultimately transform workplace culture. The different principles include eliminating waste, improving flow (this could be patients, supplies, providers), and ensuring everything being done adds value to the customer. Similar to the Model for Improvement, Lean also emphasizes the importance of frontline staff members in identifying problems and creating solutions. Again, as in other QI methodologies, there is also a focus on continuous improvement with multiple ongoing efforts occurring to improve an organization.[15] In Lean, the ultimate goal is a perfect process, which by definition is valuable (for the customer), capable (produces a good result reliably), adequate (minimal delays), available, flexible, and linked to continuous flow.[16]

Project Design and Execution
As with every QI methodology, having a comprehensive understanding of the baseline system is essential with Lean. Because Lean focuses on eliminating waste and errors, there are some unique tools that can help identify waste in current processes. It is important to first become familiar with the different kinds of waste that may exist; "DOWNTIME" is a helpful acronym used to remember them. **Table 1** provides further explanations and examples.[2,17]

A Lean project then flows through a "roadmap" as detailed in **Box 2**.[18] The focus is on identifying value and tracking it through a system such that waste can be eliminated and that value can be prioritized. The A3 described below is a structured way to do this.

Lean assessment tools. A Lean project is often tracked through a living document known as an "A3," named after the paper size, as this paper was often literally carried around on factory floors at the Toyota Motor Company. An A3 Report can help keep a project comprehensive and organized while also being accessible to all people involved in a process.[2] It can also be a helpful organizational tool in other methodologies. A template for an A3 is provided in **Fig. 9.**

We will demonstrate additional specific tools with a neonatology project as an example: the process of transporting an infant off the unit for an MRI and eliminating waste in this system.

Going to the gemba or a "go and see". The purpose of a gemba walk is to observe every single step of the process one is attempting to change as a "fly on the wall." Ideally, the observer takes notes on all of the steps, supplies, and people involved

Table 1	
DOWNTIME acronym to remember some of the different kinds of waste	
Waste	**Definition/Examples**
Defects	Error, duplicate work, checking, inspection and incorrect information
Overproduction	Preparing more than is necessary, more information than can be processed
Waiting	Waiting for something to arrive or for something to be done
kNowledge wasted (non-utilized talent)	Not utilizing utilized staff efficiently, ideas that are lost, not allowing people to practice at the full extent of their license
Transportation	Moving material or people for the next stop in the process
Inventory	Excess supply that is never utilized
Motion	Unnecessary human movement
Extra processing	Items performed that do not add value, duplicated effort, documenting the same item in multiple places

> **Box 2**
> **Steps of lean roadmap**
>
> Steps of lean roadmap
> 1. Specify the value desired by the customer.
> 2. Identify the value stream for each product and challenge all of the wasted steps currently necessary to provide it.
> 3. Make the product flow continuously through the remaining value-added steps.
> 4. Introduce pull between all steps where continuous flow is not possible.
> 5. Manage toward perfection so that the number of steps and the amount of time and information needed to serve the customer continuously fall.

as well as the duration of each step. Using the above example, a member of the project team would go on multiple patient trips to MRI without having a role in patient care, and instead, note the steps of the process in objective detail.

Process mapping and value stream mapping. A process map is a way of visually depicting the "gemba walk." It allows a team better understand and share with others how complicated a process is. There are many different types of process maps, including spaghetti diagrams, SIPOC (Supplier, Input, Process, Output, Customer) Charts, and swim-lane diagrams.[19] **Fig. 10** shows an example of a swim-lane diagram depicting the process of taking an NICU patient off the floor for MRI. In this example, the swim-lane format allows for different locations to be depicted while also noting steps and personnel. Lanes do not have to be locations; they could be people,

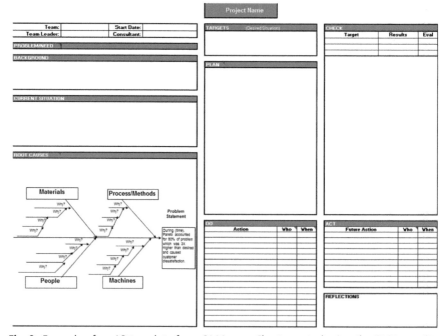

Fig. 9. Example of an A3 template from QI Macros. Charts created using the QI Macros statistical process control (SPC) Software for Excel developed by Jay Arthur, (888) 468 to 1537 www.qimacros.com.

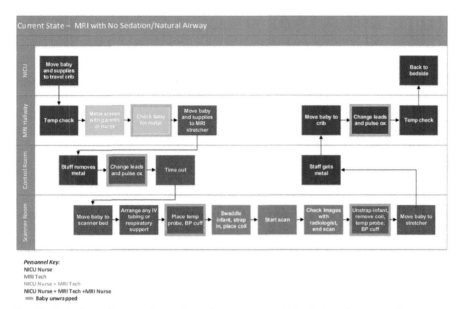

Fig. 10. Swim-lane diagram (a version of a process map) depicting the steps of a neonate going for an MRI. (*From* Coughlin K, Posencheg MA. Quality improvement methods - Part II. J Perinatol. 2019;39(7):1000 to 1007. https://doi.org/10.1038/s41372-019-0382-1.)

departments, or some combination of these things, depending on the project. From a process map (or in place of a process map), one can create a value stream map, which again requires information from "going to the gemba." **Fig. 11** is another example from the project on removing waste in the MRI process. A value stream map notes each major step in the process, and underneath also includes the amount of time needed and whether this time is "value-added" or "non-value added".[17] With this information, a team can identify where there is waste and what percentage of the process is waste (ie, where there is the most waste).

Other Lean assessment tools. There are many other assessment tools that can be applied in Lean, including time-value analyses, fishbone diagrams (or Ishikawa diagrams), root cause analysis, and tools for investigating the "voice of the customer."[19] Discussing these tools in detail is beyond the scope of this article, although several are highlighted below in examples from the literature.

Lean activity tools. Once a process is understood in detail and waste is identified, one can move toward identifying the appropriate change ideas.

A *Kaizen* event, or a Rapid Process Improvement Workshop, is a common first step. In a Kaizen, key stakeholders meet and spend (ideally) one or several days reviewing the system using the tools above and brainstorming ways to add value and eliminate waste. Classically, the ideas from a Kaizen are implemented immediately and then adjusted as needed by the team; it encourages continuous and rapid improvement.[2]

The 5-S method may be used if the goal involves creating an organized, safe, high-performing workplace. 5-S stands for: sort, simplify, standardize, shine (or sweep), and self-discipline. Another concept is leveled production or *heijunka,* which seeks to better manage fluctuations in demand by managing demand or increasing the flexibility of production.[2,16]

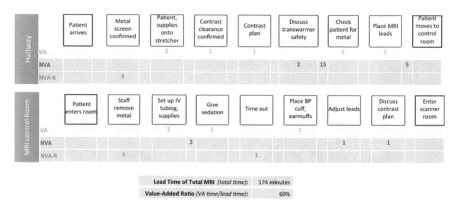

	Patient arrives	Metal screen confirmed	Patient, supplies onto stretcher	Contrast clearance confirmed	Contrast plan	Discuss transwarmer safety	Check patient for metal	Place MRI leads	Patient moves to control room
VA			2	1	1		1	1	
NVA						2	15		5
NVA-R		3							

	Patient enters room	Staff remove metal	Set up IV tubing, supplies	Give sedation	Time out	Place BP cuff, earmuffs	Adjust leads	Discuss contrast plan	Enter scanner room
VA			1	1		1			
NVA			2				1	1	
NVA-R		1		1					

Lead Time of Total MRI *(total time)*:	174 minutes
Value-Added Ratio *(VA time/lead time)*:	60%

Fig. 11. A portion of a value stream map for a neonate undergoing an MRI with sedation. NVA, non-value added; NVA-R, non-value added but required time; VA, value added. Time is noted (in minutes) for each step. (*From* Coughlin K, Posencheg MA. Quality improvement methods - Part II. J Perinatol. 2019;39(7):1000 to 1007. https://doi.org/10.1038/s41372-019-0382-1.)

Examples from the Literature

Lean is not used as frequently as the Model for Improvement in Pediatrics, however, there are still many common problems where it is very applicable and valuable.

Kenaley and colleagues used Lean Six Sigma methodology to decrease time to parents' first hold in the NICU. They utilized the tools of process mapping, a fishbone diagram, and a parent survey to better understand the current state.[20] The fishbone diagram is shown in **Fig. 12**. They then used a 5-S tool, impact control matrix, a barrier and aids chart, and failure modes effect analysis to identify opportunities for improvement. After implementing their bundle, they significantly reduced their median time to first hold.

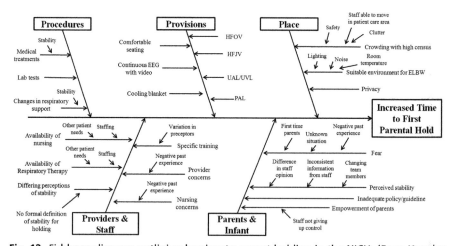

Fig. 12. Fishbone diagram outlining barriers to parent holding in the NICU. (*From* Kenaley KM, Rickolt AL, Vandersteur DA, Ryan JD, Stefano JL. An intervention to decrease time to parents' first hold of infants in the Neonatal Intensive Care Unit requiring respiratory support. J Perinatol. 2020;40(5):812 to 819.)

Rounding is also a process that can be susceptible to inefficiencies. Atul and colleagues designed a Lean project that significantly decreased rounding time by identifying and eliminating non-value-added activities. This also led to earlier discharge from the unit. To do this, they practiced "going to the gemba," shadowing the rounding process in detail. They then performed a time-value analysis, shown in **Fig. 13**, and were able to show a reduction in waste.[21]

Six Sigma Methodology

History
Six Sigma entered the industry as a measurement method for managing product variation in the 1920s with Walter Shewhart, who demonstrated that at three sigma from the mean, a process requires correction. The term "Six Sigma" actually came from Motorola in the 1980s, whose engineers developed a new methodology to measure defects.[22] Six Sigma methodology is often combined with Lean. It has been suggested that the two function well together as Lean can focus on productivity and culture while Six Sigma has additional tools that help uncover the unseen roots of problems.[23]

The goal of Six Sigma is to reduce process output variation such that there are no more than 3.4 defects per million opportunities, which is equivalent to six process standard deviations from the mean (hence the name).[22] This technically applies to a process with one specification limit, however, visually it is easier to appreciate the concept with a bell curve that has upper and lower specification limits. A secondary goal of Six Sigma is to improve profits, effectiveness, and efficiency to meet the customer's needs (not unlike Lean).[24] Although Six Sigma was not initially designed for health care, with the current state of rising costs, often decreasing reimbursements,

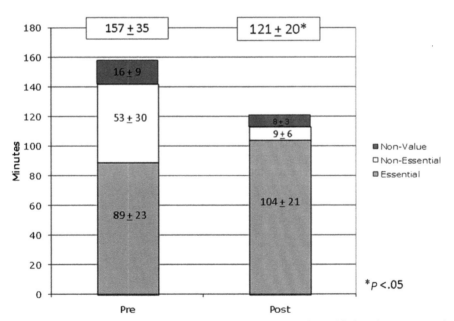

Fig. 13. A Time-Value Analysis comparing essential to non-value added and non-essential time in the rounding process before and after project interventions. (*From* Vats A, Goin KH, Villarreal MC, Yilmaz T, Fortenberry JD, Keskinocak P. The impact of a lean rounding process in a pediatric intensive care unit. Crit Care Med. 2012;40(2):608 to 617.)

and wide variation in practice, the application of Six Sigma practices is quite relevant.[25]

The Methodology

The three core practices associated with implementation are Six Sigma role structure, Six Sigma structured improvement procedure, and Six Sigma focus on metrics. The role structure is also known as the "belt system." Training leads to getting a "belt," with a color that correlates with increasing expertise (green belt, black belt, master black belt, and champion). A team is assembled, ideally consisting of people with different levels of training who then have different responsibilities in the project and the organization, as shown in **Fig. 14**.[24] The two main methods for improvement are DMAIC (define, measure, analyze, improve, control) and DMADV (define, measure, analyze, design, verify). DMAIC is used for process improvement whereas DMADV is more so for process or product design. Given the focus of this article, we will preferentially elaborate on DMAIC.[26]

Project Design and Execution

Many organizations used a combined Lean Six Sigma approach to quality, with the valid argument that elimination of waste and removal of defects through standardization are overlapping goals that can both lead to improved efficiency, lower cost, and higher value.[27] For clarity, we will review some Six Sigma-specific tools below, but again, one can appreciate the synergy with Lean.

DMAIC. DMAIC leads a team from defining a problem to implementing solutions and establishing best practices, and finally, making sure the solutions stay in place. DMAIC stands for Define, Measure, Analyze, Improve, Control. **Table 2** elaborates on each step with specific action items.[22,24] As noted above, many steps overlap with other methodologies.

Suppliers, Inputs, Process, Outputs, and Customers Chart. Fig. 15 is a template of one of the more commonly used tools, an SIPOC chart. SIPOC stands for Suppliers, Inputs, Process, Outputs, and Customers. It can be helpful to ensure that all parts of a process are accounted for and, if desired, can function similarly to a swim-lane process map.

The 5 Whys. The "5 Whys" helps determine the root cause of a problem. After identifying a problem, the team asks why it occurred. If the answer to this question does not identify the root of the problem, then the team asks "why" again. This question is classically asked five times to uncover the underlying issue. Typically, there is good clarity

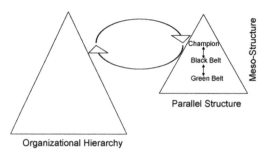

Fig. 14. Representation of Six Sigma structure with the belt system. (*From* Schroeder RG, Linderman K, Liedtke C, Choo AS. Six Sigma: Definition and underlying theory. Journal of Operations Management. 2008;26(4):536 to 554.)

Table 2
Explanation of "DMAIC" acronym for the project planning in six sigma

DMAIC	Explanation and Examples
Define	Develop problem statement goals, milestone, and process map
Measure	Collect data to quantitate problems, identify input and output measure, develop operational definitions, collect baseline data
Analyze	Consider pareto charts, fishbone diagrams, time-value analysis, SIPOC chart, create a narrowed/prioritized lists of root cause
Improve	Design experiments, develop situation, consider a Failure Mode Effects Analysis (FMEA), create an implementation plan
Control	Monitor improvements, develop standards and procedures, verify benefits, track with SPC charts

by the 5th "Why," but it can be asked even more times if necessary. The final answer is where interventions should likely be applied. "The five Whys" is also a tool used in Root Cause Analyses and does not need to be limited to Six Sigma.

Examples from the Literature
Although there are few examples published using Six Sigma in neonatology, it is a well-described methodology in health care, particularly with process optimization and resource management.[28] Specific examples could include improving patient throughput in the emergency department while also increasing patient satisfaction, or reducing hospital costs. Practically speaking, most projects in health care combine tools from Lean and Six Sigma.

Gleich and colleagues tackled the problem of ineffective and inefficient transfers from the operating room to the pediatric intensive care unit (PICU) using Lean and Six Sigma methodology. They observed the baseline process, performed value stream mapping, and tracked handoff error reduction. With the introduction of a new transfer process, they had a significant decrease in handoff errors and decreased transfer time. They also improved staff satisfaction.[29]

An excellent example of applying DMAIC to an inefficient process is seen in the work by Prajapati and Suman, who clearly outline a more streamlined approach for managing patients with jaundice in a rural setting. They effectively use a charter, process map, and fishbone diagram to come up with targeted interventions that improve the process.[30]

S	I	P	O	C
Suppliers	Inputs	Process	Outputs	Customers
Who supplies the materials/input? Who is involved?	What resources are needed or provided by supplier? Materials or information.	What steps or activities are carried out to create value for the customer?	What products or services are created by or result from the process?	Who are the customers?

Fig. 15. An SIPOC chart can help break out the components of a system to more easily identify where the defects might be.

Other Methodologies

Total Quality Management

Total Quality Management (TQM) was born out of the work of W. Edwards Deming, Joseph Juran, and Philip Crosby, with momentum in the United States largely in the 1980s and 1990s and originating with the US Navy. Not surprisingly, it has some overlap with Lean. TQM is defined as an ongoing process where management takes the necessary steps to make sure everyone in the organization is trained to establish and achieve standards that meet the needs of the customer.[31] Many of the TQM practices are applicable and have been used in health care, including process management, management commitment, and organizational culture,[32] however, not much has been published using this methodology in health care since the 1990s.

Evidence-Based Practice for Improving Quality

The Evidence-Based Practice for Improving Quality (EPIQ) method for continuous quality improvement was first published by Lee and colleagues in 2009 through a project carried out by the Canadian Neonatal Network (CNN).[33] The method is based on three pillars: the use of evidence from published literature, the use of data from participating hospitals to identify hospital-specific practices for targeted intervention, and the use of a national network to share expertise. EPIQ builds on existing quality improvement methods and uses many of the same tools associated with the Model for Improvement and Lean, such as pareto charts, rapid cycle tests of change, process maps, and control charts. However, rather than adopting a "package" of practices from a hospital with good outcomes, it enables sites to select specific practice changes and implementation tools that are more pertinent or targeted. The authors argue this is potentially more efficient and cost-effective.

The group conducted a prospective cluster-randomized randomized controlled trial (RCT) to reduce nosocomial infections and bronchopulmonary dysplasia in preterm infants born in 12 hospitals in the CNN to evaluate the efficacy of the EPIQ method. In their study, they showed that quality improvement using EPIQ led to a reduction in bronchopulmonary dysplasia (BPD) and that it may reduce nosocomial infections.[33] The EPIQ approach is well-suited for an area with regionalized NICUs, as the CNN tasked different groups to perform evidence reviews on various topics, from which recommendations and consensus were created and implementation was then dependent on the local context. The group has also acknowledged the importance of adequate QI training and unit culture in achieving success.[34,35]

Achieving success and the power of people

The different QI methodologies outlined previously specifically address three of the four domains of Deming's System of Profound Knowledge. They appreciate that systems create our outcomes in health care and embrace changes in the system to drive improvement. Each methodology understands the system or problem in its own unique way. Likewise, each methodology has its unique way to learn about its systems and utilize that knowledge for improvement. Data in each of these methods are presented in a time-series fashion to understand the type of variation seen in their data. A comparison of the three main methodologies covered is included in **Table 3**. The fourth domain of Deming's System of Profound Knowledge, psychology or the human side of change, is one area not specifically addressed by the different methodologies. Given its importance, specific attention is being paid to it here.

	Model for Improvement	Lean	Six Sigma
Table 3 Comparison of the project flow in the three most commonly used methodologies, the Model for Improvement, Lean, and Six Sigma			
Identify the problem or goal	SMART Aim	Define value for the customer (or patient)	Define - Defects and projects goal
Establish "theory" of the problem	Driver diagram	Fishbone diagram	Measure - Collect data to quantify problem
Understand the system in detail	Define measures (outcome, process balancing)	"Go to the gemba, Process mapping" and value stream mapping	Analyze - SIPOC chart, Pareto chart
Identify and apply change ideas	PDSA cycles	Kaizen event to identify areas for improvement	Improve - create implementation plan
Track data and adjust as needed over time	Measure data over time using run charts or SPC	Implement changes altogether, make adjustment as needed	Control - monitor with SPC, develop standards and procedures

Note that all move through a similar thought process and there is overlap in the tools used.

Team Formation

No matter which methodology is used, a project should begin with the formation of a multidisciplinary team that is representative of all of the different roles that touch the issue being addressed. The importance of a team of key stakeholders that actually work in the day-to-day system one is attempting to change is essential. A team comprised solely of leadership or administrators will likely overlook or fail to appreciate valuable details in the process and achieving buy-in from staff may also become more challenging. In addition to the frontline care providers, it is similarly critical to involve the families of our patients.

The Psychology of Change

Although all of the methodologies listed above have discussed the importance of involving people in the process of improvement, it has been suggested that maybe they do not go far enough. The IHI produced a white paper entitled, The Psychology of Change, to address this issue.[36] The authors cite, "Improvement Science has given health care improvers the framework and the skills to understand variation, study systems, build learning, and determine the best evidence-based interventions ("what") and implementation strategies ("how") to achieve the desired outcomes. Yet, health care improvers worldwide still struggle with the adaptive side of change, which relates to unleashing the power of people ("who") and their motivations ("why") to advance and sustain improvement—two commonly cited reasons for the failure of improvement initiatives."

To sustain improvement initiatives, they suggest that it is imperative that team leaders "activate agency" in the frontline staff that are so important in improvement efforts. This means that they must help people gain the ability to choose to act with purpose. They theorize that the way to accomplish this is by addressing these five inter-related domains.

- Unleashing Intrinsic Motivation

- Co-Designing People-Driven Change
- Co-Producing in Authentic Relationships
- Distributing Power
- Adapting in Action

Although the details of these domains are beyond the scope of this article, suffice it to say that without doing a better job of embracing and improving the human side of change, even the most thorough improvement efforts will not be sustained.

SUMMARY

The history of quality improvement and its movement from industry into health care is a vast topic. With so many different methodologies and tools, it can be overwhelming to decide where to start. We recommend looking at the resources and tools used at one's institution as well as developing a keen understanding of the aim or problem to be solved. One can then refer to the different approaches in this article and decide which one makes the most sense. It is considered a best practice to embrace one methodology in an organization so there is familiarity in language and approach. However, there may be instances where combining aspects of more than one methodology adds value. Regardless of the methodology chosen, a thorough and structured approach to problem definition, creation of change ideas that are tested and implemented, continuous tracking of data, and effective teamwork will result in quality improvement for our patients.

DISCLOSURE

Katherine Coughlin is the recipient of a grant from Chiesi USA, to execute a local quality improvement effort to reduce chronic lung disease. No aspects of that project or grant are discussed in the article. Michael Posencheg is on the contract faculty of the Institute for Healthcare Improvement and receives stipends for quality improvement methodology teaching.

REFERENCES

1. Edwards Deming W. Out of the Crisis. Cambridge, MA: MIT Press; 1986.
2. Scoville RLK. Comparing lean and quality improvement. IHI White Paper. Cambridge, Massachusetts: Institute for Healthcare Improvement; 2014.
3. Langley GJ, Moen RD, Nolan KM, et al. *The improvement guide: a practical approach to enhancing organizational performance.* 2nd ed. San Francisco, CA: Jossey-Bass; 2009.
4. Science of Improvement: Establishing measures. Boston, Massachusetts: Institute for Healthcare Improvement, Available at: www.IHI.org. Accessed on March 20, 2023.
5. de Bono E. Six thinking Hats: the multi-million bestselling guide to running better meetings and making faster decisions. Westminster, London, England: Penguin; 2017.
6. Provost LPMS. The healthcare data guide: learning from data for improvement. San Francisco, CA: Jossey-Bass; 2011.
7. Perla RJ, Provost LP, Murray SK. The run chart: a simple analytical tool for learning from variation in healthcare processes. BMJ Qual Saf 2011;20(1):46–51.
8. Schwartz SP, Rehder KJ. Quality improvement in pediatrics: past, present, and future. Pediatr Res 2017;81(1–2):156–61.

9. Coughlin K, Posencheg M, Orfe L, et al. Reducing variation in the management of apnea of prematurity in the intensive care Nursery. Pediatrics 2020;145(2). https://doi.org/10.1542/PEDS.2019-0861.

10. Glenn T, Price R, Culbertson L, et al. Improving thermoregulation in transported preterm infants: a quality improvement initiative. J Perinatol 2021;41(2):339–45.

11. Black J.R., Miller D. and Sensel J., The Toyota way to healthcare excellence : increase efficiency and improve quality with lean, Health Adminstration Press; Chicago IL.

12. Sloan T, Fitzgerald A, Hayes KJ, et al. Lean in healthcare– history and recent developments. J Health Organisat Manag 2014;28(2):130–4.

13. Hallam CRA, Contreras C. Lean healthcare: scale, scope and sustainability. Int J Health Care Qual Assur 2018;31(7):684–96.

14. Flynn R, Newton AS, Rotter T, et al. The sustainability of Lean in pediatric healthcare: a realist review. Syst Rev 2018;7(1). https://doi.org/10.1186/s13643-018-0800-z.

15. Rotter T, Plishka C, Lawal A, et al. What is lean management in health care? Development of an operational definition for a cochrane systematic review. Eval Health Prof 2019;42(3):366–90.

16. Going Lean in Healthcare. IHI Innovation Series white paper. Cambridge, MA: Insitute for Healthcare Improvement; 2005.

17. Coughlin K, Posencheg MA. Quality improvement methods – Part II. J Perinatol 2019;39(7). https://doi.org/10.1038/s41372-019-0382-1.

18. Womack JP, Jones DT. Lean thinking: banish waste and create wealth in your corporation. New York: Simon & Schuster. 2003. Available at: https://books.google.com/books/about/Lean_Thinking.html?id=l8hWAAAAYAAJ. 396. Accessed July 4, 2022.

19. George ML, Rowlands D, Price M, et al. The lean six sigma pocket toolbook. Lean Six Sigma Pocket Toolbook 2005;55–62.

20. Kenaley KM, Rickolt AL, Vandersteur DA, et al. An intervention to decrease time to parents' first hold of infants in the Neonatal Intensive Care Unit requiring respiratory support. J Perinatol 2020;40(5):812–9.

21. Vats A, Goin KH, Villarreal MC, et al. The impact of a lean rounding process in a pediatric intensive care unit. Crit Care Med 2012;40(2):608–17.

22. Schroeder RG, Linderman K, Liedtke C, et al. Six sigma: definition and underlying theory. J Oper Manag 2008;26(4):536–54.

23. Smith B. Lean and six sigma–a one-two punch. Qual Prog 2003;36(4):37–41. Available at: https://www.proquest.com/magazines/lean-six-sigma-one-two-punch/docview/214773431/se-2?accountid=34798.

24. Al-Qatawneh L, Abdallah AAA, Zalloum SSZ. Six sigma application in healthcare logistics: a framework and A case study. J Healthc Eng 2019;2019. https://doi.org/10.1155/2019/9691568.

25. Besunder JB, Super DM. Lean Six Sigma: trimming the fat! Effectively managing precious resources. Crit Care Med 2012;40(2):699–700.

26. Cronemyr P. DMAIC and DMADV - differences, similarities and synergies. Int J Six Sigma Compet Advant 2007;3(3):193–209.

27. Polk DO. Lean six sigma, innovation, and the change acceleration process can work together. Physician Exec 2011;37(1):38–42. Available at: https://www.proquest.com/scholarly-journals/lean-six-sigma-innovation-change-acceleration/docview/846786725/se-2?accountid=34798.

28. Deblois S, Lepanto L. Lean and Six Sigma in acute care: a systematic review of reviews. Int J Health Care Qual Assur 2016;29(2):192–208.

29. Gleich SJ, Nemergut ME, Stans AA, et al. Improvement in patient transfer process from the operating room to the PICU using a lean and six sigma-based quality improvement project. Hosp Pediatr 2016;6(8):483–9.

30. Prajapati D, Suman G. Six sigma approach for neonatal jaundice patients in an Indian rural hospital - a case study. Int J Health Care Qual Assur 2019;36–51, ahead-of-print(ahead-of-print).

31. Miller WJ. A working definition for total quality management (TQM) researchers. J Qual Manag 1996;1(2):149–59.

32. Faisal T, Rahman Z, Azam M. Best practices of total quality management implementation in health care settings. Health Mark Q 2011;28(3):232–52.

33. Lee SK, Aziz K, Singhal N, et al. Improving the quality of care for infants: a cluster randomized controlled trial. CMAJ (Can Med Assoc J) 2009;181(8):469–76.

34. Cronin CMG, Baker GR, Lee SK, et al. Reflections on knowledge translation in Canadian NICUs using the EPIQ method. Healthc Q 2011;8–16, 14 Spec No 3.

35. Lee SK, Aziz K, Singhal N, et al. The Evidence-based Practice for Improving Quality method has greater impact on improvement of outcomes than dissemination of practice change guidelines and quality improvement training in neonatal intensive care units. Paediatr Child Health 2015;20(1):e1–9.

36. Hilton KAA. IHI psychology of change framework to advance and sustain improvement boston, Massachusetts. IHI White Paper 2018.

Sustaining Improvement Initiatives: Challenges and Potential Tools

Asaph Rolnitsky, MSc HQ, MD[a],*, Chaim M. Bell, MD, PhD[b]

KEYWORDS

- Sustainability • Quality • Improvement • Change • Neonatology

KEY POINTS

- Change in human behavior is difficult to achieve due to resistance and reversal.
- A significant proportion of quality improvement (QI) initiatives do not sustain.
- Characteristics of leadership, resources, process, and change can contribute to the sustainability of successful change.
- Several tools to plan for, promote, and sustain QI interventions are available and presented.

"After victory, tighten your helmet cord." Japanese proverb

INTRODUCTION

It is a common observation that many quality improvement (QI) interventions fade gradually over time, as many organizational changes occur.[1] Studies quantified sustainment as around a typical 40%.[2] Like many processes, successful implementation and initial encouraging outcomes do not always translate to sustained effort or sustained improvement.[2] There is accumulating evidence that the more laborious the process, and the more limited its impact, the higher the risk becomes of abandoning it or allowing it to fade away gradually.[3,4] Moreover, as with research on negative outcomes or errors of omission, the extent of the phenomenon is underreported, thereby limiting rigorous studies. Indeed, by definition, proper evaluation of sustainability requires longitudinal observation over time. This contrasts with a QI intervention that can span a relatively short period. Assessing sustainability naturally examines a

---

[a] DAN Women and Babies Program, Newborn and Developmental Paediatrics, University of Toronto, Sunnybrook Health Sciences Centre, 2075 Bayview Avenue, Toronto, Ontario M4N 3M5, Canada; [b] University of Toronto, Mount Sinai Hospital Suite 426 600 University Avenue Toronto, ON M5G 1X5, Canada
* Corresponding author. NICU, M4 wing, Sunnybrook Health Sciences Centre, 2075 Bayview Avenue, Toronto, Ontario M4N 3M5, Canada
E-mail address: asaph.rolnitsky@sunnybrook.ca

Clin Perinatol 50 (2023) 307–320
https://doi.org/10.1016/j.clp.2023.01.001
0095-5108/23/© 2023 Elsevier Inc. All rights reserved.

phenomenon that is frequently less measurable, not clearly defined, and often not reproducible to clinicians.

Like most QI sciences and methods, most evidence regarding sustaining improvement is from the fields of cognitive sciences, management, manufacturing, and engineering. These findings were then imported and applied to implementation in health care. Deming's "Theory of Profound Knowledge"[5] already established the foundations of change within the contexts of knowledge, systems, variation, and psychology.[6] For example, we know that culture is a key component[7] in the success of QI work, a component that is not within the "clinical" realm, but important.

A clinical example can be quite illustrative. Suppose a team implements an antimicrobial stewardship program to reduce antibiotic prescription in a neonatal intensive care unit (NICU). This process involves daily updates on antibiotic usage rates (AUR), expected length of therapy for each baby, and confirming the plan at the bedside. The process is successful, reducing antimicrobial use by 30% and is presented at a conference. All too often, as time progresses and some team members move to other roles, the previous strict adherence to protocol deteriorates. Thereafter, more days after the intervention may pass and eventually, the stewardship program may no longer be properly functioning or is abandoned within a year or two.

This review aims to detail what successfully maintains processes, the causes of sustainability failures, the evidence behind them, systemic efforts to sustain improvement, and suggested mechanisms to maintain improvement efforts when planning a QI intervention. Of note, sustainability here refers to continuation or maintenance and not sustainability in the financial, environmental, and societal context, which by itself is an emerging topic in QI literature.[8–10]

This review focuses on processes after the change has occurred, and the intervention has achieved its target or is in the desired direction toward its intended result. The processes before the aim, the changes, and the measurements are reviewed elsewhere in this journal.

DEFINITION

Sustainability of a change can be defined as a new 'steady state' when the change (improvement in QI interventions) becomes the new norm, involving better outcomes, and new standardized processes and behavior. The United Kingdom's National Health Service defines sustainability as "When new ways of working and improved outcomes become the norm. Not only have the process and outcome changed, but the thinking and attitudes behind them are fundamentally altered and the systems surrounding them are transformed in support. In other words, it has become an integrated or mainstream way of working rather than something 'added on'."[11]

Even when it seems that the concept is clear and the definition of sustainability is intuitive, the literature on the topic is variable. Moore and colleagues[12] studied the themes behind the definition of sustainability in this context in 200 publications, and suggest the definitions of sustainability as (1) after a defined period, (2) the program, clinical intervention, and/or implementation strategies continue to be delivered and/or (3) individual behavior change (ie, clinician, patient) is maintained; (4) the program and individual behavior change may evolve or adapt although (5) continuing to produce benefits for individuals/systems. Lennox and colleagues[13] analyzed the definition of sustainability in 62 QI projects. Their analysis shows that 86% defined sustainability as a continuation of the program and 44% defined it as continuing health benefits. A minority defined it as built capacity (19%), adaptation or development (16%), or cost recovery (3%). Wiltsey Stirman et al.[3] reviewed 125 studies on sustainability and found variable definitions and partial reporting of sustained results. In their analysis, even when sustainment was a defined, measured outcome, 34% showed a reduction in sustainment parameters, irrespective of the clinical outcomes.

We can summarize and define sustainability as *a shift of mindset, a change in systems, and a continuation of the new processes despite challenges and variations*. As mentioned, sustaining improvement does require adaptability and the capacity to adjust as the systems develop. Sustainability of QI interventions specifically is the focus of this review.

In our example, an alternate, sustained scenario is presented: The antimicrobial stewardship program continues to function. As new team members come and go, others are assigned to lead it. The stewardship protocol continues and becomes the norm in daily rounds. Within a year no one "does it differently" and despite changes in patient complexity, and infection clusters, the program continues, with similar AURs and even a few months of superior performance. When planning revised NICU clinical workflow, the program was considered integral to usual care and the program would never be canceled or abandoned.

On Change

Understanding sustainability requires learning about change theory. The fields of behavioral science, management, and leadership psychology have studied the matter of change itself,[14] its drivers and obstacles, and also examined why changes revert to a previous state. Lewin's theory of change,[15] and other later models use the concept of "freezing" to describe the establishment of new norms and their continuation. Lewin and subsequent researchers discussed "resisting forces" to changes and its four components: (1) real project difficulties (in our example—a surge in infections, convincing staff to "go back to longer therapy"); (2) management commitment limits (in our example—perhaps conflict between clinical decision makers and managers); (3) significant disagreements that were deemed manageable in the planning process (in our example—"culture-negative sepsis" in a sick baby and clinicians insisting antibiotics be continued despite stewardship guidelines); and (4) lack of system thinking, thus fixing individual issues but not system problems (in our example—attempting to reduce antibiotic use but not reducing unneeded septic evaluations).

Summarizing works by Lewin,[15] Buchanan,[16] Stouten,[4] Pettigrew[17], and others,[18–22] we can collate the main factors that enable or limit change. Those can be "hard" factors such as time, resources, and measurable benefits, or "soft" factors such as culture, motivation, leadership, and perceived values. The factors can be mapped to system layers—from individual factors to organizational ones as detailed in **Table 1**.

From the table, we can anticipate characteristics of human behavior, system, and organizational context, and the process itself to contribute to change acceptance or risk of changes decline. Learning the proposed process from different participants' perspectives, planning for staff engagement, and proper leadership selection, can mitigate some of the barriers to change success.

Why Changes Fail?

After implementing a change in a system, we know that many decline or revert to the previous state. Kotter's explanation of failed organizational transformations provides some insight into barriers to sustained changes. Studying failures of change in a cohort of 100 major organizations, he identified and described potential causes: (1) not planning to remove obstacles; (2) not planning for and demonstrating short-term wins; (3) declaring success too early; and (4) not anchoring change by (a)

Table 1
Contributing factors to successful organizational changes

Level	Characteristic	Influencers
Micro (individual) level	Predisposition toward changes	Dispositional employability
		Flexibility, adaptiveness
		Tolerance for uncertainty
		Positive change orientation
		Optimism
		Perceived control
		Workplace autonomy
		Perceived value
		Anxiety
		Fear of measurement
		Fear of isolation from an organization due to difference
	Motivational	Favorableness (anticipated benefit)
		Commitment to the organization
		Stress mitigation
		Perceived inevitability
	Fairness	Interpersonal justice
		Anticipatory justice beliefs
		Transparency, information
		Role modeling
	Identification	Identification with the organization
		Creating translational identity
Meso-level	Social ties and quality of relationship	Trust in peers
		Support from the higher level
		Training change agents
		Middle managers
		Quality interpersonal connection
		Change leaders from own group
	Emergent processes of change (small-scale changes)	Organizational routines
		Small local changes
		Negotiating policy
	Shared goals and beliefs	Shared vision
		Group-level shared beliefs
	Resources required	Time allocation
		Staffing requirement
		Measurable results
Macro level	Leadership competency	Management effectiveness
		Change leaders with complimentary competencies
		Social skills of change agents
		Managerial coping (positive self-concept and risk tolerance)
	Trust in leaders	Trust and reliance
	Change nature	Change bundles
		Process mechanisms
		Context within the organization
		Specific, targeted intervention (ie, Revision of professional roles for performance outcomes; teamwork for clinical outcomes, and so on)

(continued on next page)

Table 1 (continued)		
Level	Characteristic	Influencers
	Readiness for change	Employees' commitment to the organization
		Organizational history
		Jobs that promote initiative, independent thinking, decision making
		Supporting individual-level motivation

Modified from Stouten J, Rousseau DM, De Cremer D. Successful Organizational Change: Integrating the Management Practice and Scholarly Literatures. Acad Manag Ann. 2018;12(2):752-788.

demonstrating a link between the change and the improvement and (b) selecting and connecting the next generation of staff with the process for continuity. Kotter emphasizes different perspectives on the effect of sustainability. Linking to system theory, he details leadership, management, political/policy drives, organizational (and individual) culture, and time allowed for the changes to be embedded. Other researchers have described the tendency of changes to decay as well as the interconnected human behavior, organizational behavior, and mechanisms of change to promote sustainability. The sustainment effort is part of the process of achieving the changes and reaching their targets.

Characteristics of Successful, Sustained Interventions

So, what makes a change last? There are several analyses describing successful, sustained, QI implementations. We found several common characteristics and themes, organized in **Table 2** with their references and summarized below. We divided them into four main categories, partially in agreement with Laur and colleagues,[2] who use Concept, Capacity, and Competencies as the three main categories of their analysis.

1. Leadership: The theme of leadership was the most often recurring in all studies on the topic. Clear leadership involvement, from the design, through the intervention, to the results, and continued maintenance of the effort, and having a clear vision of QI work and its continuous sustainment, were all associated in all studies as important characteristics of sustained improvement, or lack of which to lack of successful sustained improvement.
2. Change and its effectiveness: A frequently noted characteristic of successful implementation is the change itself or the conceptual change in the day-to-day practice. Studies showed that evidence-based, effective, and clinically meaningful interventions were more likely to sustain.
3. Capacity: Numerous elements of capacity, or system capability of making the change, were demonstrated as important for sustainment. Those are
   a. Resources availability in reference to *dedication of time for QI work, using QI tools* for the intervention and its sustainment, *dedicated funding and its continuous flow* as required, and *supply of equipment* when applicable.
   b. Availability of staff in general, *dedicated staff* for the interventions, and *dedicated staff for sustainment* as enablers of continuous success.
   c. Quality of *work and workload* considerations were associated in some studies with the success or failure of sustainability of the intervention. *Added workload* was considered a barrier to success, and *high quality of work*, or *high value* of the work, supported engagement and continuous success.

Table 2
Themes indicating enablers of quality improvement sustainability

		References
Leadership	Leadership involvement	25–35
	Leadership characteristics	17,20,36
	Clear vision	30
	Accountability	26,29,30,33
Change	Evidence-based	3,13,23,28,31,37
	Effective	3,13,17,20,31,37
	Conforming to client's needs	36
Capacity/Resources	Dedication of time for QI work	2,30,32
	Funding	25,30,31,38
	Equipment/resources	30,33,37,38
	Availability of staff, dedicated staff	25,30,32,36
	Quality of work, workload	35,37,38
	Members' engagement	28,29,31,33,35,38
	Accountability of staff	26,29,30,33
	Education and QI training	2,13,23,24,26,28,30,32,34,36,38
Process	Planning for sustainment	2,13,29,32
	Standardization	23,31,36
	Stakeholder's involvement	3,13,32
	Alignment with systems priorities	13,17,20,23,31,33,37
	Adaptation to changes	2,3,13,23,27,28,30,31,34
	Communicating results	25–27,32–34
	Continuous analysis	3,13,23,25–27,30,37,38
	Collaboration, partnerships, and communication	2,3,13,25,29,31,37
	Engagement	23,28,29,31,33,35,37,38
	Reducing barriers, resistance, fear	30,32,35,36
	Staff continuity	23,26,37
	Incentives, rewards	23,32

d. Accountability is frequently mentioned as important for sustained outcomes. accountability of staff, leadership, and dedicated QI leaders is a driver for continuous successful intervention.

e. Education and QI training are mentioned as important for prolonged sustainability. *Staff knowledge* of QI or QI *methods*, and *continuous education* on the project, its methods, or its outcomes, contributed to sustained success.

4. Process

Many process-related elements were identified as contributors to successful sustainment. Those elements are usually within the content of the project or its execution.

a. Planning for sustainment in the form of documented strategy, *standardization* of interventions with clear design for sustainment, using *tools and forcing functions*, alignment with strategies, and standardized interventions were established enablers of sustainability.

b. Alignment with priorities at local, organizational, or national levels enabled better engagement and sustainment. This is a recurring theme and important theme that overlaps with the personal engagement factors.

c. Adaptation to changes—a frequent theme in analyses showed that adaptation of the intervention to required system needs or the required clinical needs over time enables better participation, better engagement, and prolonger sustainability. Lack of adaptation or rigidity can cause disengagement.

   d. Results—Studies show that demonstrating results, *communicating* the results to the involved participants and the organization, and publicly, *transparently* sharing them are associated with sustained success. Some studies suggest that *visual displays* as aids were particularly important.

   e. Continuous *analysis, continuous measurement*, and adaptation of measures as applicable enabled adaptation and sustainable outcomes.

   f. Stakeholders—involving stakeholders in different levels of the organization and different stages of the interventions are crucial to its continuous success. Stakeholders' withdrawal was associated with loss of support, engagement, and loss of outcomes benefits. This theme is recurring in the majority of the studies.

   g. Collaborations, partnerships, and communication—interventions require multi-professional teamwork, sometimes at the organizational level, and sometimes across systems, jurisdictions, and even at international levels. Continuation of communication, networking, and team relationships enabled continuous work and fruitful adaptation in studies on sustainability.

   h. Engagement, reducing barriers, resistance, and fear—the project participants' engagement, approval, and acceptance of the change are frequently counted as major enablers of sustainment. Studies showed that early engagement and cooperation support sustainability, and that remaining barriers and resistance are counterproductive and predictor of future decline.

   i. Staff *continuity*—reduced staff turnover was associated with increased sustainment and maintained project processes.

   j. Incentives, rewards are mentioned only in a minority of the studies but sometimes can be potential motivators to increase engagement and staff support.

To summarize this section, several studies evaluated the characteristics of successful QI interventions, and others that also analyzed the characteristics of those which failed. Although both types of studies have limitations and methodology differences, several themes are clearly repeating. The themes of leadership involvement, continuous education, availability of resources, adaptability of the process and the outcomes, alignment with the organization's aim, communication with others, and sharing results are the main running threads in both health care quality QI interventions, and general business, management, and organizational change studies. Most prominently present are the personal aspects of the works, emphasizing that the main driving forces behind successful changes are the human behavioral factors, and only to a lesser degree the resources and technical needs. In our antimicrobial stewardship example, the successful implementation and sustainment were attributed to effective and deeply involved leadership by the team leader—a pharmacist who presented results, kept the staff educated, demonstrated results, and kept collaboration with different stakeholders. In parallel, the project fitted the organization's aims, and although the change was conceptually hard to accept initially, it continued and sustained. In our antimicrobial stewardship example, we found that successful sustainment was dependent on the leadership and commitment of the champion, but we also found that the habituation of the new processes was maintained mainly due to forcing functions, continuous education, and because the processes and updated outcomes were routinely reviewed and transparently communicated to the team.

SUSTAINABILITY MODELS, FRAMEWORKS, AND TOOLS

What tools are available to assist the sustainability of QI interventions? Several published QI frameworks and models are available in the health care literature, with sustainability of the QI intervention as their target.

The UK National Health Services sustainability model[39] is one of the most commonly applied frameworks. It includes three main components for sustainability evaluation: Staff, Organization, and Process. Each contains several subcomponents—10 in total—that when placed in the template, allow for the QI professional to act as a planner, maintainer, or adjustor of the processes when the sustainment declines. In other words, this is a generic process review and audit tool of the sustainability components irrespective of the clinical and QI processes and outcomes. The framework components are quantified, calculated, and plotted on a radar chart, to provide visual aids to the current state compared with the optimal or desired state. The strength of this model is the ability to provide a quantifiable measure of sustainability measures and to track changes.[40] The radar chart, however, is not always intuitive to interpret and may be less useful for general users. Still, this tool can be extremely useful and productive for the leading QI staff.

The second widely-used framework is the one from the Institute for Healthcare Improvement (IHI).[41] The whitepaper is grounded in Juran's trilogy of quality planning, quality control, and QI. It is focused on elements of high-performance management, and details a driver diagram for sustainment, the primary drivers of which are the trilogy components. The primary drivers are driving quality control, managing QI, and establishing a culture of high-performance management. For each primary driver, they list secondary drivers and recommended actions, such as standardized processes, integration, problem-solving policy, and feedback. The framework strength is the aim for engagement of higher organization levels, but its weakness is the lack of measurable elements to provide sustainment indicators. Nevertheless, the widespread use and important contribution of the IHI as an organization, make this model a valuable and readily accessible tool. IHI also provided a sustainability toolkit[42] for their 5 Million Lives campaign. In the aid, they detail the components of sustainability and offer best practices to consider adopting, to enhance sustainability. We find that some of the suggested best practices are too general and may be difficult to implement as a sole sustainment element. For example, suggesting that everyone in a hospital will be educated on a certain intervention is ideal, but may be impractical. Nevertheless, their toolkit gives valuable examples from clinical units for each proposed practice, thus putting the title in real-life experience and proving the utility of many of them. The toolkit has no measurable indicators, but of potential use is the IHI Sustainability Planning Worksheet, one of the QI education toolkits, and lists five categories for sustainment planning, and some proposed actions under each one.[43] This functions as a useful checklist for sustainability drivers.

A very detailed model for evidence-based practice implementation was suggested by Aarons and colleagues,[44] based on public mental health services. Their work covers all parts of change practices, initially based on the reach, efficacy, adoption, implementation, maintenance (RE-AIM) model of health care change implementation,[45] but also includes in depth a suggestion for sustainability planning. In their sustainment component, they account for outer contexts—sociopolitical (leadership, policies), funding, and academic collaboration; and inner contexts—organizational characteristics (leadership, network, alignment with practices), monitoring and support, and staffing. This model does not offer quantifiable measures but provides an evidence-based change model and is useful in understanding a broader perspective of change management in health care.

Gruen and colleagues[46] performed a systematic review of sustainability studies in health care programs and proposed a framework for "Sustainability Science". Their framework is constructed from the interaction between the health issue, the intervention's characteristics, and their drivers. This is included within a defined context or culture and with effects from economic forces, politics, quality cycle steps, and the changes in the health problem. They also proposed a model for planning a sustained program, by asking questions that target system components, the interactions between the aforementioned elements, and the outcomes. They described their model as an ecosystem of complex interactions within the system. They noted that their proposed model was not validated but they found it useful when applied to certain case studies.

Other models, by Robert and colleagues,[34] Buchanan and colleagues,[16] Health Quality Ontario[47] Agency for Healthcare Research and Quality,[48] Stirman and colleagues,[3] Burke and colleagues,[49] and Schreier and colleagues[31] should be acknowledged, each aiming at different aspects of the sustainment enablers or the framework of the change, but are beyond the scope of this review.

Although each model has strengths and limitations, all take the most important drivers of sustainability that we reviewed. We recommend that early planning for project sustainment should be an integral part of the QI intervention itself,[31] especially if the change is of large scale and involves multiple collaborators. Behavioral sciences confirm that promoting a sustained change requires that the QI team take a preemptive approach[13,21,30,31,33] or expect a decline in their processes.

TO SUMMARIZE THIS SECTION, WE WILL ANSWER TWO QUESTIONS
Question 1: I Want to Plan My Quality Improvement Intervention to Last. What Should I Do?

We suggest the following considerations when embarking on a new QI intervention.

1. Meticulous planning of the process with a multidisciplinary team that would engage many involved team members
2. Including standardized and routinized tools, such as forcing functions or standardized order sets
3. Adequate allocation of staffing, hours, and resources on a long-term basis
4. Careful selection of leaders and team members with QI knowledge and personal skills to lead and maintain good communication and cooperation
5. Proper education on the benefits of the intervention and its alignment with the organization's goal
6. Involving stakeholders at an early stage and at interim intervals
7. Planning for process reevaluation with timed analyses
8. Presentations of results in visual aids that are transparent and clear
9. Allowing for a margin of adaptation of the aims, measures, and resources along the intervention and beyond

In an attempt to make a useful planning, auditing, and measuring tool, we propose a tool (**Fig. 1**) that includes the main elements of sustainability that were suggested in the previous studies, including categories (by colors, of systems, individuals, policies, patient centeredness, the QI project characteristics, and resources) and contributors that can be quantified or visually scaled, drawn on the arrows. The sustainment is measured and labeled in the central circle and the tool can be updated regularly (**Fig. 2**).

Question 2: I Have Already Implemented a Quality Improvement Change in My Organization. What Should I Do Now?

After the QI intervention is started or completed, we suggest routine steps to assist in the successful sustainment of the improved outcomes.

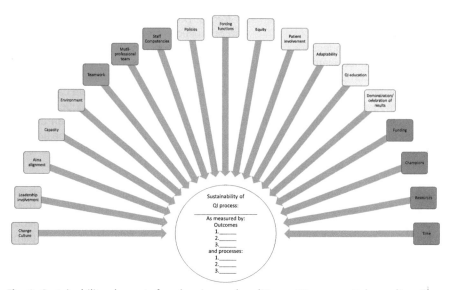

Fig. 1. Sustainability elements for planning and auditing a QI process. Color coding: Blue, project environment and leadership; Red, staff and team interactions; Green, change assurance; Yellow, patient centeredness; Light blue, process characteristics and maintenance; Purple, resources.

1. Maintain a leadership that is involved and accountable. This can be at any level as long as the leader is engaged and effective for the team.
2. Allocate dedicated time for QI work. This can be for comprehensive work or for short interim analyses.

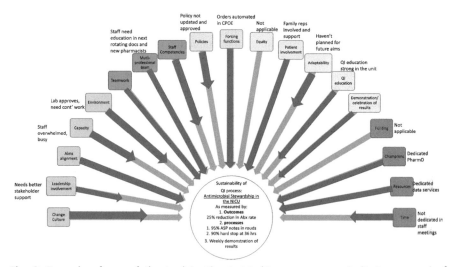

Fig. 2. Example of use of the tool in **Fig. 1**. Markings on arrows indicate measure of completeness or compliance. In this example, family involvement is at 100%, but policy elements are 30% only. Color coding: Blue, project environment and leadership; Red, staff and team interactions; Green, change assurance; Yellow, patient centeredness; Light blue, process characteristics and maintenance; Purple, resources.

3. Allocate funding, equipment/resources, and staff, as applicable. When in need, use stakeholders to support the required resources demonstrating the sustainment and its needs, as well as the clinical benefits.
4. Maintain core staff continuity, even if minimal, to prevent gaps and allow transitions.
5. Evaluate workload and intervene accordingly.
6. Maintain members' engagement through continuous education, QI refreshers, and communicating results honestly and transparently. Demonstrating challenges can help more than concealing them.
7. Standardize processes and incorporate work into policies with adaptation and flexibility to changes in the organizational or clinical settings.
8. Keep stakeholder's involved and updated. This can be one of the forcing functions of the work.
9. Adapt to changes as needed and communicate changes transparently and collaboratively. Adhering rigidly to obsolete processes will maintain work but may not sustain the improvement.
10. Continuous analysis or results—outcomes, as well as previously agreed sustainment measures, will help you reroute when needed.
11. Communicate results frequently to the team and collaborators. A fresh set will see processes that the team may be desensitized to.
12. Maintain collaborations or partnerships through updates and discussions. Learn from better performers and adopt processes as needed.

SUMMARY

QI interventions involve changes in the involved team's behavior, but resistance to changes and reversal to previous habits commonly cause a lower success rate in the longer term. Sustainment of successful interventions is best planned at the intervention's design stage and should then pursue with periodic reevaluations. Our tool and other models are available to facilitate planning and routine auditing of the progress to ensure its sustainability. Successful sustainment involves active leadership, capacity for resource allocation, alignment of the process with the systems, frequent adjustments, audits, and communication of the results to the involved members. Open collaboration and discussion about the process and the results are important enablers of prolonged, sustained changes that would benefit patients and improve effectiveness in health care.

DISCLOSURE

The authors have nothing to disclose and no funding or financial support was given for this manuscript.

REFERENCES

1. Beer M, Nohria N. Cracking the code of change. Harv Bus Rev 2000;78(3): 133–41.
2. Laur C, Corrado AM, Grimshaw JM, et al. Trialists perspectives on sustaining, spreading, and scaling-up of quality improvement interventions. Implement Sci Commun 2021;2(1):35.
3. Wiltsey Stirman S, Kimberly J, Cook N, et al. The sustainability of new programs and innovations: a review of the empirical literature and recommendations for future research. Implement Sci 2012;7(1):17.

4. Stouten J, Rousseau DM, De Cremer D. Successful organizational change: integrating the management practice and scholarly literatures. Acad Manag Ann 2018;12(2):752–88.
5. Deming WE. The new economy for industry, government, education. Cambridge (MA): Mass Inst of Technology; 1993.
6. Deming WE. The new economics for industry, government, education. Cambridge, MA: MIT Press; 2018.
7. Kaplan HC, Brady PW, Dritz MC, et al. The influence of context on quality improvement success in health care: a systematic review of the literature. Milbank Q 2010;88(4):500–59.
8. Mortimer F, Isherwood J, Wilkinson A, et al. Sustainability in quality improvement: redefining value. Future Heal J 2018;5(2):88–93.
9. Mortimer F, Isherwood J, Pearce M, et al. Sustainability in quality improvement: measuring impact. Future Heal J 2018;5(2):94–7.
10. Spooner R, Stanford V, Parslow-Williams S, et al. Concrete ways we can make a difference": a multi-centre, multi-professional evaluation of sustainability in quality improvement education. Med Teach 2022;44:1116–24.
11. OLD, S., 2010. Institute for Innovation and Improvement Sustainability - Model and Guide, Hospice UK. United Kingdom. Available at: https://policycommons. net/artifacts/1674733/institute-for-innovation-and-improvement-sustainability/ 2406382/. Accessed February, 28, 2023.
12. Moore JE, Mascarenhas A, Bain J, et al. Developing a comprehensive definition of sustainability. Implement Sci 2017;12(1):1–8.
13. Lennox L, Maher L, Reed J. Navigating the sustainability landscape: a systematic review of sustainability approaches in healthcare. Implement Sci 2018;13(1):27.
14. Grol R, Baker R, Moss F. Quality improvement research: understanding the science of change in health care. BMJ Qual Saf 2002;11(2):110–1.
15. Lewin K. Field theory in social science: selected theoretical papers. New York: Greenwood Press; 1975.
16. Buchanan D, Fitzgerald L, Ketley D, et al. No going back: a review of the literature on sustaining organizational change. Int J Manag Rev 2005;7(3):189–205.
17. The management of strategic change. In: Andrew P, editor. Long Range Plan 1989;22(6):136. Blackwell (1987), 370 pp., £29.95 (hardback).
18. Rimmer M. Reinventing competitiveness: achieving best practice in Australia. Pitman; 1996. Available at: https://books.google.ca/books?id=F8RpPQAACAAJ.
19. Jacobs RL. Institutionalizing organizational change through cascade training. J Eur Ind Train 2002;26(2/3/4):177–82.
20. Garman AN. Patrick Dawson. Understanding organizational change: the contemporary experience of people at work. Pers Psychol 2005;58(2):537.
21. Senge P, Kleiner A, Roberts C, et al. The dance of change: The challenges to sustaining momentum in learning organizations. Published online 1999.
22. Sirkin HL, Keenan P, Jackson A. The hard side of change management. Harv Bus Rev 2005. Available at: https://hbr.org/2005/10/the-hard-side-of-change-management. Accessed June 23, 2022.
23. Staines A, Thor J, Robert G. Sustaining improvement? The 20-year Jönköping quality improvement program revisited. Qual Manag Health Care 2015;24(1): 21–37.
24. Øvretveit J, Staines A. Sustained improvement? Findings from an independent case study of the jönköping quality program. Qual Manag Healthc 2007;16(1): 68–83.

25. Bray P, Cummings DM, Wolf M, et al. After the collaborative is over: what sustains quality improvement initiatives in primary care practices? Jt Comm J Qual Patient Saf 2009;35(10):502-AP3.

26. Santos P, Joglekar A, Faughnan K, et al. Sustaining and spreading quality improvement: decreasing intrapartum malpractice risk. J Healthc Risk Manag J Am Soc Healthc Risk Manag 2019;38(3):42–50.

27. Baker D, Quinn B, Ewan V, et al. Sustaining quality improvement: long-term reduction of nonventilator hospital-acquired pneumonia. J Nurs Care Qual 2019;34(3):223–9.

28. Kacholi G, Mahomed OH. Sustainability of quality improvement teams in selected regional referral hospitals in Tanzania. Int J Qual Health Care 2020;32(4):259–65.

29. Khurshid Z, De Brún A, Martin J, et al. A systematic review and narrative synthesis: determinants of the effectiveness and sustainability of measurement-focused quality improvement trainings. J Contin Educ Health Prof 2021;41(3):210–20.

30. Verma P, Moran JW. Sustaining a quality improvement culture in local health departments applying for accreditation. J Public Health Manag Pract JPHMP 2014; 20(1):43–8.

31. Scheirer MA, Dearing JW. An agenda for research on the sustainability of public health programs. Am J Public Health 2011;101(11):2059–67.

32. Compas C, Hopkins KA, Townsley E. Best practices in implementing and sustaining quality of care. A review of the quality improvement literature. Res Gerontol Nurs 2008;1(3):209–16.

33. Parand A, Benn J, Burnett S, et al. Strategies for sustaining a quality improvement collaborative and its patient safety gains. Int J Qual Health Care J Int Soc Qual Health Care 2012;24(4):380–90.

34. Robert G, Sarre S, Maben J, et al. Exploring the sustainability of quality improvement interventions in healthcare organisations: a multiple methods study of the 10-year impact of the "Productive Ward: releasing Time to Care" programme in English acute hospitals. BMJ Qual Saf 2020;29(1):31–40.

35. Cranley LA, Hoben M, Yeung J, et al. SCOPEOUT: sustainability and spread of quality improvement activities in long-term care- a mixed methods approach. BMC Health Serv Res 2018;18(1):174.

36. Dale B, Boaden R, Wilcox M, et al. Sustaining continuous improvement: what are the key issues? Qual Eng 1999;11(3):369–77.

37. Devi R, Martin GP, Banerjee J, et al. Sustaining interventions in care homes initiated by quality improvement projects: a qualitative study. BMJ Qual Saf 2022. https://doi.org/10.1136/bmjqs-2021-014345. bmjqs-2021-014345.

38. Belostotsky V, Laing C, White DE. The sustainability of a quality improvement initiative. Healthc Manage Forum 2020;33(5):195–9.

39. Maher L, Gustafson D, Evans A. Sustainability model and guide. UK: NHS Institute for Innovation and Improvement; 2009.

40. Silver SA, McQuillan R, Harel Z, et al. How to sustain change and support continuous quality improvement. Clin J Am Soc Nephrol CJASN 2016;11(5):916–24.

41. Scoville R, Little K, Rakover J, et al. Sustaining improvement. Boston, MA: Inst Healthc Improv White Pap; 2016.

42. 5 Million Lives Campaign. Getting Started Kit: Sustainability and Spread. Published online 2008.

43. Sustainability Planning Worksheet. Published online 2019. ihi.org/QI.

44. Aarons GA, Hurlburt M, Horwitz SM. Advancing a conceptual model of evidence-based practice implementation in public Service sectors. Adm Policy Ment Health Ment Health Serv Res 2011;38(1):4–23.

45. Glasgow RE, Vogt TM, Boles SM. Evaluating the public health impact of health promotion interventions: the RE-AIM framework. Am J Public Health 1999;89(9): 1322–7.
46. Gruen RL, Elliott JH, Nolan ML, et al. Sustainability science: an integrated approach for health-programme planning. Lancet 2008;372(9649):1579–89.
47. Heath Quality Ontario. Implementing and sustaining changes-Primer. Available at: http://www.hqontario.ca/Portals/0/documents/qi/qi-implementing-and-sustaining-changes-primer-en.pdf. Accessed July 22, 2022.
48. A model for sustaining and spreading safety interventions. Agency for Healthcare Research and Quality. Available at: https://www.ahrq.gov/hai/cauti-tools/guides/sustainability-guide.html.
49. Burke RE, Mheen PJM van de. Sustaining quality improvement efforts: emerging principles and practice. BMJ Qual Saf 2021;30(11):848–52.

Challenging Cases in Statistical Process Control for Quality Improvement in Neonatal Intensive Care

Munish Gupta, MD, MMSc[a],*, Lloyd P. Provost, MS[b],
Heather C. Kaplan, MD, MSCE[c]

KEYWORDS

- Control chart • Statistical process control • Quality improvement
- Quality improvement methods

KEY POINTS

- Statistical process control methods allow rigorous time-series data analysis to support quality improvement efforts.
- Nontraditional statistical process control methods may be needed to analyze properly quality improvement data in selected situations.
- These situations include skewed continuous data, autocorrelation, small persistent changes in performance, confounders, and workload or productivity measures.

INTRODUCTION

Measurement over time is critical for quality improvement (QI). Statistical process control (SPC) methods were developed to facilitate rigorous analysis of time-series data, based on both statistics and pragmatism. SPC has become widely accepted as an optimal approach for examining and understanding QI data, in health care broadly and in the neonatal intensive care unit (NICU).[1–6]

As the use of SPC has spread, situations increasingly arise in which common SPC charts are not effective and more advanced or specialized SPC approaches may be required. In this review, we provide several examples of these challenging cases and review more advanced SPC approaches. We intentionally focus on examples from NICU QI efforts. We will review the following: (1) approaches to nonsymmetrically distributed

[a] Beth Israel Deaconess Medical Center, 330 Brookline Avenue, Boston, MA 02215, USA;
[b] Associates in Process Improvement, 2000 Red Hawk Road, Wimberly, TX 78676, USA;
[c] Cincinnati Children's Hospital Medical Center, 3333 Burnet Avenue, Cincinnati, OH 45229, USA
* Corresponding author.
E-mail address: mgupta@bidmc.harvard.edu

Clin Perinatol 50 (2023) 321–341
https://doi.org/10.1016/j.clp.2023.02.004
0095-5108/23/© 2023 Elsevier Inc. All rights reserved.
perinatology.theclinics.com

or highly skewed continuous data; (2) approaches to autocorrelation; (3) use of Cumulative Sum (CUSUM) or Exponentially Weighted Moving Average (EMWA) control charts to detect small, persistent changes in systems; (4) methods for addressing confounders with SPC charts; (5) and workload or productivity measures, in which discrete data may be better considered continuous for SPC analysis. This review illustrates SPC examples for these situations, although a full understanding of these more advanced concepts will likely require consulting resources that are more comprehensive.

CONTROL CHARTS FOR HIGHLY SKEWED CONTINUOUS DATA

The special situation of nonsymmetrically distributed or highly skewed continuous data is encountered frequently in neonatal QI. For example, common measures such as length of stay (LOS), ventilator days, or time to complete an activity such as kangaroo care, first oral feeding with colostrum, or antibiotic administration are often highly skewed. Several examples are shown in **Fig. 1**.

I-charts (also called X or XmR charts) and Xbar-S charts are the most commonly used SPC charts for continuous data, and the calculations used for plotting the centerline and control limits assume that the distribution of the measure is normal (or approximately normal). Skewness in the data may affect the validity of these charts and affect the application of probability-based rules for detecting special cause variation. Specifically, the use of control charts for continuous data with skewed distributions increases the risk of a type 1 error (false-positive signal of special cause). Xbar charts are generally more robust to a variety of types and distributions of data because the Central Limit Theorem assures that the averages of any distribution will approach a symmetric (normal) distribution, as the number of averaged values increases.[7] However, S-charts are more sensitive to the underlying distribution of the data and highly skewed data can result in the S-chart having false evidence of special cause variation. Furthermore, in the cases where S-charts are affected by skewed data, the resulting Xbar chart may not be useful, as the calculation of the limits for an Xbar chart is based on centerline of the S-chart. I-charts that plot individual values are particularly sensitive to the shape of the distribution of the data, and highly skewed data can make these charts ineffective for learning.

There are several conditions when highly skewed data make interpretation and learning from an Xbar-S or I-charts difficult, including the following: (1) when the calculated control limit is less than 0 for a measure where this is not possible; (2) much more than 50% of the data are below the average; (3) when the S-chart has a large number of unexplained special causes occurring due to extreme (but not unexpected) values that occur regularly in a process; (4) and when there are multiple false signals of

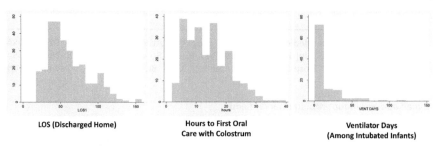

LOS (Discharged Home)   Hours to First Oral
Care with Colostrum   Ventilator Days
(Among Intubated Infants)

Fig. 1. Histograms of multiple skewed NICU measures.

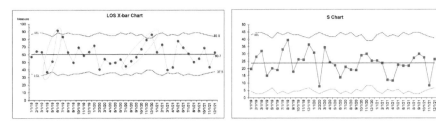

Fig. 2. Xbar and S-chart of NICU LOS (nontransformed).

special cause variation.[4] In cases where skewed data are not affecting learning, typical I-charts or Xbar-S charts can be created. However, in cases where learning is affected, likely due to increased false-positive signals of special cause variation, data can be transformed to create a more symmetric distribution before plotting on a control chart. There are several different transformations that can create a more symmetric distribution including square root transformation, reciprocal (1/X), or logarithmic transformation. To determine the optimal transformation, it is helpful to look at the histogram visually to identify the most symmetric appearing distribution. In addition, it is helpful to compare the mean and median and select the transformation where the mean and median values are closest (given that the mean equals the median in symmetrically distributed data). It is also possible to use software to compute statistical tests that test the normality of a given data set based on skewness (a measure of asymmetry or direction of outliers) and/or kurtosis (a measure of how often outliers occur) of the data.[8]

Example: Neonatal Intensive Care Unit Length of Stay

NICU LOS is a frequent target for QI initiatives. Because LOS data are continuous, QI efforts frequently use an I-chart or Xbar-S charts. As previously shown, NICU LOS data are typically skewed. **Fig. 2** shows NICU LOS analyzed with Xbar-S charts; these charts seem robust enough to allow for sufficient interpretation and learning without transformation. However, an I-chart of the same data, shown in **Fig. 3**, is less robust, with several false-positive special cause signals, a lower control limit of less than 0 (which is not possible), and more than 50% of the data below the average. Consequently, learning from this chart is limited.

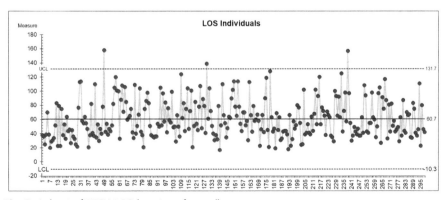

Fig. 3. I-chart of NICU LOS (nontransformed).

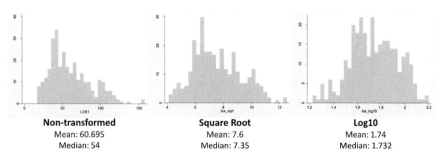

Non-transformed
Mean: 60.695
Median: 54

Square Root
Mean: 7.6
Median: 7.35

Log10
Mean: 1.74
Median: 1.732

Fig. 4. Histogram of NICU LOS data nontransformed and with square root and logarithmic transformations.

When an S-chart or I-chart is significantly affected by skewed data, transforming the data can create a more symmetric distribution. **Fig. 4** shows histograms of LOS data nontransformed and then with square root and logarithmic transformations. Both transformations show a more symmetric distribution, with the logarithmic transformation showing the most symmetric.

After transforming the data, the control chart can be created with the limits and centerline calculated using the transformed data. **Table 1** shows the difference between the values for the data point and upper and lower control limits for both the original and transformed data set for a selection of the LOS datapoints. Examining the control chart of the transformed data can be helpful for identifying special cause; **Figs. 5** and **6** show Xbar-S and I-charts using the log-transformed data. However, because it can be difficult to interpret a control chart where the units are on a nontraditional scale (eg, logarithmic scale), typically, the centerline and upper and lower control limits are reverse transformed to the original units. For an I-chart, the resulting control chart plots the original data points but with the centerline and control limits calculated based on the transformed data and then reverse transformed, as shown in **Fig. 7**. For the Xbar-S charts, however, the individual data points that are plotted are not the same as the original points because when the data are transformed before calculating the subgroup averages, the reverse

Table 1
Data and control limits for length-of-stay metric (Xbar chart), original, log transformed, and back transformed

	Original Data			Log Transformed Data			Back Transformed Data		
	Data Point	UCL	LCL	Data Point	UCL	LCL	Data Point	UCL	LCL
01/01/2019	57.3	86.8	34.6	1.74	1.93	1.55	55.0	85.3	35.2
02/01/2019	64.6	88.8	32.6	1.76	1.95	1.53	57.5	88.2	34.1
03/01/2019	63.4	88.8	32.6	1.75	1.95	1.53	56.2	88.2	34.1
04/01/2019	37	86.8	34.6	1.54	1.93	1.55	34.7	85.3	35.2
05/01/2019	51.3	83.9	37.5	1.67	1.91	1.57	46.8	81.2	37.0
06/01/2019	91.6	88.8	32.6	1.95	1.95	1.53	89.1	88.2	34.1
07/01/2019	83.5	86.8	34.6	1.89	1.93	1.55	77.6	85.3	35.2
08/01/2019	63.14	88.8	32.6	1.72	1.95	1.53	52.5	88.2	34.1

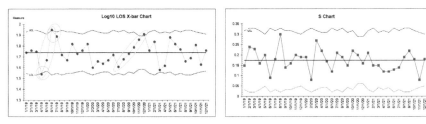

Fig. 5. Xbar and S-chart of NICU Log10 LOS (transformed).

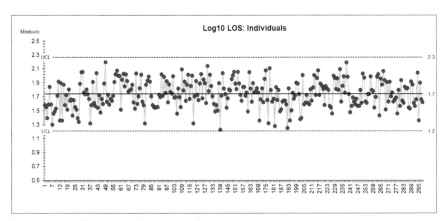

Fig. 6. I-chart of NICU LOS (transformed).

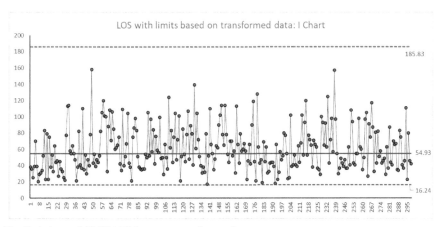

Fig. 7. I-chart of NICU LOS (reverse transformed).

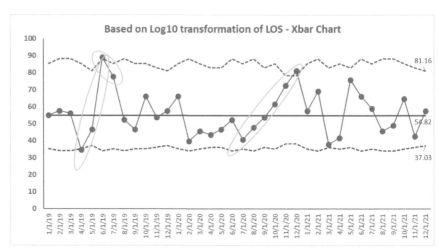

Fig. 8. Xbar of NICU Log10 LOS (reverse transformed).

transformation produces a value that is closer to the subgroup median than the subgroup mean. **Fig. 8** shows the reverse transformed Xbar-S charts; in this chart, for example, the point for 01/01/2019 is 55.0, whereas the original value on the Xbar-S charts in **Fig. 2** was 57.3. The point on the reverse transformed chart is closer to the median of the January 2019 LOS values (median = 53, data not shown) than the average (average = 57.3). As would be expected, the transformed Xbar-S charts are robust to the skewness of the data, and **Fig. 2** (nontransformed) and **Figs. 5** and **8** (transformed) are similar with consistent special cause signals. On the other hand, the I-chart is somewhat sensitive to the skewed data with multiple "false" special cause signals on **Fig. 3** (nontransformed) that are no longer present on the transformed charts in **Figs. 6** and **7**.

Work published by the Ohio Perinatal Quality Collaborative examining changes in LOS among infants with neonatal opioid withdrawal syndrome provides an example of how transformation can be used to create control charts when the data are significantly skewed.[9,10] There are numerous other examples in the perinatal QI literature that use control charts for LOS data without considering transformation.[11–14] In a California Perinatal Quality Care Collaborative QI initiative to decrease NICU LOS, while the team transformed the data using lognormal mixed models for their frequentist statistical analyses, the participating teams found that I-charts without transformation were sufficient for learning.[15]

Recommendations

- If continuous data are skewed, try to use Xbar-S charts with large subgroup sizes. These charts are less sensitive to skewed distributions than I-charts.
- If your data are skewed with evidence of false-positive special cause signals on either the S-chart or I-chart, transform the data to create a more symmetric distribution and more helpful control chart.
- Although transformation of data and creation of a control chart using transformed data can be done manually to enable creation of charts in SPC programs, it can be helpful to engage with a data analyst or statistician if this is necessary.

AUTOCORRELATED DATA

Traditional SPC charts rely on the assumption of independent data points, meaning the data from one subgroup do not influence data from subsequent groups. If a process is in statistical control, any given data point is best predicted by the average of all the data points. Measures based on subgroups of patients will typically meet this definition of independence. For example, average admission temperature of very-low-birth-weight (VLBW) infants in a given month in a given NICU is likely better predicted by the performance in that NICU for the past year rather than the average temperature the previous month. If the process is stable, performance in a given month does not have particular predictive value for performance the next month. In this example, if only common cause variation is present, variation within subgroups is comparable with variation between subgroups.

In some cases, measurement of certain processes can result in interdependence of data points, such that data for one subgroup influence the next group. For example, if an NICU is tracking length of rounds, the average length of rounds for a given week is likely better predicted by the average the previous week rather than the average length over the past year. In this example, variation within each subgroup is less than variation between subgroups.

Data that are not independent from subgroup to subgroup are autocorrelated. Autocorrelation can be positive (successive data points are more likely to be similar) or negative (successive data points are more likely to be dissimilar); in health care, positive autocorrelation is much more common. Autocorrelation affects the reliability of control charts in at least 2 aspects. First, rules for detecting special cause variation that rely on patterns seen across more than one sequential data point are not valid for nonindependent subgroups; this includes the common shift and trend rules, as well as rules identifying 2 out of 3 points near the outer control limit and 15 consecutive points close to the centerline. Second, for continuous data, autocorrelation will affect the calculation of control limits due to the unusual variation within subgroups, with falsely narrowed control limits resulting in false-positive signals of special cause variation.

A common approach to assess for autocorrelation in a data set is to calculate a correlation coefficient and examine the extent of correlation through a scatterplot. To create the scatterplot, each data point is plotted on one axis with the next subsequent data point on the other axis. A regression line is fitted to the data, giving an r-squared value as an estimate of goodness of fit. The square root of this value, r, is the correlation coefficient. Modeling studies of control charts using generated data have shown that rates of false-positive signals tend to be modest with correlation coefficients less than 0.4 to 0.5 and are substantially elevated with coefficients higher than 0.8.[16] The Health Care Data Guide suggests that control charts can likely still be used if correlation coefficient is less than 0.5 and should not be used if correlation coefficient is greater than 0.8; if coefficient is between 0.5 and 0.8, then autocorrelation should be at least considered as control charts are interpreted.[4]

Complicated adjustments have been applied to statistical process control charts to attempt to correct for autocorrelation, but at present, these techniques have limited practical applicability, particularly in health care.[16] In situations where data are truly autocorrelated, definitive solutions to using control charts are limited.[17] Several reasonable approaches that follow may help. First, altering the sampling strategy may reduce the impact of autocorrelation. For example, length of rounds compared month to month would likely be less affected by autocorrelation than length of rounds compared daily or weekly. Second, rules applied to detect special cause variation can be limited to only the occurrence of data points outside the outer control limits, as these signals depend on only one data point and therefore not affected by autocorrelation. For attribute data control charts, the standard control limit calculations are not affected by autocorrelation. For continuous data control charts, an adjustment to the control limit calculation can compensate for autocorrelation; this is done by multiplying the calculated control limit by $1/(sqrt(1-r^2))$.[4] Of note, even after adjusting control limits, only the single point outside the outer control limit rule should be used to identify special cause variation. Third, visual inspection of a simple time-series graph of the data can still provide insight, without the additional run chart or control chart elements such as centerline and control limits; marked changes or astronomical data points likely will still indicate opportunities for learning.

Although autocorrelation can be a significant problem for certain NICU QI metrics, it is important to note that most cases of nonindependence of data are due to true special cause variation. With a change in process, subgroups in the period of special cause variation will tend to be more similar to each other than subgroups in the period of common cause variation. Thus, in some cases, data that seem autocorrelated may be revealing special cause variation that has not been recognized.

Example: Ventilator Days Per Patient Day

Reducing ventilator use is a common target of NICU respiratory QI efforts. Average ventilator days per patient can be a useful measure but is limited by lags in data timeliness due to long LOS and can be disproportionately affected by individual patient outliers. Measuring ventilator days by patient census may offer greater insight into changing patterns of performance over time. **Fig. 9** shows a U-chart of ventilator

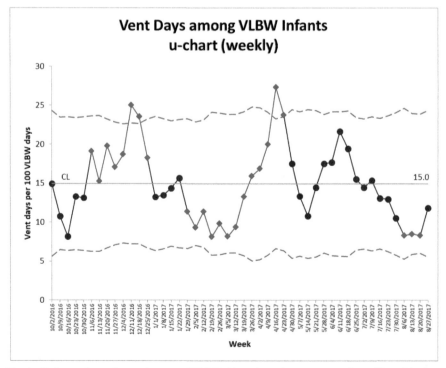

Fig. 9. U-chart of ventilator days per 100 VLBW patient days, measured weekly, with standard health care rules used to indicate special cause variation (*red*).

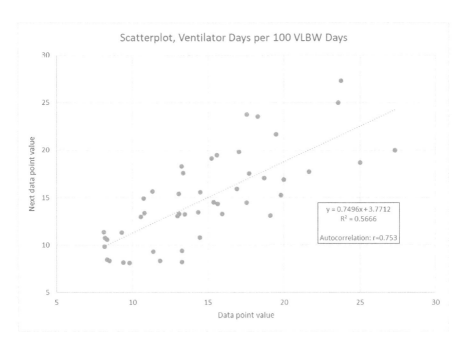

Fig. 10. Scatterplot of ventilator days per 100 VLBW days; each data point plotted with next data point.

days per 100 VLBW infant days for an NICU, measured weekly. Multiple patterns of special cause variation are present, which could reflect true special cause variation. However, the pattern of cyclical shifts in the data is unusual. **Fig. 10** shows a scatterplot of the data points from **Fig. 9**, with each data point plotted with the next sequential point. The correlation coefficient ("r") is 0.753, suggesting a concerning degree of autocorrelation.

Autocorrelation may not be surprising with the measurement strategy of examining ventilator days per patient day weekly. Longer intervals may be less affected by autocorrelation. **Fig. 11** shows U-charts of the same data measured biweekly or monthly, using only one point beyond outer control limits to indicate special cause variation. Although similar general patterns are present, the persistence of special cause

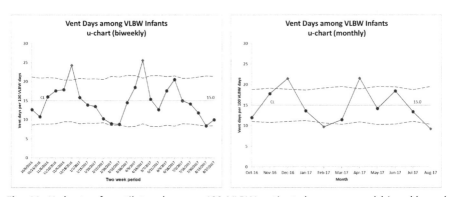

Fig. 11. U-charts of ventilator days per 100 VLBW patient days, measured biweekly and monthly, with only one point beyond outer control limits used to indicate special cause variation (*red*).

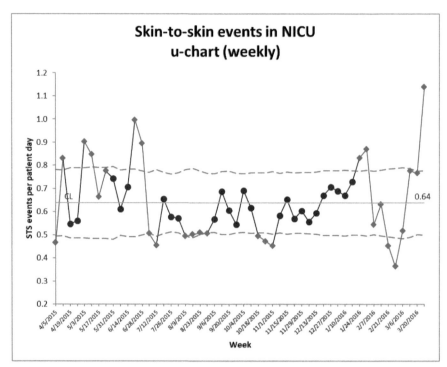

Fig. 12. U-chart of skin-to-skin (STS) events per patient day, measured weekly, with standard health care rules used to indicate special cause variation (*red*).

variation at selected time points may indicate true differences in performance that may warrant investigation.

Example: Skin-To-Skin Events per Patient Day

Increasing skin-to-skin (STS) is a common goal of NICU family-centered care efforts. STS rates could theoretically have a similar pattern of autocorrelation, as the likelihood of infants in an NICU receiving STS in a given day likely predicts the likelihood of STS the next day. **Fig. 12** shows a U-chart of STS events per patient day in an NICU, measured weekly. Multiple indicators of special cause variation are seen, and the cyclic pattern of the data could be suggestive of autocorrelation. However, the scatterplot of this data, shown in **Fig. 13**, reveals a correlation coefficient of 0.043, suggesting autocorrelation is not a significant contributor. In this case, other reasons should be sought to explain the special cause variation seen in the U-chart (see later discussion).

Recommendations

- Remember that the most common cause of nonindependence of data is true special cause variation due to process change; therefore, first start with initial investigation and discussion of the special cause signals.
- If autocorrelation is suspected, determine correlation coefficient ("r") on a scatterplot of each data point plotted with subsequent data point to assess degree of autocorrelation.
- If autocorrelation is present:
  - Consider alternative measurement strategies to limit impact of autocorrelation.

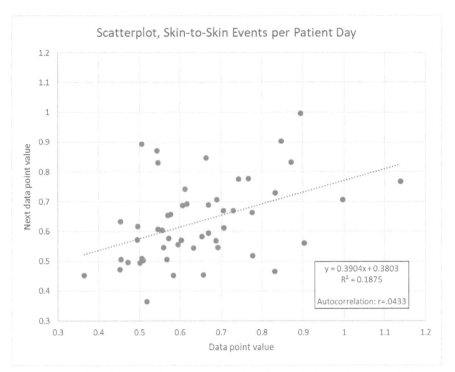

Fig. 13. Scatterplot of skin-to-skin events per patient day; each data point plotted with next data point.

- Use control charts with only a point beyond the outer control limits to identify special cause variation, with standard control limits for attribute-data charts and adjusted control limits for continuous data charts.
- Use a simple time-series graph and assess visually for marked or unexpected changes in data or unusual data points.

DETECTING SMALL PROCESS CHANGES

At times in QI, traditional control charts (eg, I-chart, P-chart, or U-chart) are not sensitive enough to detect change, particularly when the subgroup sample size is less than recommended. Using a CUSUM or EMWA control chart can be helpful in more quickly detecting small changes in performance.

The CUSUM statistic is the sum of the differences in individual measurements from a target value, which often defaults to the average of all available data points or a historical average. Each point on the chart indicates the cumulative deviation from the target. The centerline is zero, and we expect a stable process to move randomly around the centerline. When special cause variation is present, the CUSUM slopes upward or downward and will cross the control limit.[4] The National Pediatric Cardiology Learning Network effectively used a CUSUM chart to show improvement in mortality during the interstage period (after stage 1 palliation) for infants with hypoplastic left heart syndrome.[18] Although the CUSUM chart has been shown to be the statistically optimal chart for fast detection of small changes, it can be confusing and counterintuitive to interpret; therefore, we prefer the use of the EWMA chart.

The EWMA chart was introduced as an SPC methodology in the 1960s.[19] An EWMA plots a single data point at each time point that reflects the (weighted) moving average of the measure. Unlike the CUSUM chart, the metric of interest is plotted in its original measure unit on an EWMA chart, making it easier to interpret. The most weight is given to the current data, less to the immediately past data, and less still to more historical data using an exponential weighting approach. For example, if 50% of the weight is given to the most recent data point, then 25% is given to the prior point ($0.5*0.5 = 0.25$) and 6.25% to the point before that ($0.5^3 = 0.0625$). The exponential factor is defined by lambda (λ) and usually ranges from 0.1 to 0.3. A large value of λ (eg, $\lambda = 1$) places more weight on the most current data, and the EWMA will look similar to an I-chart. On the other hand, smaller values of λ place more emphasis on historical data. The appropriate λ should be selected based on the baseline rate and the desired magnitude of the change to be detected. There are several tables that can be used to select an appropriate value. The EWMA chart can be used with either attribute or variable (continuous) data. Although the calculations for the EWMA chart are based on parameters from a continuous, symmetric distribution, the chart is robust to a variety of data distributions.[4] The details of calculating the EMWA statistical and control limits are beyond the scope of this article; formulas can be found in SPC textbooks and some SPC software have existing programs to create EMWA charts. Similar to other control charts, a point outside the control limits indicates special cause variation; unlike other control charts, other rules for detecting special cause or nonrandom patterns cannot be applied. The centerline in an EWMA chart can be either a target value or the average. Although the EMWA is not as effective at detecting small absolute changes (<10%) as the CUMSUM chart, it still outperforms a traditional Shewhart chart (eg, P-chart) and is more intuitive than the CUMSUM chart.[20]

Example: Nosocomial Infection

A recent example related to a QI effort to reduce the percent of infants with a nosocomial infection demonstrates the utility of an EMWA chart. Using their Vermont Oxford Network (VON) time-series data, a center plotted the percentage of infants discharged with nosocomial infection on a P-chart using monthly data (**Fig. 14**). By the fall of 2019, the team had made several changes and qualitatively thought that they were seeing a

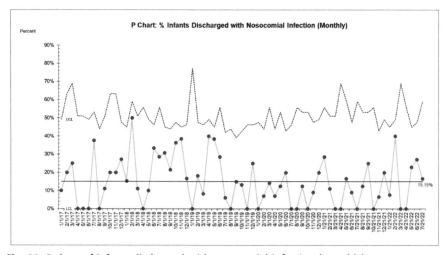

Fig. 14. P-chart of infants discharged with nosocomial infection (monthly).

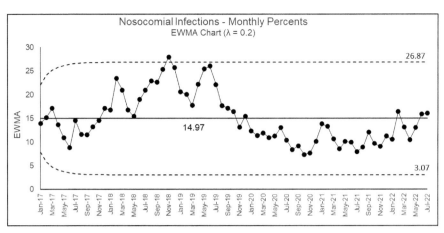

Fig. 15. EWMA chart of infants discharged with nosocomial infection (monthly).

reduction in the number of infants experiencing infections, yet there was no evidence of special cause variation to suggest that their changes were resulting in improvement. Of note, this chart has more than 25% of the plotted values at zero, which can be a sign of an ineffective P-chart. Because of their relatively small monthly subgroup sizes with a desire to quickly detect small changes, they created an EMWA chart that showed evidence of special cause variation with a peak in infections in September 2018 (**Fig. 15**). Based on this signal and the pattern of points subsequently, they phased the EWMA chart into 2 periods (**Fig. 16**) with the second phase starting in July 2019. This chart indicates 2 stable periods with the infection rate reducing from 19.9 to 11.0. Although this improvement can also be seen on a quarterly P-chart (**Fig. 17**) that has the recommended subgroup sizes to produce a useful chart (n > 20 in this example), the EMWA chart allowed the team to learn more quickly. Although use has been limited in the past, there are increasing reports of EMWA charts in the medical literature.[21–24]

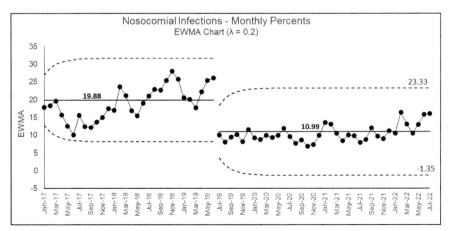

Fig. 16. EWMA chart of infants discharged with nosocomial infection (monthly) with phase change.

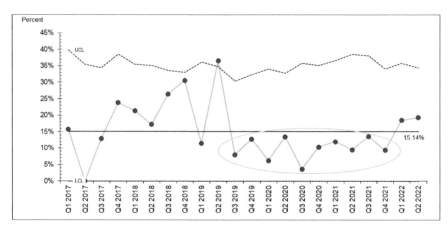

Fig. 17. P-chart of infants discharged with nosocomial infection (quarterly).

Recommendations

- Continue to use traditional control charts to track outcomes; however, consider simultaneously creating a EWMA chart if it is important to identify small process changes quickly, particularly with limited subgroup sizes.
- Sometimes the number of events limits learning on a traditional control chart on a weekly or monthly basis. An EWMA chart can be useful in this situation.

ADDRESSING CONFOUNDERS AND COVARIATES IN CONTROL CHARTS

One of the main goals of a Shewhart chart is to help distinguish between common cause and special cause variation. Special cause variation is unpredictable variation resulting from a cause that is not an inherent part of the process. Common cause variation is intrinsic to the process over time and affects all outcomes of the process. Normal fluctuations in factors such as patient volume and staffing levels can be responsible for common cause variation. In classic epidemiologic terminology, the variables responsible for common cause variation are described as "confounders" or "covariates."[25] Historically, control charts have not been adjusted for covariates or confounders. However, as the application of SPC has evolved and SPC methods are being used in more complex circumstances, there has been greater interest in considering how multiple factors (confounders and covariates) work together to influence a process.[4]

The first step that should be undertaken when considering confounders or covariates is to understand the relationship between the variables of interest. For continuous outcome data, this can be accomplished by creating a scatterplot to graphically display the relationship between the presumed confounder and outcome of interest and then performing regression analysis to quantify the relationship. The relationships of interest can be examined by individual patient (**Fig. 18**) for measures being plotted on an I-chart or by averages calculated by week, month, or other period (**Fig. 19**) for measures being plotted on Xbar-S charts. For attribute data, logistic regression can be used to examine the relationship between the presumed confounder and outcome of interest.

Classically, a confounder is a variable that is associated with both the dependent and independent variable. Because we are examining data over time, time is always a key independent variable in statistical process control. Therefore, when we think

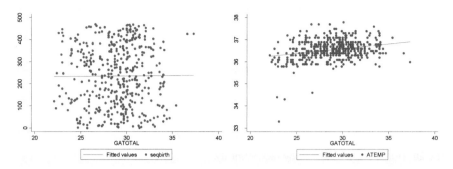

Fig. 18. Scatterplots of gestational age versus time and gestational age versus admission temperature (individual infant).

about confounders in the context of control charts, we are looking for factors that are associated with both time and the measure of interest. In theory, confounders can mask or suggest a false association between our changes and the measure. Despite this concern, in our experience, NICU systems are generally stable over time with respect to potential confounder variables. As seen in **Fig. 18**, there is no association between time (sequential births) and the key confounder of gestational age. In instances where confounding is present, however, there are methods for creating adjusted control charts, which are beyond the scope of this review article.[4,26]

Because covariates are related to one measure but not the other (eg, related to the outcome measure but not time), they typically do not require adjustment. However, covariates can inform QI measure analysis using rational subgrouping. Rational subgrouping involves organizing data by similar subgroups to create a situation where there is only common cause variation within a subgroup and any cases of special cause variation are occurring between subgroups. Subgroups of data are typically created based on grouping across important variables such as gestational or birthweight category, sex, severity of illness, race, diagnosis, or treatment approach.

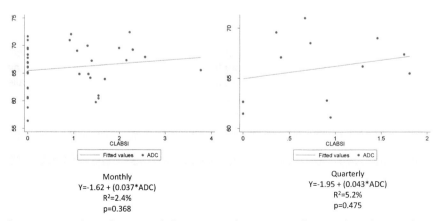

Monthly
Y=-1.62 + (0.037*ADC)
R^2=2.4%
p=0.368

Quarterly
Y=-1.95 + (0.043*ADC)
R^2=5.2%
p=0.475

Fig. 19. Scatterplots of average daily census and CLABSI rate (by month and quarter).

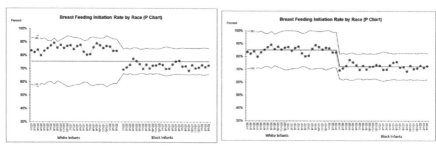

Fig. 20. Human milk initiation by race/ethnicity.

Fig. 20 demonstrates 2 P-charts for breastfeeding initiation among term infants, with the subgroups ordered first by race (white and black infants) and then by time. Examining breastfeeding initiation rates by subgroup identifies an important disparity in outcomes that would otherwise be masked in a traditional control chart; this disparity can become an important target of QI efforts.

Rational ordering is analogous to rational subgrouping but is used in the specific case of an I-chart where the subgroup size is one. **Fig. 21** demonstrates 2 I-charts for admission temperature grouped by birthweight category. Again, grouping by birthweight category demonstrates a particular problem with admission hypothermia among infants weighing less than 750 g that would have been masked in a traditional I-chart. Examining QI measures using rational subgrouping or ordering can be very helpful in identifying ideas for change and understanding the causal mechanisms in a process.

Recommendations

- If you are interested in considering how multiple factors work together to influence a process or outcome, start by making scatterplots to understand the relationship between the variables of interest.
- If there is evidence of a confounder that is associated with both time and the metric plotted on your control chart, consider creating an adjusted control chart; this will likely require engagement with a statistician.
- Identify important covariates that may influence whether your changes are resulting in improvement and explore those covariates using rational subgrouping.

DISCRETE DATA TREATED AS CONTINUOUS

The power of SPC charts for determining common and special cause variation come from control limits. The calculation of control limits depends on the type of data and the appropriate measure of common cause variation for that type of data (called

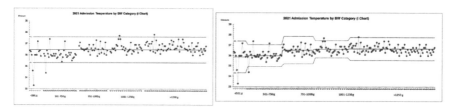

Fig. 21. Admission temperature by birthweight category (I-chart).

"sigma"). Commonly, data are categorized as either attribute or continuous. Attribute data are discrete integers or whole numbers and include both classification and count data. Classification data have 2 possible responses, usually yes or no. P-charts based on the sigma from a binomial distribution are typically used to analyze classification data. Count data measures several events or incidents, most typically unwanted events such as errors or defects. U-charts or C-charts with sigma based on the Poisson distribution are typically used to analyze count data. Continuous data are measures that can be recorded on a scale and generally do not have to be a whole number. I-charts and Xbar-S charts are used for analysis of continuous data with sigma based on the variation of the actual data.

However, in some cases, discrete whole number data, despite representing counts of events, are best treated as continuous for SPC charts. These are typically measures of *workload* or *production*. Unlike discrete measures that examine random or unexpected events, such as infection rates or unplanned extubations, measures of workload or production reflect a systematic process and examine events that are expected to happen. The former should be analyzed with P-charts, U-charts, or C-charts; the latter require I-charts or Xbar-S charts.[4]

The statistical explanations for this distinction come from assumptions underlying the common attribute charts. Two parameters, mean and variation, describe continuous data and are used for I-charts and Xbar-S charts; the mean measures the central tendency of the data, and the standard error measures the variability or dispersion of the data. Conversely, only one parameter, the mean value, describes both the central tendency and the dispersion for the binomial distribution (used for P-charts) and the Poisson distribution (used for U-charts and C-charts).[27] The binomial and Poisson distributions are described by one parameter because they are based on the assumption that events being measured have a consistent likelihood of occurring throughout the sample period, leading to expected patterns of variability; the mean value can thus measure the central tendency of the data and predict its dispersion. Control limits for attribute charts are based on this theoretical dispersion of the data rather than measured variation.[27]

In health care, count measures may not meet the assumptions of equal probability underlying the binomial and Poisson distributions.[28] In these situations, the control limits calculated by P-charts, U-charts, and C-charts incorrectly describe the distribution of the data; this will often apply to workload or productivity measures; as the events being counted are expected to happen (as compared to relatively infrequent events), the probability of those events not happening is unlikely to be consistent throughout the sample period. Visually, in cases where discrete data do not follow typical binomial or Poisson distributions, attribute control charts will show unusual data patterns, such as wide control limits with data points clustered around the centerline or narrow control limits with many data points beyond the outer limits.[27,29] Although these patterns could sometimes reflect special cause variation, for workload and productivity measures, they more likely reflect inappropriate calculation of control limits. When this occurs, I-charts can be used instead of attribute charts. The control limits for I-charts are based on measured variation in the data (the moving range) rather than predicted dispersion and thus will more accurately identify common and special cause variation.[27,29] I-charts can be constructed using each sample's value as individual data points, such as the monthly proportion, monthly count, or monthly rate.

To avoid difficulties in determining which measures reflect workload or production data, some investigators have proposed that I-charts can always be used in place of attribute charts.[27] However, I-charts have limitations. I-charts do not consider the

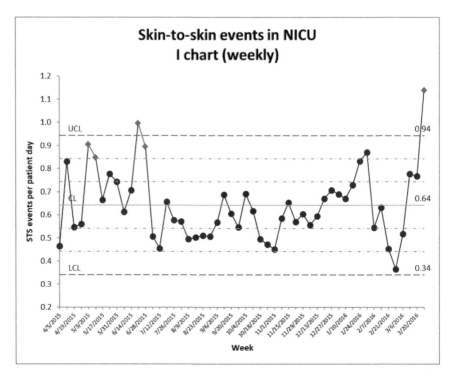

Fig. 22. X-chart of skin-to-skin (STS) events per patient day, measured weekly, with standard health care rules used to indicate special cause variation (*red*).

sample size (denominator) of each subgroup and for less frequent events, may be less sensitive than attribute charts for detecting special cause variation. In addition, I-charts are unable to account for differences in sample size from point to point, which can influence understanding variation. I-charts are also sensitive to skewed data distributions (see earlier discussion). Although I-charts would be the appropriate analysis for measures of workload or productivity, traditional attribute charts would be better suited for most other discrete measures.

Examples: Skin-To-Skin Events Per Patient Day

In **Fig. 12**, a U-chart examined STS events per patient day in an NICU. The chart showed multiple instances of special cause variation, with many data points well beyond the outer control limits. This pattern suggests that the control limits may be inappropriately narrow; as STS events can be considered a measure of activity or productivity in the unit, their rate may be better analyzed as a continuous measure with an I-chart. **Fig. 22** shows the I-chart; the calculated limits seem more appropriate for the data patterns, and the instances of special cause variation may be more likely to reflect true changes in performance warranting investigation.

Example: Antibiotic Utilization Rate

Antibiotic stewardship is an ongoing important improvement goal for neonatal intensive care. Antibiotic use is commonly tracked as the antibiotic utilization rate (AUR) of antibiotic days per patient days. As antibiotic usage in an NICU is somewhat expected, the distribution of AURs may not follow typical attribute measure patterns.

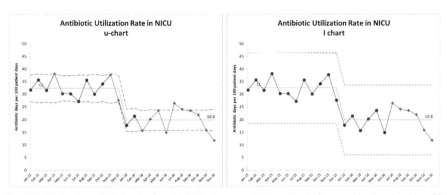

Fig. 23. U-chart and X-chart of antibiotic days per 100 patient days, with standard health care rules used to indicate special cause variation (*red*).

Fig. 23 shows AURs for an NICU graphed as a U-chart and as an I-chart. Although a change in performance is evident in both charts, the U-chart shows multiple points beyond the outer control limits and inappropriately narrow control limits. A Laney U-prime chart is likely not indicated; patient days in this data set are from 800 to 1200 per month, well less than the threshold of 3000 commonly used to indicate the need for a prime chart.[4] Instead, the I-chart, considering this measure as continuous, still shows the change in performance but with control limits that seem to more accurately describe the dispersion in the data.

Recommendations

- Most discrete measures should be considered attribute data and analyzed using P-charts, U-charts, and C-charts.
- For measures of productivity or workload, where events are not infrequent but rather are planned and expected to happen, consider using I-charts of individual data points, particularly if attribute charts show control limits that seem inappropriately wide or narrow.

SUMMARY

Effective QI depends on rigorous analysis of time-series data through methods such as SPC. As use of SPC has become more prevalent in health care, QI practitioners must also be aware of situations that warrant special attention and potential modifications to common SPC charts, including those described in this review. Developing greater SPC proficiency will allow our neonatology QI community to improve the rigor of our improvement efforts and thereby achieve better outcomes for our newborns and their families.

DISCLOSURE

The authors have nothing to disclose.

ACKNOWLEDGMENTS

We gratefully acknowledge our many colleagues in neonatology who have collaborated and learned with us as we continue our quality improvement journey. We specifically thank Dmitry Dukhovny, Michelle-Marie Peña, and Wendy Timpson for sharing data used in this article.

REFERENCES

1. Berwick DM. Controlling variation in health care: a consultation from Walter She-whart. Medical care 1991;29(12):1212–25.
2. Benneyan JC, Lloyd RC, Plsek PE. Statistical process control as a tool for research and healthcare improvement. Qual Saf Health Care 2003;12(6):458–64.
3. Mohammed MA, Worthington P, Woodall WH. Plotting basic control charts: tuto-rial notes for healthcare practitioners. Qual Saf Health Care 2008;17(2):137–45.
4. Provost LP, Murray SK. The health care data guide : learning from data for improvement. 2nd edition. Hoboken, NJ: John Wiley & Sons; 2022. volumes cm p.
5. Gupta M, Kaplan HC. Using statistical process control to drive improvement in neonatal care: a practical introduction to control charts. Clin Perinatol 2017; 44(3):627–44.
6. Lloyd RC. Navigating in the turbulent sea of data: the quality measurement journey. Clin Perinatol 2010;37(1):101–22.
7. Rosner B. Fundamentals of biostatistics. 8th edition. Boston, MA: Cengage Learning; 2016. p. 927.
8. Mishra P, Pandey CM, Singh U, et al. Descriptive statistics and normality tests for statistical data. Ann Card Anaesth 2019;22(1):67–72.
9. Walsh MC, Crowley M, Wexelblatt S, et al. Ohio perinatal quality collaborative im-proves care of neonatal narcotic abstinence syndrome. Pediatrics 2018;141(4): e20170900.
10. Kaplan HC, Kuhnell P, Walsh MC, et al. Orchestrated testing of formula type to reduce length of stay in neonatal abstinence syndrome. Pediatrics 2020;146(4): e20190914.
11. Ponder KL, Egesdal C, Kuller J, et al. Project Console: a quality improvement initiative for neonatal abstinence syndrome in a children's hospital level IV neonatal intensive care unit. BMJ Open Qual 2021;10(2):e001079.
12. Welch CD, Check J, O'Shea TM. Improving care collaboration for NICU patients to decrease length of stay and readmission rate. BMJ Open Qual 2017;6(2): e000130.
13. Mansfield SA, Ryshen G, Dail J, et al. Use of quality improvement (QI) methodol-ogy to decrease length of stay (LOS) for newborns with uncomplicated gastro-schisis. J Pediatr Surg 2018;53(8):1578–83.
14. Asti L, Magers JS, Keels E, et al. A quality improvement project to reduce length of stay for neonatal abstinence syndrome. Pediatrics 2015;135(6):e1494–500.
15. Lee HC, Bennett MV, Crockett M, et al. Comparison of collaborative versus single-site quality improvement to reduce NICU length of stay. Pediatrics 2018;142(1): e20171395.
16. Borckardt JJ, Nash MR, Hardesty S, et al. How unusual are the "unusual events" detected by control chart techniques in healthcare settings? J Healthc Qual 2006;28(4):4–9.
17. Carey RG. Improving healthcare with control charts : basic and advanced SPC methods and case studies. Milwaukee, WI: ASQ Quality Press; 2003. p. 194.
18. Anderson JB, Beekman RH 3rd, Kugler JD, et al. Improvement in interstage sur-vival in a national pediatric Cardiology learning Network. Circ Cardiovasc Qual Outcomes 2015;8(4):428–36.
19. Roberts SW. A comparison of some control chart procedures. Technometrics 1966;8(3):411–30.

20. Neuburger J, Walker K, Sherlaw-Johnson C, et al. Comparison of control charts for monitoring clinical performance using binary data. BMJ Qual Saf 2017; 26(11):919–28.
21. Baldewijns G, Luca S, Vanrumste B, et al. Developing a system that can automatically detect health changes using transfer times of older adults. BMC Med Res Methodol 2016;16:23.
22. Cook DA, Coory M, Webster RA. Exponentially weighted moving average charts to compare observed and expected values for monitoring risk-adjusted hospital indicators. BMJ Qual Saf 2011;20(6):469–74.
23. Morton AP, Whitby M, McLaws ML, et al. The application of statistical process control charts to the detection and monitoring of hospital-acquired infections. J Qual Clin Pract 2001;21(4):112–7.
24. Steiner SH, Grant K, Coory M, et al. Detecting the start of an influenza outbreak using exponentially weighted moving average charts. BMC Med Inform Decis Mak 2010;10:37.
25. Gordis L. Epidemiology. 5th edition. Philadelphia, PA: Elsevier/Saunders; 2014. p. 392.
26. Berkowitz D, Chamberlain J, Provost LP. Addressing challenges of baseline variability in the clinical setting: lessons from an emergency department. Pediatr Qual Saf 2019;4(5):e216.
27. Wheeler DJ. So you want to use a p-chart? Quality Digest Daily 2021;1–9. https://www.qualitydigest.com/inside/statistics-column/so-you-want-use-p-chart-100421.html.
28. Hanley JA, Bhatnagar S. The "Poisson" distribution: history, reenactments, adaptations. Am Statistician 2022;76(4):363–71.
29. Fang Y., C-chart, X-Chart, and the katz family of distributions, J Qual Technol, 35 (1), 2003, 1–15.

Integrating Implementation Science with Quality Improvement to Improve Perinatal Outcomes

Jennifer Callaghan-Koru, PhD, MHS[a],*, Azadeh Farzin, MD, MHS[b],
Erick Ridout, MD[c], Geoffrey Curran, PhD[d]

KEYWORDS

- Implementation science • Implementation research • Quality improvement
- Implementation strategies • Model for Improvement

KEY POINTS

- Implementation science is a developing interdisciplinary field in health research with a goal of accelerating the translation of research evidence into routine clinical practice.
- Models and frameworks developed within implementation science, such as the Behavior Change Wheel, can provide theoretic and empirical grounding to support clinical practice change within quality improvement (QI) work.
- Partnerships between implementation researchers and clinicians engaged in perinatal QI can support the translation of implementation research evidence into useable tools to enhance QI.

INTRODUCTION

The substantial lag in medicine between the generation of new evidence and the implementation of that evidence in routine clinical care has been well-documented.[1] In perinatology, examples of persistent evidence-to-practice gaps include incorporating the latest evidence in optimizing neonatal resuscitation,[2] blood transfusion practices during the neonatal period,[3] and antenatal corticosteroids.[4] Quality improvement (QI) initiatives, such as the Vermont Oxford Network, have made great

[a] Department of Internal Medicine, University of Arkansas for Medical Sciences, 1125 North College Avenue, Fayetteville, AR 72703, USA; [b] Pediatrix of Maryland/Adventist Healthcare, 9901 Medical Center Drive, Rockville, MD 20850, USA; [c] American Academy of Pediatrics, 1380 East Medical Center Drive, St George, UT 84790, USA; [d] Department of Pharmacy Practice, University of Arkansas for Medical Sciences, 4301 West Markham Street, Little Rock, AR 72205, USA
* Corresponding author.
E-mail address: jck@uams.edu
Twitter: @JCalKoru (J.C.-K.)

Clin Perinatol 50 (2023) 343–361
https://doi.org/10.1016/j.clp.2023.01.002
perinatology.theclinics.com

gains in reducing the evidence-to-practice gap.[5,6] Examples of widespread improvements include reductions in nosociomial infections[7] and improved screening and treatment for retinopathy of prematurity.[8]

Although laudable improvements have been made, the pace of improvements in perinatal care can be slow.[9,10] Among hospitals participating in the Vermont Oxford Network, it took between 4 and 8 years for all hospitals to reach selected quality improvement benchmarks for very low birth weight (VLBW) infants.[11] Similarly, 7 years after the initial guidelines recommended delayed cord clamping (DCC) for all gestational ages, 15% of neonatology practices did not have a policy supporting DCC and one-third of neonatologists did not report delaying clamping for at least 60 seconds.[12] This improvement lag leaves many patients out of the benefits of clinical evidence. Given that the patient populations left out of improvements are often disproportionately from minority and low-income communities,[13,14] accelerating the implementation of clinical evidence will also contribute to reducing perinatal disparities.

Implementation science was developed by researchers with an interest in closing the gap between clinical evidence and routine clinical practice. Implementation science has coalesced as a distinct field in the last 20 years, with major milestones including the launch of the journal *Implementation Science* in 2006,[15] the first Annual Conference on the Science of Dissemination and Implementation in Health in 2008,[16] and publication of National Institutes of Health (NIH) funding opportunities specific to dissemination and implementation research (NIH program announcement PAR-06–039, issued October 2005).

As implementation science has matured, there is increasing recognition that the field often operates too separately from the real-world work of implementation in clinical settings, including the practice of quality improvement.[17–20] The limited dialogue between implementation researchers and quality improvement practitioners has resulted in missed opportunities for clinicians engaged in quality improvement to apply the tools and lessons of implementation science, and for implementation scientists to ensure that they are developing measures and tools that are useable by those same clinicians. To promote better integration of implementation science with quality improvement in perinatology, the objectives of this article are (1) to provide an overview of the concepts of implementation science for perinatal clinical providers, particularly those involved in QI work and (2) to describe strategies for better aligning implementation science and QI efforts for mutual benefit.

AN OVERVIEW OF IMPLEMENTATION SCIENCE CONCEPTS FOR QUALITY IMPROVEMENT PRACTITIONERS IN PERINATOLOGY

Implementation science is an interdisciplinary field that draws on multiple social sciences for its foundations, including behavioral and psychological science, organizational science, public health, and economics.[21,22] The most commonly cited definition of the field, from the introductory editorial to the journal *Implementation Science*, is "the scientific study of methods to promote the systematic uptake of research findings and other evidence-based practices into routine practice."[15] Within this broad scope, Mitchell and Chambers further describe implementation science as focusing on three areas: (1) the study of techniques for effective dissemination and receipt of research evidence; (2) the study of processes for incorporating new practices into routine clinical care; and (3) the study of strategies for intervening on determinants (e.g., barriers and facilitators) for delivery of new practices in routine care.[23]

An emphasis of implementation science during its first decade was on the development and codification of models, frameworks, and theories to undergird research in the field.[17,24] The proliferation of these conceptual frameworks has contributed to perceived complexity and difficulty for newcomers to grasp the field.[24,25] As a result, Curran developed a simple explanation of implementation science oriented around a model evidence-based practice, denoted as "THE THING" (**Box 1**). We can replace "THE THING" with any intervention or practice of interest. Using a perinatal example, we can consider the clinical practice of "eat, sleep, console" (ESC) for management of opioid-exposed newborns[26,27] as "THE THING." An effectiveness study would assess whether ESC improved clinical outcomes, such as length of stay and morphine use. In contrast, an implementation research study would assess how to "best help" neonatal intensive care units (NICUs) and clinicians to provide ESC care ("do the thing"). Such a study might focus on identifying the barriers to providing ESC or on developing and testing implementation strategies to promote or support the provision of ESC care. The outcomes for an implementation research study of ESC care could include what proportion of NICUs have adopted the care model, what proportion of eligible newborns receive it, and whether ESC is provided with fidelity ("how much and well they do the thing").

Although familiarity with all of the conceptual frameworks and theories that have been developed within implementation science is not realistic or necessary for the quality improvement (QI) practitioner, understanding the different types of frameworks and their functions is helpful orientation. The three categories of implementation frameworks that may be most applicable for perinatal QI teams are process models, determinant frameworks, and evaluation frameworks. *Process models* "describe or guide" the process of implementing evidence-based practices.[28] Some process models, like the Knowledge to Action Framework,[29] recommend steps common to successful implementation efforts, whereas others, like the Exploration, Preparation, Implementation, Sustainment framework, describe stages of implementation activities.[30] *Determinants frameworks* delineate and group the factors that influence the processes and outcomes of implementation.[28] Studies of "barriers" and "facilitators" of implementation are typically guided by a determinants framework like the Consolidated Framework for Implementation Research. Lastly, *evaluation frameworks* conceptualize outcomes that can be measured to assess the success of implementation efforts.[28] Evaluation frameworks typically define a category of outcome, such as reach or fidelity, which must be operationalized for the particular clinical practice under study.

Box 1
"Implementation science made too simple"

- The intervention/clinical practice/innovation is THE THING

- Effectiveness research looks at whether THE THING works

- Implementation research looks at how best to help people/places DO THE THING

- Implementation strategies are the *stuff we do* to try to help people/places DO THE THING

- Main implementation outcomes are HOW MUCH and HOW WELL they DO THE THING

Adapted from Curran GM. Implementation science made too simple: a teaching tool. Implement Sci Commun. 2020;1:27. Published 2020 Feb 25.

Table 1
Recommended implementation science resources for QI practitioners

Category of Resource	Name of Resource	Considerations for Use
Introductions to implementation science	*Implementation Science at a Glance*	This publication from the National Cancer Institute[74] was written to provide clinical and public health practitioners with an overview of implementation science concepts and how they relate to the practice of implementing evidence-based interventions.
	The "subway line" of translational research	The "subway line" schematic was developed to assist researchers with classifying study goals within the continuum of translational research.[75] Although the subway line is focused on explaining research concepts, it can be useful for QI practitioners who want to understand the objectives and methods of implementation research.
Process frameworks	Exploration, Preparation, Implementation, Sustainment (EPIS) framework	The EPIS framework is a comprehensive framework that describes implementation processes in four distinct phases—exploration, preparation, implementation, and sustainment—and also includes determinants of implementation related to the outer context, inner context, innovation, and bridging factors.[30] A website (episframework.com) provides detailed information on the framework, including worksheets and tools to guide implementation at each phase.
	Knowledge to Action (K2A) framework	The K2A framework describes the process of translating research evidence into "products" (eg, programs, policies, toolkits, strategies) for dissemination, adoption, and institutionalization.[76] A strength of the K2A framework is the specification of supporting structures necessary to implement new programs or practices at each step. The Centers for Disease Control and Prevention created a planning guide for using the K2A that explains each step in the process and lists planning questions for different stakeholders, including implementers/QI practitioners.[77]

Determinants frameworks	The Behavior Change Wheel (BCW)	The BCW consolidates 19 frameworks of behavior change at three levels: determinants of behavior (capability, opportunity, and motivation); intervention functions to change behavior; and policies that support intervention delivery.[53] The BCW is particularly suited for considering determinants of implementation at the individual level, such as why healthcare providers do or do not use a new clinical practice. A website (behaviorchangewheel. com) provides definitions for the constructs in the wheel, with greater detail available in the book, *The Behavior Change Wheel: A Guide to Designing Interventions*, and related journal articles.[78]
	The Consolidated Framework for Implementation Research (CFIR)	Perhaps the most widely used determinants framework, the CFIR is particularly suited to considering contextual barriers and facilitators at the organizational level. A robust supporting website (cfirguide.org) provides operational definitions for constructs, interview guides, and related literature to support implementation research. The CFIR recently underwent a revision that incorporated the capability-opportunity-motivation constructs for individual behavior.[78]
Implementation strategy taxonomies	The Expert Recommendations for Implementing Change (ERIC) Compilation of Implementation Strategies	Widely cited within the implementation literature, the publications from the ERIC compilation include 73 strategies with definitions that representing a broad range, from public policy changes to individual-level feedback.[54,55] The CFIR developers have also created a tool to map CFIR determinants to implementation strategies from the ERIC compilation (available at: https://cfirguide. org/choosing-strategies), but this tool is not yet mature for easy use.
	The BCW	As with determinants, the BCW is also a resource for identification of strategies. When considering the behavior of clinical practice change, the middle layer of the Wheel includes "intervention functions" that are equivalent to implementation strategies, whereas the outer layer presents implementation strategies at the policy level.

(continued on next page)

Table 1
(continued)

Category of Resource	Name of Resource	Considerations for Use
Implementation outcomes frameworks	Taxonomy of Outcomes for Implementation Research (the "Proctor framework")	The taxonomy published by Proctor et al. defines seven core implementation outcomes (acceptability, appropriateness, feasibility, adoption, penetration, cost, fidelity, and sustainability).[60] The taxonomy maps these outcomes to other terms and suggests measurement methods.
	RE-AIM Framework	Originally introduced in 1999, RE-AIM stands for Reach, Effectiveness, Adoption, Implementation, and Maintenance.[79] A website (www.re-aim.org) provides tools for its use. RE-AIM has also undergone revisions to incorporate equity, sustainability, and a determinants framework.[80]
Other resources	Implementation Research Logic Model (IRLM)	A one-page, semi-structured tool, the IRLM guides users to specify clinical interventions, determinants of implementation (according to CFIR domains), implementation strategies, and the outcomes to be measured.[68] The simplicity with which the IRLM incorporates implementation science frameworks makes it a particularly useful tool for QI practitioners. The IRLM also prompts users to specify the "mechanisms" by which they expect their chosen implementation strategies to improve outcomes. Although particularly important in research contexts,[81] considering mechanisms may also be useful for QI teams in the thoughtful development of implementation strategies.

Table 1 presents a list of recommended process models, determinants frameworks, outcomes frameworks, and other resources for getting started with implementation science. This is by no means a comprehensive list, as there are numerous frameworks to choose from.[25] Nor are the listed resources necessarily the best suited for addressing any particular research or improvement challenge. Rather, these are tools that the authors have used themselves and have found to be useful within perinatal and other clinical settings. The list is also limited to two resources in each category, in order to make it manageable. Those who are new to implementation science are often cautioned against getting "bogged down" in selecting the optimal theory or framework[31]—the perfect should not be the enemy of the good when it comes to the benefits of using an empirically-based theory or framework to guide improvement work. Later sections of this article provide examples of how perinatal QI teams might apply these resources in their own projects.

A VISION FOR INTEGRATING IMPLEMENTATION SCIENCE WITH PERINATAL QUALITY IMPROVEMENT

The principal concern of implementation science is to contribute *generalizable knowledge* about the implementation of evidence-based practices into routine health care or services.[19,32,33] Implementation science prioritizes the rigorous methods to ensure that studies can validly answer the hypothesis that they were designed to answer. A null finding (eg, that an implementation strategy is not effective in improving use of an evidence-based practice in a particular context) is an equally valuable contribution to the evidence base as is a positive finding confirming a study's hypothesis. Recent debates in the field have questioned whether it is necessary for a practice to have a robust evidence base (eg, demonstrated effectiveness in a randomized controlled trial) to be the subject of an implementation research study.[17] Such a prerequisite prevents implementation science from engaging when rapid change is required (eg, adjusting clinical practices in response to public health emergencies like the COVID-19 pandemic) and from prioritizing patient and community perspectives.[17] In the context of multisite QI initiatives, studies of the implementation of policies or practices that have less robust evidence (eg, best practices not yet supported by effectiveness trials) may still contribute important generalizable knowledge about implementation.

Improvement science, which has its origins in the industrial management work of Shewart and Deming (originators of the Plan-Do-Study-Act cycle) and the later Model for Improvement,[34] has been characterized as straddling research and change management.[35] Improvement science emphasizes systematic data-driven tests of change within a system.[35,36] QI initiatives following improvement science approaches have a goal of achieving local improvements. It is expected that QI teams will continue conducting multiple tests of change until they achieve a preset target. Although there is overlap in the goals of implementation science and QI, implementation science's focus on generalizable knowledge contrasts with improvement science's focus on achieving local or system change.[37]

Despite the contrasts, both implementation science and QI can benefit from better integration. From the perspective of implementation scientists, partnership with quality improvement initiatives can bridge the growing gap between implementation evidence and implementation practice.[32,38] As depicted in **Fig. 1A**, the goal of implementation science is to address the challenges with incorporating *clinical* research evidence into routine care—the evidence–practice gap—by generating evidence about implementation of clinical evidence. However, implementation scientists

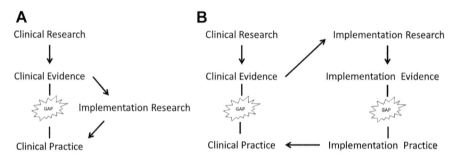

Fig. 1. The goals and reality for implementation science. (*A*) The goals for implementation science's contributions: bridging the evidence–practice gap. (*B*) The reality of implementation science's contributions without better integration with practice: recreating an evidence–practice gap for implementation.

are increasingly recognizing that unless that implementation evidence is able to be put into use by implementation practitioners, they may be paradoxically creating a parallel evidence–practice gap for *implementation* evidence (**Fig. 1**B).[20,39] Partnerships with quality improvement practitioners are needed to ensure that the growing body of implementation evidence supports routine implementation in clinical settings.

QI practice, in turn, can benefit from the evidence generated by implementation science. Substantial investments are being made in the development of implementation science methods and extending their application to new clinical areas, including perinatology. For example, the National Institute for Child Health and Development's initiative, Implementing a Maternal Health and Pregnancy Outcomes Vision for Everyone, recently published funding opportunities for both implementation research studies and an implementation science hub/resource center.[40,41] Perinatal research and QI efforts are also beginning to incorporate implementation science methods and concepts.[42–45]

INTEGRATING IMPLEMENTATION SCIENCE WITH PERINATAL QUALITY IMPROVEMENT: STEPS FOR QI PRACTITIONERS

Improvement science offers frameworks to guide the work of perinatal QI practitioners. Perhaps the most commonly used is the Model for Improvement. Originally developed by Langley and colleagues, the Model for Improvement recommends that practitioners answer three questions as a foundation of any QI initiative: (1) what are we trying to accomplish? (2) how will we know that a change is an improvement? and (3) what changes can we make that will result in the improvement?[34] These three questions ask practitioners to define the aim of the initiative, measure to assess progress, and potential changes.[46] Practitioners then test potential changes following a Plan-Do-Study-Act cycle.[34,36] This model is promoted by organizations such as the Institute for Healthcare Improvement[46] and has been widely adopted by QI practitioners.

Applying an implementation science lens to the Model for Improvement can lead us to expand on how "changes" are conceptualized. Implementation scientists would distinguish between the clinical practice changes and other activities that are intended to help providers successfully make that change in clinical practice. Using the terminology from **Box 1**, the clinical practice change is "the thing" and the activities to support the clinical practice change are considered implementation strategies that "help" providers "do the thing." One reason to draw this distinction is that clinical practices, particularly those with a strong evidence base, often have core components that cannot change without compromising efficacy.[47] However, the strategies that we use to help providers make a change in their clinical practice may be highly adaptable without impacting the efficacy of those practices. For example, the recommended course of corticosteroids for pregnant women at risk of imminent preterm delivery between 24 and 34 weeks gestation is a clinical intervention with clear administration guidelines.[48] Although deviations from the corticosteroid administration guidelines are not recommended,[48] QI teams might use a variety of strategies to help providers follow those guidelines—from establishing formal policies to entering standard order sets in the electronic health record or auditing unit performance. With this distinction between clinical practice changes and implementation strategies, we can add two more implementation-specific questions to the Model for Improvement for health care settings (**Box 2**): (1) how can we help providers to make clinical practice changes? and (2) how will we know if our help is working?

When following the Model for Improvement, the "Aim" and "Patient Outcome Measure" are driven by the clinical challenges and goals faced by particular health care settings. In contemporary clinical contexts, QI teams can often rely on clinical guidelines, systematic reviews, and individual trial results for evidence regarding which clinical practice changes to make. In some cases, clinical challenges without a tested solution may necessitate locally developed clinical innovations, as was the case with our earlier example of the ESC protocol. In many other cases, an effective clinical practice is already known, and the change the QI team needs to make is in better implementing that practice in their setting. With the clinical practice defined, our implementation science-informed revision to the Model for Improvement directs us to the two implementation questions. The following steps for QI practitioners provide

---

Box 2
Implementation science-informed additions to the Model for Improvement for health care settings

What are we trying to accomplish?
 (AIM)

 ⇓

How will we know that a change is an improvement?
 (PATIENT OUTCOME MEASURE)

 ⇓

What *clinical practice* changes can we make that will result in improvement?
 (CLINICAL PRACTICE CHANGE)

 ⇓

How can we help providers to make the clinical practice changes?
 (IMPLEMENTATION STRATEGIES)

 ⇓

How will we know if our strategies to help are working?
 (IMPLEMENTATION OUTCOME MEASURE)

Note: Additions to the Model for Improvement noted in with asterisks and bold type.

suggestions and examples for using implementation science-based resources to answer those questions in perinatal QI projects.

Step 1 for QI Practitioners: Systematically Consider Determinants of Implementation

The first addition to the Model for Improvement asks, "how can we help providers to make the clinical practice changes?" In other words, what implementation strategies can we use to support and incentivize providers to change? To select appropriate implementation strategies for an improvement effort, it is first necessary to understand the barriers and facilitators for change. This is consistent with the increasing recognition among implementation researchers that implementation strategies need to be tailored to the determinants of implementing a particular clinical practice change within a particular context.[49] Identifying barriers and facilitators for implementation is similar to developing a driver diagram for a QI initiative. However, QI teams typically start with a blank template, and brainstorm factors to include in their driver diagrams.[50,51] Within implementation science, there has been an emphasis on developing and using common determinants frameworks, to enable generalizable learning across individual settings. An implementation determinants framework can be a good guide for Qi teams assessing the implementation barriers and facilitators for their initiative; rather than starting with a blank template that runs the risk of overlooking critical determinants when planning their initiative, teams can start with a menu of empirically derived possibilities.

To illustrate the advantages of using a theoretically-informed implementation science framework, we can apply one of the recommended determinants frameworks from **Table 1** to a common QI challenge in perinatology, improving human milk feeding for VLBW infants.[52] Human milk feeding is an evidence-based practice for reducing

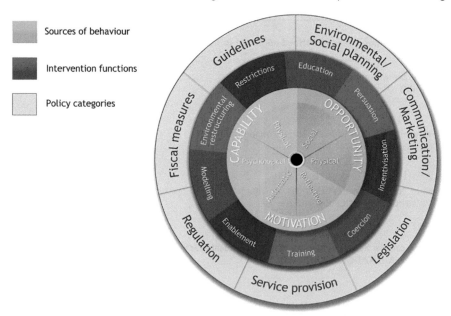

Fig. 2. The behavior change wheel. (Michie S, Atkins L, West R. (2014) The Behaviour Change Wheel: A Guide to Designing Interventions. London: Silverback Publishing. www. behaviourchangewheel.com.)

the risk of necrotizing enterocolitis as well as other complications, yet many NICU patients do not receive human milk and there are disparities by region and patient race.[52] The Behavior Change Wheel (BCW) (**Fig. 2**) can help QI teams think through the individual-level factors prohibiting human milk for VLBW infants. At the center of the wheel are the three drivers of individual behaviors in the model—capability, opportunity, and motivation—derived from existing theories.[53]

By considering the capability, opportunity, and motivation of individuals involved when brainstorming drivers of change, QI teams are more likely to identify the full range of barriers to human milk feeding. For birth mothers, they might identify a lack of opportunity—both social, in terms of support from family for frequent milk expression, and physical, in terms of access to the needed space within the NICU for pumping.[52] Some mothers may also have physical capability barriers due to medical morbidities that delayed lactogenesis and/or reduced milk production. For providers, they might identify a lack of psychological capability among staff in terms of knowledge about breastfeeding, the proper use of an electric pump, skin-to-skin care, and oral colostrum care, and a lack of motivation among physicians to provide the needed counseling and ongoing communication for families on the important known benefits of human milk. For the hospital system, they might identify a lack of physical opportunity to provide pasteurized donor human milk for when mother's own milk is not available and to ensure access to an electric pump for birth mothers after discharge.[52]

Step 2 for QI Practitioners: Use Targeted Strategies to Address Determinants of Clinical Practice Change

With a thorough understanding of the barriers to changing a clinical practice, QI teams are ready to select implementation strategies to help providers make the practice change. Several compilations or taxonomies of implementation strategies have been created, including the two recommended in **Table 1**: the BCW and the Expert Recommendations for Implementing Change (ERIC) list.[54,55] Referring to implementation strategy lists or taxonomies can be helpful for QI teams to consider the range of implementation strategies, including both those that they are familiar with and others that they have not yet tried. There is a general consensus in the implementation science literature that implementation strategies should be selected to address the barriers and leverage the facilitators for implementation that are specific to the given clinical setting.[56] Despite this consensus, and some preliminary work in this area,[57] there are few well-developed tools to facilitate the selection of implementation strategies.

The BCW, from our earlier example, is one of the most mature tools currently available for selecting implementation strategies, particularly when considering barriers and facilitators to implementation at the individual level. The middle and outer layers of the wheel list intervention and policy categories—both equivalent to types of implementation strategies—to support behavior change.[53] The middle layer strategies are those that are feasible for a QI team to use, and the wheel also "links" categories of strategies that address specific COM-B determinants of behavior. For example, education strategies (defined as "increasing knowledge or understanding") are recommended to address psychological capability and reflective motivation, whereas incentivization (defined as "creating an expectation of reward") is recommended for both types of motivation.[53]

To model implementation strategy selection using the BCW, we can consider another example of a common perinatal QI challenge, improving neonatal resuscitation. Effective neonatal resuscitation requires communication and teamwork.[58] After assessing the determinants of implementing neonatal resuscitation protocols on their unit, a QI team might identify key barriers of psychological capability (eg, providers do not know how to communicate effectively in an emergent situation) and physical opportunity (eg, the right providers are not in the delivery room to implement the protocol). Using the BCW, the QI team can consider and select one or more strategies that address psychological capability (education, training, or enablement) as well as one or more strategies that address physical opportunity (restriction, environmental restructuring, or enablement). Following the Model for Improvement, the QI team can then implement small test of change of these strategies for addressing implementation barriers.

Step 3 for QI Practitioners: Assess Implementation Outcomes

This step aligns with the last question in our revised Model for Improvement, "how will we know if our strategies to help are working?" Implementation outcomes are the measures used in implementation science to evaluate implementation strategies. In fact, improving implementation outcomes is a prerequisite for improving patient outcomes, because implementation outcomes measure "how much" and "how well" providers are making the clinical practice change (see **Box 1**).[24] Evaluation frameworks define the range of implementation outcomes that can be considered, and commonly used evaluation frameworks include the Reach, Effectiveness, Adoption, Implementation, and Maintenance (RE-AIM) framework [59] and Proctor and colleagues' Taxonomy of Implementation Outcomes[60] (see **Table 1**). Implementation outcomes that are common to both frameworks, and often tracked in perinatal QI projects, include reach (ie, the proportion of patients that receive the clinical practice) and fidelity (ie, the extent to which the clinical practice was delivered according to protocol). The Proctor framework is notable for the inclusion of early implementation outcomes—acceptability, feasibility, and appropriateness—that reflect individuals' perceptions of a clinical practice and are expected to influence the other implementation outcomes.[60]

For an example application of implementation outcomes to strengthen perinatal QI, we can use the POKE Project. The POKE Project is a clinical practice change developed in the NICU at Intermountain St. George Regional Hospital, St George, Utah, to evaluate every intervention, including those deemed as "routine," to determine if they added value, eliminating those that failed to add value, and ultimately, protecting the newborn from experiencing non-value-added care (termed POKEs).[61,62] The POKE Project is an example of de-implementation or stopping the use of harmful or unsupported clinical practices.[63] The QI team at Intermountain used a variety of strategies to "help" providers reduce the number of POKEs, such as team huddles, intentional empowerment of every member of the care team to actively contribute, surfacing the "voice of patient" from the eHR, and frequent caregiver recognition.[61] To assess whether these strategies improved clinical practice and patient outcomes, they tracked the daily count of POKEs for patients (voice of patient) as the lead measure and the incidence of central line-associate blood stream infections as the lagging measure.

The success of the POKE project relied on the ability of the QI team to overcome a key barrier to this practice change—provider motivation. De-implementation of ingrained clinical practices requires a challenging mindset shift and can be a more difficult change than implementing a new practice.[64] NICUs that replicate the POKE project may benefit from assessing early implementation outcomes to gauge providers' perceptions about the changes they are being asked to make. Although validated measures have been developed,[65] a formal assessment of early implementation outcomes is often not feasible or practical within perinatal QI projects.

Alternatively, QI teams can informally leverage the concepts of acceptability, feasibility, and appropriateness, by gauging providers' opinions about the clinical practice change during discussions on the unit. Gauging the changes in early implementation outcomes can help QI teams determine whether their POKE project strategies are working to change providers' mindset, which determines their clinical practice.

INTEGRATING IMPLEMENTATION SCIENCE WITH PERINATAL QUALITY IMPROVEMENT: STEPS FOR IMPLEMENTATION SCIENTISTS

Although this article is focused on the ways that QI teams can take advantage of the developments within implementation science to support their own work, an equal share of the work of integration should be undertaken by implementation scientists. Just as we recognize that clinical interventions need to be designed with routine implementation in mind,[66] implementation researchers need to consider the implications and practicality of their work for routine implementation and QI. The first step that could help us align our research with quality improvement is to ask QI leaders about their needs. We need to understand what implementation challenges they face, in order to design studies that address those challenges. The second step we can take is to develop and test tools that QI teams can use to apply evidence regarding effective implementation routinely in their work. Many of the measures that have been developed for contextual assessments of barriers and facilitators are too lengthy for routine use,[67] and some implementation strategies designed for clinical settings are too resource intensive for QI. An example of a broadly useable tool resulting from implementation research is the Implementation Research Logic Model (IRLM) (see **Table 1**; **Fig. 3**).[68] This template guides researchers and QI practitioners to consider the determinants of implementation (based on the Consolidated Framework for Implementation Research [CFIR]), specify the clinical intervention as well as the implementation strategies the QI team will use, and define implementation outcomes and patient outcomes for evaluating the project or study.[68] All that one needs to begin using the IRLM is a basic familiarity with the underlying implementation science frameworks.

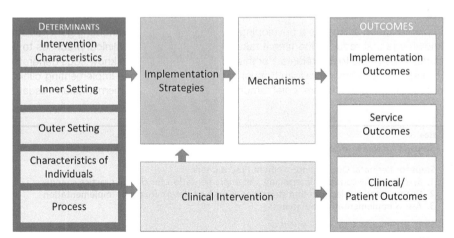

Fig. 3. The implementation research logic model. (*Adapted from* Smith JD, Li DH, Rafferty MR. The Implementation Research Logic Model: a method for planning, executing, reporting, and synthesizing implementation projects. Implement Sci. 2020;15(1):84. Published 2020 Sep 25.)

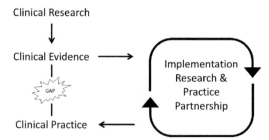

Fig. 4. A solution of closing both the clinical and implementation evidence gaps: implementation science-quality improvement partnerships.

A third step for implementation researchers is to partner with formal QI initiatives to generate implementation evidence and incorporate that evidence into the design of future initiatives (**Fig. 4**). Perinatal quality collaboratives (PQCs) are an example of formal, multisite QI initiatives that provide an opportunity for partnership. Several implementation research studies embedded in PQCs have been published.[69–72] Implementation strategies that have been associated with stronger implementation of clinical practice in these studies include involving multiple disciplines in the QI team[71] and developing a written implementation plan.[70] This evidence can be used to strengthen future PQCs in multiple ways, such as providing tools to support planning or requiring participating hospitals to form an interdisciplinary team. Another model is establishing implementation laboratories within health care organizations that are able to deploy and modify implementation strategies at scale.[73] A challenge for these partnerships is that traditional research funding cycles operate on a longer timeline than QI initiatives—funding decisions on NIH grants takes up to 9 months, and most of the applications are not funded on the first submission. New funding opportunity mechanisms may be needed to fully realize the potential of implementation research–quality improvement partnerships.

SUMMARY

Implementation science is a developing field with a goal of contributing generalizable knowledge that reduces the time it takes for evidence-based clinical practices to be routinely available to all patients. For this goal to be realized, the knowledge generated through implementation research must itself be used by those implementing clinical practices, QI practitioners chief among them. To date, implementation research

---

Box 3
Steps to integrate implementation science with perinatal quality improvement

Steps for Perinatal Quality Improvement Practitioners:
1. Systematically consider determinants of implementation for clinical practice changes
2. Use targeted implementation strategies to address determinants of implementation
3. Assess implementation outcomes

Steps for Implementation Scientists:
1. Ask quality improvement practitioners about their needs
2. Develop and test tools for applying implementation science knowledge routinely
3. Incorporate implementation science evidence into the structure of large quality improvement initiatives

evidence has not been adequately accessible and useable for QI practitioners—the different vocabulary and proliferation of theories and frameworks of implementation science can be daunting for busy clinicians. This article seeks to clarify how implementation science can add value in QI projects by presenting a framework that links the Model for Improvement with implementation strategies and methods as well as actionable steps for QI practitioners. Through the proposed steps, implementation science frameworks can give QI teams a robust starting point for identifying barriers to clinical practice change in the local context, selecting strategies to address them, and measuring the success of those strategies.

This article also calls for partnerships between QI practitioners and implementation scientists to better integrate the two fields (**Box 3**). Meaningful partnerships can lead to co-creation of tools and approaches that translate implementation research evidence into QI practice. Realizing the potential of implementation science to close the clinical evidence-to-practice gap requires stronger engagement with the routine work of implementation, and clinicians leading quality improvement can be a critical partner in that effort.

ACKNOWLEDGEMENTS

The authors would like to thank Dr Munish Gupta for his helpful review and recommendations.

DISCLOSURES

Dr J. Callaghan-Koru has worked as a paid consultant for the Alliance for Innovation in Maternal Health. The authors have no other conflicts to disclose.

REFERENCES

1. Morris ZS, Wooding S, Grant J. The answer is 17 years, what is the question: understanding time lags in translational research. J R Soc Med 2011;104(12): 510–20.
2. Whitesel E, Goldstein J, Lee HC. Quality improvement for neonatal resuscitation and delivery room care. Semin Perinatol 2022;46(6):151629.
3. Keir A, Grace E, Stanworth S. Closing the evidence to practice gap in neonatal transfusion medicine. Semin Fetal Neonatal Med 2021;26(1):101197.
4. Edwards EM, Greenberg LT, Profit J, et al. Quality of care in US NICUs by race and ethnicity. Pediatrics 2021;148(2). e2020037622.
5. Pai VV, Lee HC, Profit J. Improving uptake of key perinatal interventions using statewide quality collaboratives. Clin Perinatol 2018;45(2):165–80.
6. Pearlman SA. Advancements in neonatology through quality improvement. J Perinatol 2022;42(10):1277–82.
7. Payne NR, Barry J, Berg W, et al. Sustained reduction in neonatal nosocomial infections through quality improvement efforts. Pediatrics 2012;129(1):e165–73.
8. Prakalapakorn SG, Greenberg L, Edwards EM, et al. Trends in retinopathy of prematurity screening and treatment: 2008–2018. Pediatrics 2021;147(6). e2020039966.
9. Manuck TA, Fry RC, McFarlin BL. Quality improvement in perinatal medicine and translation of preterm birth research findings into clinical care. Clin Perinatol 2018;45(2):155–63.
10. Zupancic JAF. Broadening the scope and scale of quality improvement in neonatology. Semin Fetal Neonatal Med 2021;26(1):101228.

11. Horbar JD, Edwards EM, Greenberg LT, et al. Variation in performance of neonatal intensive care units in the United States. JAMA Pediatr 2017;171(3): e164396.

12. Leslie MS, Greene J, Schulkin J, et al. Umbilical cord clamping practices of U.S. obstetricians. J Neonatal Perinatal Med 2018;11(1):51–60.

13. Boghossian NS, Geraci M, Lorch SA, et al. Racial and ethnic differences over time in outcomes of infants born less than 30 Weeks' gestation. Pediatrics 2019;144(3):e20191106.

14. Ravi D, Iacob A, Profit J. Unequal care: racial/ethnic disparities in neonatal intensive care delivery. Semin Perinatol 2021;45(4):151411.

15. Eccles MP, Mittman BS. Welcome to implementation science. Implement Sci 2006;1(1):1.

16. Chambers D, Simpson L, Neta G, et al. Proceedings from the 9th annual conference on the science of dissemination and implementation. Implement Sci 2017; 12(1):48.

17. Beidas RS, Dorsey S, Lewis CC, et al. Promises and pitfalls in implementation science from the perspective of US-based researchers: learning from a pre-mortem. Implementation Sci 2022;17(1):1–15.

18. Metz A, Jensen T, Farley A, et al. Is implementation research out of step with implementation practice? Pathways to effective implementation support over the last decade. Implementation Research and Practice 2022;3. 26334895221105584.

19. Ovretveit J, Mittman B, Rubenstein L, et al. Using implementation tools to design and conduct quality improvement projects for faster and more effective improvement. Int J Health Care Qual Assur 2017;30(8):755–68.

20. Westerlund A, Sundberg L, Nilsen P. Implementation of implementation science knowledge: the research-practice gap paradox. Worldviews Evid Based Nurs 2019;16(5):332–4.

21. Kislov R, Pope C, Martin GP, et al. Harnessing the power of theorising in implementation science. Implement Sci 2019;14(1):103.

22. Weiner BJ, Lewis CC, Sherr K. Introducing implementation science. In: Weiner B, Lewis C, Sherr K, editors. *Practical implementation science*. New York, NY: Springer Publishing; 2023. p. 1–21.

23. Mitchell SA, Chambers DA. Leveraging implementation science to improve cancer care delivery and patient outcomes. J Oncol Pract 2017;13(8):523–9.

24. Curran GM. Implementation science made too simple: a teaching tool. Implementation Science Communications 2020;1(1):4.

25. Tabak RG, Khoong EC, Chambers DA, et al. Bridging research and practice: models for dissemination and implementation research. Am J Prev Med 2012; 43(3):337–50.

26. MacMillan KDL. Neonatal abstinence syndrome: review of epidemiology, care models, and current understanding of outcomes. Clin Perinatol 2019;46(4): 817–32.

27. Wachman EM, Grossman M, Schiff DM, et al. Quality improvement initiative to improve inpatient outcomes for Neonatal Abstinence Syndrome. J Perinatol 2018;38(8):1114–22.

28. Nilsen P. Making sense of implementation theories, models and frameworks. Implement Sci 2015;10:53.

29. Field B, Booth A, Ilott I, et al. Using the Knowledge to Action Framework in practice: a citation analysis and systematic review. Implementation Sci 2014; 9(1):1–14.

30. Aarons GA, Hurlburt M, Horwitz SM. Advancing a conceptual model of evidence-based practice implementation in public service sectors. Adm Policy Ment Health 2011;38.
31. Hamm RF, Iriye BK, Srinivas SK. Implementation science is imperative to the optimization of obstetric care. *Am J Perinatol*. Published online December 2020;15.
32. Leeman J, Rohweder C, Lee M, et al. Aligning implementation science with improvement practice: a call to action. Implementation Science Communications 2021;2(1):99.
33. Curran GM, Bauer M, Mittman B, et al. Effectiveness-implementation hybrid designs: combining elements of clinical effectiveness and implementation research to enhance public health impact. Med Care 2012;50.
34. Langley GJ, Moen RD, Nolan KM, et al. The improvement guide: a practical approach to enhancing organizational performance. San Francisco, CA: John Wiley & Sons; 2009.
35. Lemire S, Christie CA, Inkelas M. The methods and tools of improvement science. N Dir Eval 2017;2017(153):23–33.
36. Perla R, Provost L, Parry G. Seven propositions of the science of improvement: exploring foundations. Qual Manag Health Care 2013;22(3):170–86.
37. Lane-Fall MB, Fleisher LA. Quality improvement and implementation science: different fields with aligned goals. Anesthesiol Clin 2018;36(1):xiii–xv.
38. Check DK, Zullig LL, Davis MM, et al. Improvement science and implementation science in cancer care: identifying areas of synergy and opportunities for further integration. J Gen Intern Med 2021;36(1):186–95.
39. Rapport F, Smith J, Hutchinson K, et al. Too much theory and not enough practice? The challenge of implementation science application in healthcare practice. J Eval Clin Pract 2021;15.
40. National Institutes of Health. NOT-OD-22-125: notice of special interest (NOSI): IMPROVE initiative: implementation science to advance maternal health and maternal health equity. Available at: https://grants.nih.gov/grants/guide/notice-files/NOT-OD-22-125.html. Published 2022. Accessed September 14, 2022.
41. National Institutes of Health. RFA-HD-23-037: maternal health research centers of excellence implementation science hub/resource center (U24 clinical trial optional). Available at: https://grants.nih.gov/grants/guide/rfa-files/RFA-HD-23-037.html. Published 2022. Accessed September 14, 2022.
42. Kaplan HC, Walsh KE. Context in implementation science. Pediatrics 2022; 149(Supplement 3). e2020045948C.
43. Guyatt S, Ferguson M, Beckmann M, et al. Using the Consolidated Framework for Implementation Research to design and implement a perinatal education program in a large maternity hospital. BMC Health Serv Res 2021;21(1):1077.
44. Coutts S, Woldring A, Pederson A, et al. What is stopping us? An implementation science study of kangaroo care in British Columbia's neonatal intensive care units. BMC Pregnancy Childbirth 2021;21:52.
45. Quinn JM, Gephart SM, Davis MP. External facilitation as an evidence-based practice implementation strategy during an antibiotic stewardship collaborative in neonatal intensive care units. Worldviews Evid Based Nurs 2019;16(6):454–61.
46. Institute for Healthcare Improvement. How to improve | IHI - Institute for healthcare improvement. Available at: https://www.ihi.org:443/resources/Pages/HowtoImprove/default.aspx. Accessed October 26, 2022.
47. Greenhalgh T, Robert G, Macfarlane F, et al. Diffusion of innovations in service organizations: systematic review and recommendations. Milbank Q 2004; 82(4):581.

48. Committee on Obstetric Practice. Committee opinion No. 713: antenatal cortico-steroid therapy for fetal maturation. Obstet Gynecol 2017;130(2):e102–9.

49. Powell BJ, Beidas RS, Lewis CC, et al. Methods to improve the selection and tailoring of implementation strategies. J Behav Health Serv Res 2017;44(2): 177–94.

50. Institute for Healthcare Improvement. QI essentials toolkit: driver diagram. Boston, MA: Institute for Healthcare Improvement; 2017.

51. Center for Medicare and Medicaid Innovation. Defining and using aims and drivers for improvement: a how-to guide. Baltimore, MD: Centers for Medicare & Medicaid Services; 2013.

52. Parker MG, Stellwagen LM, Noble L, et al. Promoting human milk and breastfeed-ing for the very low birth weight infant. Pediatrics 2021;148(5). e2021054272.

53. Michie S, van Stralen MM, West R. The behaviour change wheel: a new method for characterising and designing behaviour change interventions. Implement Sci 2011;6(1):42.

54. Powell BJ, Waltz TJ, Chinman MJ, et al. A refined compilation of implementation strategies: results from the Expert Recommendations for Implementing Change (ERIC) project. Implement Sci 2015;10(1):21.

55. Waltz TJ, Powell BJ, Matthieu MM, et al. Use of concept mapping to characterize relationships among implementation strategies and assess their feasibility and importance: results from the Expert Recommendations for Implementing Change (ERIC) study. Implement Sci 2015;10(1):109.

56. Chambers DA, Glasgow RE, Stange KC. The dynamic sustainability framework: addressing the paradox of sustainment amid ongoing change. Implement Sci 2013;8(1):117.

57. Waltz TJ, Powell BJ, Fernández ME, et al. Choosing implementation strategies to address contextual barriers: diversity in recommendations and future directions. Implement Sci 2019;14(1):42.

58. Brogaard L, Hvidman L, Esberg G, et al. Teamwork and adherence to guideline on newborn resuscitation-video review of neonatal interdisciplinary teams. Front Pediatr 2022;10:828297.

59. Glasgow RE, Harden SM, Gaglio B, et al. RE-AIM planning and evaluation frame-work: adapting to new science and practice with a 20-year review. Front Public Health 2019;7. Available at: https://www.frontiersin.org/article/10.3389/fpubh. 2019.00064. Accessed May 11, 2022.

60. Proctor E, Silmere H, Raghavan R, et al. Outcomes for implementation research: conceptual distinctions, measurement challenges, and research agenda. Adm Policy Ment Health 2011;38(2):65–76.

61. Profit J, Scheid A, Ridout E. First, do No harm: value-driven patient safety in the neonatal intensive care unit. PSNet Collection. Available at: https://psnet.ahrq. gov/perspective/first-do-no-harm-value-driven-patient-safety-neonatal-intensive-care-unit. Published online 2019. Accessed November 1, 2022.

62. Harrison M, Lee T. Short-term loss, long-term gain: encouraging bottom-up ideas that revise the value equation. NEJM Catalyst Innovations in Care Delivery. Avail-able at: https://catalyst.nejm.org/doi/full/10.1056/CAT.20.0046. Published online February 11, 2020. Accessed November 1, 2022.

63. Prasad V, Ioannidis JP. Evidence-based de-implementation for contradicted, un-proven, and aspiring healthcare practices. Implement Sci 2014;9(1):1.

64. Norton WE, Chambers DA. Unpacking the complexities of de-implementing inap-propriate health interventions. Implement Sci 2020;15(1):2.

65. Weiner BJ, Lewis CC, Stanick C, et al. Psychometric assessment of three newly developed implementation outcome measures. Implement Sci 2017;12(1):108.
66. Chambers DA. Sharpening our focus on designing for dissemination: lessons from the SPRINT program and potential next steps for the field. Transl Behav Med 2020;10(6):1416–8.
67. Lewis CC, Weiner BJ, Stanick C, et al. Advancing implementation science through measure development and evaluation: a study protocol. Implement Sci 2015;10:102.
68. Smith JD, Li DH, Rafferty MR. The Implementation Research Logic Model: a method for planning, executing, reporting, and synthesizing implementation projects. Implementation Sci 2020;15(1):1–12.
69. VanGompel ECW, Perez SL, Datta A, et al. Culture that facilitates change: a mixed methods study of hospitals engaged in reducing cesarean deliveries. Ann Fam Med 2021;19(3):249–57.
70. Callaghan-Koru J, Creanga A, DiPietro B, et al. Implementation of the safe reduction of primary cesarean births safety bundle during the first year of a statewide collaborative in Maryland. Obstet Gynecol 2019. Published online.
71. Kaplan HC, Sherman SN, Cleveland C, et al. Reliable implementation of evidence: a qualitative study of antenatal corticosteroid administration in Ohio hospitals. BMJ Qual Saf 2016;25(3):173–81.
72. Vamos CA, Thompson EL, Cantor A, et al. Contextual factors influencing the implementation of the obstetrics hemorrhage initiative in Florida. J Perinatol 2017;37(2):150–6.
73. Ivers NM, Grimshaw JM. Reducing research waste with implementation laboratories. Lancet 2016;388(10044):547–8.
74. National Cancer Institute. Implementation Science at a Glance. National Cancer Institute, National Institutes of Health.
75. Lane-Fall MB, Curran GM, Beidas RS. Scoping implementation science for the beginner: locating yourself on the "subway line" of translational research. BMC Med Res Methodol 2019;19(1):133.
76. Wilson KM, Brady TJ, Lesesne C. An organizing framework for translation in public health: the knowledge to action framework. Prev Chronic Dis 2011;8(2):A46.
77. Centers for Disease Control and Prevention. Applying the knowledge to action framework: questions to guide planning. Centers for Disease Control and Prevention, U.S. Department of Health and Human Services; 2014.
78. Damschroder LJ, Reardon CM, Widerquist MAO, et al. The updated Consolidated Framework for Implementation Research based on user feedback. Implement Sci 2022;17(1):75.
79. Glasgow RE. Evaluating the public health impact of health promotion interventions: the RE-AIM framework. Am J Public Health 1999;89(9):1322–7.
80. Holtrop JS, Estabrooks PA, Gaglio B, et al. Understanding and applying the RE-AIM framework: clarifications and resources. J Clin Transl Sci 2021;5(1):e126.
81. Lewis CC, Klasnja P, Powell BJ, et al. From classification to causality: advancing understanding of mechanisms of change in implementation science. Front Public Health 2018;6:136.

Developing a Respiratory Quality Improvement Program to Prevent and Treat Bronchopulmonary Dysplasia in the Neonatal Intensive Care Unit

Lauren A. Sanlorenzo, MD, MPH[a],
Leon Dupree Hatch III, MD, MPH[b,c,d],*

KEYWORDS

- Respiratory quality improvement • Bronchopulmonary dysplasia
- Mechanical ventilation • Noninvasive ventilation

KEY POINTS

- Improvements in neonatal respiratory care have resulted in improved survival rates and lower morbidities for infants in the neonatal intensive care unit over the past several decades.
- Bronchopulmonary dysplasia (BPD), one of the most frequent targets of neonatal quality improvement activities, is a complex, multifactorial disease that often requires multiple interventions for improvement.
- Potentially modifiable drivers for improving BPD include optimal establishment of functional residual capacity, optimal use of noninvasive ventilation, minimization of mechanical ventilation, optimal use of pharmacologic therapies, optimal growth and nutrition, and the avoidance of nosocomial infections or other comorbidities of prematurity.

INTRODUCTION

Over the past several decades, advances in neonatal respiratory care have resulted in improved survival and decreased morbidity for preterm and term infants with respiratory disease requiring admission to the neonatal intensive care unit (NICU).[1–3] These

a Department of Pediatrics, Division of Neonatology, Columbia University Medical Center, 3959 Broadway Avenue, New York, NY 10032, USA; b Department of Pediatrics, Division of Neonatology, Vanderbilt University Medical Center, 4413 VCH, 2200 Children's Way, Nashville, TN 37232, USA; c Center for Child Health Policy, Vanderbilt University Medical Center, Nashville, TN, USA; d Critical Illness, Brain Dysfunction, and Survivorship Center, Vanderbilt University Medical Center, Nashville, TN, USA
* Corresponding author.
E-mail address: leon.d.hatch@vumc.org

Clin Perinatol 50 (2023) 363–380
https://doi.org/10.1016/j.clp.2023.01.003
0095-5108/23/© 2023 Elsevier Inc. All rights reserved.
perinatology.theclinics.com

advances include the introduction of exogenous surfactant, inhaled nitric oxide, improvements in mechanical ventilation (MV), and an improved understanding of the role of supplemental oxygen and pharmacologic therapies in preventing or mitigating neonatal lung injury. Given the many therapies that impact respiratory outcomes and the multifactorial nature of neonatal lung development, injury, and repair, quality improvement (QI) approaches have been increasingly used with success in NICUs to implement potentially better practices (PBPs) to improve respiratory outcomes.[4] Despite the growth of respiratory QI, bronchopulmonary dysplasia (BPD), the most frequent target for respiratory QI activities in the NICU, has remained largely unchanged in population-based cohort studies.[3,5] Given the multifactorial nature of lung growth and injury, it is likely that a multifactorial approach must also be taken to improve respiratory outcomes, such as BPD, on a large scale.

The excellent reviews of evidence-based strategies to prevent BPD[6] and completed QI reports to reduce BPD[7] have been published. Interested readers are encouraged to consult these papers for further discussion of these topics. The goal of this review is to provide neonatal QI practitioners with a potential framework for building and implementing an interdisciplinary QI program to improve respiratory outcomes in the NICU. The authors do this by drawing on available evidence for PBPs for preventing neonatal lung injury and successful single-center and collaborative QI reports. As most published neonatal respiratory QI reports have focused on prevention of BPD, the bulk of this review pertains to that topic. However, the authors also highlight QI activities that can be undertaken to improve the treatment of infants with established BPD.

KEY COMPONENTS FOR BUILDING A RESPIRATORY QUALITY IMPROVEMENT PROGRAM

Successful improvement efforts often share similar characteristics, and these characteristics are important to consider when building or reinvigorating a respiratory QI program. These characteristics include (among others) having positive organizational culture for change,[8] senior leadership support,[9–11] shared visions and framework for change,[12,13] interdisciplinary teams with subject matter and QI methodology expertise,[9] and a focus on rigorously measuring change.[8,9] Detailed discussions of these topics are discussed elsewhere, including in other articles in this issue. The authors highlight several areas as they relate to respiratory QI.

Goals, Measurement, and Data

Once the decision has been made to improve respiratory outcomes, the next step is to determine what outcomes are the measurable targets of improvement and set goals related to those outcomes.

In the NICU, BPD has been the outcome most often targeted in respiratory QI efforts.[7] BPD has features that make it an important target for improvement efforts.

1. The most common definition of BPD, supplemental oxygen use at 36 weeks postmenstrual age (PMA),[14] is easily measurable and can be tracked by QI teams without significant data burden.
2. Benchmarking data for both raw and risk-adjusted BPD rates are readily available from large collaboratives such as the Vermont Oxford Network (VON)[3] and the California Perinatal Quality Care Collaborative.[15] These data can be used to assess current results and develop goals for respiratory QI efforts.
3. Multiple PBPs to decrease BPD exist and have proven efficacious in clinical trials[6] and QI reports.[7]

4. BPD is associated with adverse long-term pulmonary[16] and neurodevelopmental outcomes.[17] Thus, preventing BPD in the NICU may result in long-lasting effects on the health of individual patients.

Despite these advantages, BPD also has some disadvantages when used as the sole metric for measuring respiratory QI efforts in preterm infants.

1. The pathogenesis of BPD is multifactorial,[18] and to ultimately improve the incidence, interventions in multiple domains may be needed.
2. Oxygen use at 36 weeks (BPD) is a binary measure. QI teams could improve important markers of pulmonary health (eg, duration of positive pressure support or duration of oxygen supplementation) but still not show improvement in the rate of BPD. More granular definitions of BPD, including the popular definition by Jensen and colleagues, allow more stratification of disease.[19] However, even these definitions represent ordinal data and may not be as amenable for measuring rapid tests of change as a continuous metric.[20]
3. Oxygen use at 36 weeks (BPD) is a lagging indicator.[21] By the time the outcome of BPD is known in each patient, important developmental windows in lung growth and development have already occurred.
4. Although oxygen use at 36 weeks PMA is a widely used metric, other respiratory outcomes such as respiratory fragility at discharge have been noted to be important metrics when parental perspectives were considered.[22]

For these reasons, QI practitioners should consider using both outcome and process measures when building a respiratory QI program. Examples of process measures which can complement oxygen use at 36 weeks PMA (BPD) include leading measures such as the percent of infants who receive first-intention noninvasive ventilation (NIV), total early oxygen exposure,[23] duration of invasive MV,[24] and duration of supplemental oxygen.[25] Additional outcome measures to be considered for respiratory QI programs include supplemental oxygen at discharge, tracheostomy and home ventilation, or hospitalizations for respiratory causes in the first year of life. Many QI teams may not have the resources necessary to gather some or all of these metrics.

Shared Vision and Framework for Change

Once measures are chosen and goals are set, the next step in building a respiratory QI program is to develop a shared vision and framework for how the program will achieve the goals. Given the breadth of knowledge on neonatal lung growth, injury, and recovery, QI practitioners may consider starting with a review of the available literature for the drivers of respiratory outcomes and PBPs to improve those outcomes that may be applicable to their NICU. QI tools such as a key driver diagram (KDD)[26] can be used to organize the applicable drivers and PBPs into one place for the team(s) to view and refine. An example of a global KDD used in one of the author's centers for preventing the composite outcome of death or BPD is shown in **Fig. 1**. Importantly, this KDD was developed using both an extensive literature review, local subject matter expertise, and a comment period, where clinicians (physicians, advanced practice providers, respiratory therapists [RTs], and so forth) could comment on each driver and help refine the vision of the program. The different teams working on each of the secondary drivers in the KDD could see how their specific QI project fed into the larger goals of the program.

Interdisciplinary Teams

Given the multifactorial nature of respiratory outcomes and the multidisciplinary nature of neonatal care, a key component of any respiratory QI program must be

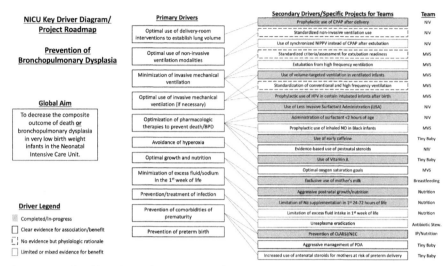

Fig. 1. Example of key driver diagram (KDD) for a unit-based quality improvement program to prevent bronchopulmonary dysplasia (BPD) in the neonatal intensive care unit (NICU). This example of KDD is used in one of the authors' NICUs to guide quality improvement (QI) efforts to prevent BPD. Primary and secondary drivers were identified by literature review and group meetings with faculty and staff in the NICU. Each secondary driver was rated based on available evidence to develop priority for targeting and was assigned to one of the existing QI teams in the NICU for implementation and testing. CLABSI, central line-associated blood stream infection; CPAP, continuous positive airway pressure; HFV, high-frequency ventilation; IP, infection prevention team; LISA, less invasive surfactant administration; MVS, mechanical ventilation safety team; NEC, necrotizing enterocolitis; NIPPV, nasal intermittent positive pressure ventilation; NIV, noninvasive ventilation team; NO, nitric oxide; PDA, patent ductus arteriosus; Stew, Stewardship.

interdisciplinary teams. For programs targeting respiratory outcomes, key members would include RTs, bedside nurses, advanced practice providers, trainees (in academic settings), physicians, parents, and NICU leadership. In units with large numbers of staff actively involved in QI, multiple teams can simultaneously target multiple primary and secondary drivers. An example of this is shown in **Fig. 1**. In this example, a total of seven teams are actively working on projects targeting drivers on the KDD. Each team has subject matter experts specific to the focus of improvement (eg, neonatal dieticians on the nutrition team, and infectious disease physicians on the antibiotic stewardship team). This use of multiple teams to target multiple drivers simultaneously may not be feasible in smaller units with fewer personnel available for QI. In these cases, QI practitioners may consider having a core team that remains together and then adding/removing content expertise with each new project as one prior study has shown that the success of QI teams is often correlated with the duration they work together.[13]

KEY DRIVERS OF BRONCHOPULMONARY DYSPLASIA AND POTENTIAL INTERVENTIONS

A large body of evidence from research studies and QI work is available to help QI teams identify potential key drivers to prevent BPD in their unit. These key drivers include optimization of noninvasive respiratory support, avoidance of ventilator-induced lung injury, evidence-based use of pharmacologic therapies, optimal growth and nutrition, avoidance of iatrogenic injury, and prevention of comorbidities associated with adverse pulmonary outcomes. For each driver, we provide ideas for QI efforts and when available, examples of successful QI reports that have targeted each specific driver. Some representative examples of QI projects targeting some of the proposed drivers above are shown in **Table 1**.

Optimal Use of Delivery Room Interventions to Establish Lung Volume

Although BPD is not formally diagnosed until 36 weeks' PMA, neonatal teams can impact respiratory outcomes starting with the first breath. Thoughtful approaches to the mode of delivery room respiratory support, timing and method of surfactant delivery, and standardized plans of care for the most premature infants are critical aspects of delivery room care.[27–29] The strategies to prevent BPD can be applied at birth to support successful transition to extrauterine life while limiting lung injury and oxidative stress. These strategies include the use of continuous positive airway pressure (CPAP), judicious use of supplemental oxygen, and surfactant therapy. Collective analysis of several landmark randomized trials from the last two decades demonstrates a statistically significant reduction in the risk for death or BPD among CPAP-treated infants compared with empirical intubation and MV after delivery.[30] The optimal initial concentration of supplemental oxygen to be used during resuscitation of preterm infants has not been clearly elucidated. However, current international recommendations suggest initiating resuscitation with low, less than 30% supplemental oxygen and targeting predefined oxygen saturation goals.[31,32] Among preterm infants who receive invasive MV, surfactant administration in the first 2 hours of life, compared with delivery after 2 hours of life, is associated with a decreased risk of BPD.[33] Excitingly, the use of less invasive surfactant administration (LISA) has been associated with lower rates of BPD.[34]

Delivery room and early respiratory focused QI have most frequently focused on the creation of tiny baby programs, golden hour initiatives, timely surfactant delivery, and optimal first-intention NIV.[35–38] Ashmeade and colleagues implemented a golden hour pathway to reduce BPD among infants born less than 28 weeks' gestational age (GA). This initiative included the creation of a standardized protocol, standardization of early respiratory support with an emphasis on CPAP use, decreased time to surfactant administration, and required proficiency of personnel who were performing delivery room intubations. The implementation of these initiatives resulted in decreased time to surfactant administration; however, no change in BPD rates was observed.[35] In a single-center tertiary NICU in Israel, Peleg and colleagues developed a comprehensive protocol implemented in the first hour of life that focused on team communication, a dedicated delivery room space, close attention to thermoregulation, and standardization of respiratory support. The respiratory guidelines included attention to adequate positive end-expiratory pressure support, limited peak inspiratory pressures, transition to the use of a T-piece resuscitator, and avoiding the use of self-inflating resuscitation devices. Retrospective analysis of nearly 200 infants in the intervention group and nearly 200 matched controls demonstrated a significant reduction in BPD rates. However, analysis of infants born ≤28 weeks at highest risk for the development of BPD did not alone have a significant reduction in the rates of BPD.[36]

Optimal Use of Noninvasive Ventilation/Minimization of Mechanical Ventilation

Enhanced use of NIV including CPAP and nasal intermittent positive-pressure ventilation (NIPPV) have transformed respiratory care in the NICU.[39] Three large randomized trials demonstrated early CPAP use, compared with intubation and surfactant delivery,

Table 1
Representative examples of quality improvement projects targeting proposed drivers for preventing bronchopulmonary dysplasia in the neonatal intensive care unit

Key Driver	Secondary Driver(s)	Interventions	Outcomes
Optimal use of delivery room interventions to establish lung volumes	• Effective facemask PPV[48]	• Formation of a "Golden Hour" team • Use of CO_2 detectors during PPV • Standardized, round mask for PPV • Standardized pressures to be given during delivery room PPV • Simulation training on troubleshooting difficulties with PPV	• Delivery room intubations decreased from 58% to 37%[a] • MV rate decreased from 85% to 70%[a] • BPD rate decreased from 26% to 13%[a]
	• Prophylactic use of CPAP after delivery to avoid mechanical ventilation[93]	• CPAP started in the delivery room for infants ≥ 26 wk' gestational age • Standardized intubation criteria	• Delivery room intubations decreased from 24% to 9% for infants ≥ 26 wk GA[a] • Delivery room CPAP increased from 0% to 70% for infants ≥ 26 wk GA[a] • BPD rate was statistically similar pre- and post-QI efforts (17% vs 8%).
Optimal use of noninvasive ventilation modalities	• Standardized noninvasive ventilation use[24]	• Standardization of CPAP use through 36 wk postmenstrual age • Standardization of algorithm for failure of weaning from CPAP and transition to nasal cannula	• Severe BPD decreased from 57% to 30% in eligible infants.[a] • Ratio of CPAP to MV days nearly doubled during the project period.
Minimization of Invasive Mechanical Ventilation	• Standardized criteria/assessment for extubation readiness[56]	• Development of a respiratory therapist-driven ventilator weaning protocol • Standardization of criteria and assessment for extubation	• Average duration of MV decreased from 18 to 6 d[a] • Extubation failure decreased from 40% to 20%[a] • Rate of BPD was unchanged.
Optimal use of invasive mechanical ventilation	• Use of VTV[25]	• Standardized diagnosis-specific MV pathways • Daily respiratory care huddle during rounds • Ventilator interface modifications to ensure easy ordering of VTV modes • Introduction of new VTV modes • Clinician education	• Use of exclusively VTV modes increased from 27% to 76%[a] • Rate of BPD was unchanged.

Optimization of pharmacologic therapies to prevent death/BPD	Use of Less Invasive Surfactant Administration (LISA)[47]	• Developed a consensus guideline for LISA use • Extensive simulation-based training for LISA • Development of a LISA kit with all needed equipment • Serial training/retraining sessions with faculty and staff on LISA	• CPAP failure rate decreased from 54% to 11%[a] • MV rate decreased from 58% to 31%[a] • Pneumothorax decreased from 8% to 1%[a] • Rate of BPD was unchanged in overall population.
	Evidence-based use of postnatal corticosteroids[76]	• Development of local guidelines for use of postnatal corticosteroids • Decision support for guidelines at multiple places in the clinical workflow • Clinician education	• Compliance with guideline use of corticosteroids increased from 71% to 96%[a] • Postnatal corticosteroid use was similar over the project. • Rate of severe BPD was unchanged.
Avoidance of hyperoxia	Optimal oxygen saturation targeting[94]	• Formation of a multidisciplinary "Oxidative Stress Initiative Committee" • Standardized guideline for supplemental oxygen management and response to hypoxia/hyperoxia • Integration of oxygen histogram review into clinical practice	• Rate of BPD was unchanged in overall population.
Optimal growth and nutrition	Aggressive postnatal growth[95]	• Development of enteral feeding guidelines • Increased protein and lipid concentrations in early parenteral nutrition • Increased speed of parenteral and enteral nutrition advancement	• Extrauterine growth failure (as defined by authors) decreased from 25% to 12%. • Rate of BPD was unchanged.

Abbreviations: BPD, bronchopulmonary dysplasia; CO_2, carbon dioxide; CPAP, continuous positive airway pressure; LISA, less invasive surfactant administration; MV, mechanical ventilation; PPV, positive pressure ventilation; QI, quality improvement; VTV, volume-targeted ventilation.

[a] Change either met special cause variation criteria or statistical significance.

resulted in a reduction in the rate of death or BPD at 36 weeks PMA.[28,40,41] These studies and others lead the American Academy of Pediatrics Committee on the Fetus and Newborn to recommend the use of early CPAP and selective surfactant administration in extremely low birth weight (ELBW) infants to reduce the risk for BPD.[42] Neonatal units often have multiple devices available to deliver noninvasive respiratory support, including CPAP, NIPPV, nasal noninvasive neutrally adjusted ventilatory assist, and high-flow nasal cannula. The modality of noninvasive support varies by center and there is significant variability in clinical practices and management strategies when using noninvasive modalities.[43]

QI work aimed at improving the use of NIV has targeted several important domains including prioritizing the use of CPAP as the primary respiratory modality in preterm infants, delineating the duration of CPAP use and a process for weaning from CPAP, and standardizing post-extubation support. As a starting point, many QI projects have focused on developing respiratory care bundles which standardize the early use of CPAP as the primary mode of NIV. As an example, Levesque and colleagues demonstrated that through the implementation of a respiratory care bundle aimed to optimize delivery of CPAP, they had high rates of compliance with the exclusive use of bubble CPAP seen in 82% of infants, which was associated with a decrease in BPD rates.[44] QI methods have been used to standardized when to wean infants from NIV. With intention to minimize inflammation from atelectasis, Bapat and colleagues developed a protocol encouraging the use of CPAP through 36 weeks' PMA unless the infant could come off CPAP without requiring more than minimal oxygen beyond 32 weeks' PMA. This group demonstrated an increase in the number of days on CPAP and a reduction in the rate of BPD from 73% in 2013 to 41% in 2018.[24] Additional areas of focus when implementing NIV include trialing different interface systems used to deliver NIV and mechanisms for assessing fit and function of the device at the bedside. Rates of skin pressure injuries related to CPAP use is an important balancing measure to consider when optimizing CPAP use as pressure injuries are a known complication of CPAP use.[45]

Optimal Use and Duration of Invasive Mechanical Ventilation

Despite increasing the use of NIV[46] and a growing number of QI reports focused on avoiding MV,[47,48] many infants will receive conventional MV or high-frequency ventilation (HFV) during their NICU hospitalization. In 2018, approximately 11% of all preterm infants (<37 weeks' GA at birth) in the United States received at least one course of MV during their birth hospitalization.[46] More than 80% of infants born less than 28 weeks' GA and nearly all infants born less than 25 weeks' GA (99%) receive MV in the NICU.[1,46] Both the use and duration of MV have been associated with adverse pulmonary outcomes.[49] Although attempting to minimize the use of MV is critical, respiratory QI programs should also focus on increasing the use of lung-protective ventilation strategies and shortening the duration of ventilation in infants who require MV.

Volume-targeted ventilation (VTV) modes have been shown to improve pulmonary (and other) outcomes compared with pressure-limited ventilation (PLV) modes.[50] In VTV modes, a target tidal volume is set by the clinician and the ventilator either increases support (peak inspiratory pressures) as respiratory mechanics worsen or reduces support as they improve. In PLV modes, a peak inspiratory pressure is set and the tidal volume varies with changes in lung mechanics or infant effort.[51] In the most recent systematic review, VTV modes were associated with lower rates of death or BPD (typical risk ratio [RR] 0.73, 95% CI 0.59–0.89), decreased rates of pneumothorax, shorter duration of MV, and fewer days of supplemental oxygen[50,52] compared with PLV. In a survey of North American neonatologists, only 42% of respondents use VTV as their primary ventilation mode compared with 47% use of PLV.[53] Given the relatively poor uptake of VTV, QI methods could be used to target the perceived barriers for VTV use.

Comparatively few respiratory QI projects have focused on improving neonatal MV.[25,54,55] In an effort to decrease BPD, Birenbaum and colleagues implemented VTV as part of a larger bundle of interventions. This group found that the use of VTV increased during the study period and the rate of BPD decreased.[55] The largest QI project solely evaluating the implementation of VTV was performed by Hatch and colleagues. This team implemented the exclusive use of VTV modes in a large referral NICU over a 3-year period (2016–2019) using common QI strategies such as implementation of standardized MV pathways, use of checklists, educational activities, and user-centered design modifications of the electronic health record and ventilator interfaces to allow easy use of VTV. The authors found that the use of VTV increased from 67% to 95% of MV hours by the end of the project. However, no significant change in the rate of BPD, duration of MV, or supplemental oxygen at discharge occurred.[25] These two projects may suggest that the impact of VTV may be greatest when paired with other interventions to decrease BPD as occurred in Birenbaum and colleagues.

Although the implementation of VTV has been shown to shorten MV duration, another commonly used strategy in QI projects to shorten MV duration has been the implementation of RT-driven ventilator weaning pathways.[37,56] The primary evidence for these interventions is robust in the adult intensive care setting,[57] though non-QI literature to support this in neonatal patients is limited.[58] Hermeto and colleagues evaluated the implementation of an RT-driven ventilator protocol in a single Canadian NICU. This ventilator protocol dictated initial and goal ventilator settings, goals for blood gas ranges, and standardized extubation criteria. After implementation of this protocol, age at first extubation attempt (from median 5 days to 1.2 days), rate of extubation failure (40% to 20%), and duration of MV (18 days to 6 days) decreased. No changes were seen in the rate of BPD.[56]

Other potential targets to optimize the use of invasive MV may include protocolized use of HFV in select populations,[59,60] extubation from HFV modes in infants receiving this therapy,[61] and the use of standard tools or screening criteria for extubation readiness. Although all of these are potential targets for MV-based QI, the primary literature supporting many of these interventions is mixed and few (if any) QI reports exist related to these interventions. Finally, unplanned extubations have been associated with increased MV duration, prolonged duration of supplemental oxygen, and higher incidence of oxygen use at 36 weeks.[62] Multiple well-designed single-center[63] and collaborative QI reports[64] exist to inform QI strategies to optimize this aspect of MV.

Optimal Use of Pharmacologic Therapies to Improve Pulmonary Outcomes

Several pharmacologic therapies have been shown to decrease BPD in preterm infants and are potential targets for respiratory QI programs. These include caffeine,[65] vitamin A,[66] and postnatal corticosteroids.[6] Although exogenous surfactant administration decreases mortality and the severity of respiratory distress syndrome, it has not been shown to decrease the incidence of survival without BPD. However, the mode[67] and timing[33] of surfactant delivery have been shown to impact BPD rates and have been a key component of QI teams working to decrease BPD.

Both caffeine and vitamin A have been shown to reduce BPD in large randomized multicenter trials.[65,66] Given the strength of these data, multiple QI reports have been published that attempted to increase the administration of these drugs.[37,68] As part of a QI collaborative supported through VON, Mola and colleagues implemented the use of vitamin A and standardized dosing of caffeine as part of a larger bundle of PBPs to decrease the incidence of BPD. This team showed that from 2002 to 2006, the median MV duration decreased from 8.5 days to 4.0 days ($P < .001$) and the rate of survival without BPD increased during the project (from 47% to 53.1%, adjusted odds ratio [aOR] 1.68 [95% CI 1.11–2.56]), though the improvement in BPD-free survival was not sustained in a follow-up period after the project completed.[37] Caffeine is widely used in ELBW infants who are most at risk for BPD. In a study from the Pediatrix database from 2010 to 2018, caffeine therapy was used in 87% of ELBW infants[69] suggesting little room for improvement by QI teams in most NICUs. One future potential area for consideration for QI teams is the timing and dosing of caffeine. In meta-analyses, early caffeine therapy (initiated before day 3 of life) and high-dose caffeine (variable definitions in each study) have pooled odds ratios that suggest beneficial effects in reducing BPD, aOR 0.69 (95% CI 0.69–0.75) and aOR 0.65 (95% CI 0.43–0.97), respectively.[70] The quality of evidence informing these meta-analyses is graded as low and QI teams should understand the data and local patterns of caffeine use before attempting to target this as a potential area for QI in their NICU. On the other hand, vitamin A use has decreased significantly over the past two decades,[69,71] in large part due to a national shortage and concerns for efficacy from some centers.[71] For NICUs with high BPD rates, QI designed to improve the administration of vitamin A may be a low-risk, evidence-based intervention to consider.

Postnatal corticosteroids (PCS) have been shown to decrease the incidence of BPD in multiple studies over the past few decades.[72] Despite this, uncertainty remains about what the optimal medication, timing of initiation, and dosing should be in order to prevent BPD without increasing adverse effects of PCS. The concern that PCS may result in worsening of neurodevelopmental outcomes in certain infants has been well-documented.[73] Potentially due to this uncertainty, few QI teams have reported projects that target PCS administration. Some projects, such as Kaempf and colleagues, have attempted to decrease the use of PCS or used PCS as an important outcome metric for other respiratory interventions.[54] Given the marked variations in PCS administration,[74] other QI work has attempted to standardize the approach to PCS. In a single-center report from 2021, Hansen and colleagues reported a QI project designed to implement guidelines for PCS use in preterm infants in a large level IV NICU. This team developed guidelines that focused on patient selection and timing of initiation using the online Neonatal Research Network BPD Calculator.[75] Once developed, they used educational interventions, just-in-time decision support emails, and guideline incorporation into existing care bundles as their implementation strategies. This team was able to improve compliance with the PCS guidelines from 71% in the baseline period to 96% after implementation. Interestingly, overall PCS use was unchanged in the two periods (33% of patient in the baseline period versus 32% in the implementation period) as was the rate of repeat PCS use. Although the incidence of BPD was not reported during the study, the rate of severe BPD (sBPD) or receipt of MV at 36 weeks' PMA remained unchanged.[76]

Finally, administration of exogenous surfactant has been a frequent target of QI teams given that both the timing and mode of administration have been associated with BPD.[33,67] Timely administration has been the focus of multiple QI reports.[37,38,77] One example of a successful QI project that was able to improve the time to surfactant administration using a novel strategy was performed by Raschetti and colleagues This team used lung ultrasound, which has growing evidence that suggests it can be used to guide some respiratory therapies,[78] to identify infants receiving NIV who may benefit from surfactant therapy before they had respiratory decompensation. This team was able to increase the number of babies who received surfactant therapy in the first 3 hours of life from 71% to 90% ($P < .001$). The overall duration of MV decreased as well after the QI interventions with no change in the BPD rate.

Mode of surfactant delivery has also been a successful target for many respiratory QI teams. Over the past decade, LISA has been reported to be associated with lower rates of BPD and less time on MV.[34,79] Conlon and colleagues successfully implemented LISA use in a level IV NICU increasing the rates from a baseline of 0% to 45% of eligible infants which aligned with a significant decrease in the use of MV among infants who received LISA.[80] Continued expansion of QI projects focused on surfactant administration, while minimizing known complications, remains an exciting area for progress in respiratory QI.

Non-respiratory Drivers of Adverse Pulmonary Outcomes

Although the primary focus of this review is to highlight potential respiratory drivers/interventions to consider when building a respiratory QI program, no QI program to improve respiratory outcomes would be complete without considering the non-respiratory drivers of optimal pulmonary outcomes. It is important to highlight that mixed or low-level evidence exists for some of these drivers. They include optimal growth and nutrition,[81] an exclusive human milk-based diet,[82] decreased sodium intake in the first postnatal week of life,[83] prevention or treatment of neonatal infection (eg, ureaplasma colonization and nosocomial infections)[84,85] and prevention or treatment of comorbidities of prematurity associated with adverse pulmonary outcomes such as patent ductus arteriosus or necrotizing enterocolitis.[86] Most of these drivers have been a target of QI teams in the NICU, though not necessarily for their association with improved pulmonary outcomes.

QUALITY IMPROVEMENT FOR INFANTS WITH ESTABLISHED SEVERE BRONCHOPULMONARY DYSPLASIA

Despite the best QI efforts, a subset of preterm infants will develop BPD and a subset of those will develop sBPD. sBPD has been defined as the requirement for ongoing needs for positive pressure ventilation at 36 weeks PMA. Infants with sBPD have lengthy NICU hospitalizations, prolonged duration of positive pressure ventilation, and may receive tracheostomy for long-term mechanical ventilatory support.[87] Given the medical complexity of this population, a critical step in management is to ensure a multidisciplinary team is formed with proper infrastructure for communication and continuity of care. Sabins and colleagues describe a QI initiative which focused on timely multidisciplinary family meetings with the goal of promoting shared decision-making.[88] Through the introduction of scheduling and documentation tools and educational initiatives, they tripled documentation of timely multidisciplinary family meetings in their NICU. For infants with established sBPD, the importance of novel QI work with the aim of improving communication, family engagement, and knowledge is of the utmost importance.

Infants with sBPD are at high risk for comorbidities including BPD-associated pulmonary hypertension and pulmonary vein stenosis (PVS).[89,90] The 2017 Pediatric Pulmonary Hypertension Network (PPHNet) developed guidelines for the diagnosis and care of infants with BPD-associated pulmonary hypertension.[91,92] The PPHNet consensus statement recommends all infants with moderate or sBPD has a comprehensive screening echocardiogram obtained at the time of BPD diagnosis (36 weeks PMA). Implementation of QI efforts, linked to the process outcome of echocardiogram within 72 hours of diagnosis could be a tangible next step to ensure these guidelines are followed in this population. PVS can become more apparent with time, as such serial echocardiograms in this population, including after discharge from the NICU, are necessary. QI methodology can be used to ensure necessary echocardiogram findings are reported in a uniform and consistent manner, including pulmonary vein gradients.

HOW TO BEGIN A QUALITY IMPROVEMENT PROGRAM TARGETING BRONCHOPULMONARY DYSPLASIA

Respiratory QI to prevent and manage BPD in the NICU is an important but difficult endeavor. For centers without a comprehensive respiratory QI program, and even for centers with a well-developed program, the most difficult challenge is often knowing how to start or reinvigorate improvement efforts. For teams that face this challenge, we offer two possible strategies. First, if the team has access to benchmarking data regarding their center's use of the PBPs listed above, a good place to start may be to identify areas in which the center's practices deviate from those of available benchmarks. For instance, if a center has a high MV rate and low rates of first-intention NIV, an early starting point in the long journey to improve respiratory outcomes may be to devote resources to increasing the use of NIV and decreasing the use of MV. Data from VON or other benchmarking collaboratives can be used to inform this approach. If benchmarking data are not readily available, a second approach is to leverage existing expertise and interest of staff who are actively involved in QI work and target drivers related to those areas of expertise. For example, if a team has a strong interest in nutrition, a good initial starting point for respiratory QI may be to target the nutritional drivers of adverse respiratory outcomes. No matter the approach, it is important for QI teams to take a systematic and patient approach to improving respiratory outcomes. In our experience, improving respiratory outcomes (particularly BPD) is one of the toughest targets for QI in the NICU given the multifactorial nature of respiratory disease and the many teams that must alter practice to improve outcomes. QI practitioners must add patience and persistence to their QI toolbox when attempting to improve respiratory outcomes in the NICU.

SUMMARY

In summary, improvements in respiratory care have resulted in improved survival and outcomes for infants in the NICU over the past three decades. To target the multifactorial nature of neonatal lung diseases and coordinate the care of multidisciplinary teams, each NICU should consider developing holistic respiratory QI programs. These programs should identify important measures of respiratory outcomes, develop goals for improvement, generate shared frameworks for the drivers of improved outcomes, and organize the available QI teams in each NICU to target as many drivers as are possible given the resources at hand. Although many QI teams have impacted BPD in preterm infants, the number of potential opportunities for improvement of respiratory outcomes continues to grow and represent an exciting area for QI practitioners in the NICU.

DISCLOSURE

Dr L.A. Sanlorenzo has nothing to disclose. Dr L.D. Hatch serves on the Scientific Advisory Board for Novonate, LLC and receives stock options as compensation for this position. No product or service related to this relationship will be discussed in the article. Dr L.D. Hatch also receives ongoing research funding from the Gerber Foundation, United States.

REFERENCES

1. Bell EF, Hintz SR, Hansen NI, et al. Mortality, in-hospital morbidity, care practices, and 2-year outcomes for extremely preterm infants in the US, 2013-2018. JAMA 2022;327(3):248–63.
2. Lee K, Khoshnood B, Wall SN, et al. Trend in mortality from respiratory distress syndrome in the United States, 1970-1995. J Pediatr 1999;134(4):434–40.
3. Horbar JD, Edwards EM, Greenberg LT, et al. Variation in performance of neonatal intensive care units in the United States. JAMA Pediatr 2017;171(3): e164396.
4. Spitzer AR. Has quality improvement really improved outcomes for babies in the neonatal intensive care unit? Clin Perinatol 2017;44(3):469–83.
5. Doyle LW, Carse E, Adams AM, et al. Ventilation in extremely preterm infants and respiratory function at 8 years. N Engl J Med Jul 27 2017;377(4):329–37.
6. Abiramalatha T, Ramaswamy VV, Bandyopadhyay T, et al. Interventions to prevent bronchopulmonary dysplasia in preterm neonates: an umbrella review of systematic reviews and meta-analyses. JAMA Pediatr May 1 2022;176(5): 502–16.
7. Healy H, Croonen LEE, Onland W, et al. A systematic review of reports of quality improvement for bronchopulmonary dysplasia. Semin Fetal Neonatal Med 2021; 26(1):101201.
8. Taylor N, Clay-Williams R, Hogden E, et al. High performing hospitals: a qualitative systematic review of associated factors and practical strategies for improvement. BMC Health Serv Res 2015;15:244.
9. Brandrud AS, Nyen B, Hjortdahl P, et al. Domains associated with successful quality improvement in healthcare - a nationwide case study. BMC Health Serv Res 2017;17(1):648.
10. Kaplan HC, Provost LP, Froehle CM, et al. The Model for Understanding Success in Quality (MUSIQ): building a theory of context in healthcare quality improvement. BMJ Qual Saf 2012;21(1):13–20.
11. Weiner BJ, Shortell SM, Alexander J. Promoting clinical involvement in hospital quality improvement efforts: the effects of top management, board, and physician leadership. Health Serv Res 1997;32(4):491–510.
12. Dye ME, Pugh C, Sala C, et al. Developing a unit-based quality improvement program in a large neonatal ICU. Jt Comm J Qual Patient Saf 2021;47(10):654–62.
13. Mills PD, Weeks WB. Characteristics of successful quality improvement teams: lessons from five collaborative projects in the VHA. Jt Comm J Qual Saf 2004; 30(3):152–62.
14. Beam KS, Aliaga S, Ahlfeld SK, et al. A systematic review of randomized controlled trials for the prevention of bronchopulmonary dysplasia in infants. J Perinatol 2014;34(9):705–10.
15. Lapcharoensap W, Gage SC, Kan P, et al. Hospital variation and risk factors for bronchopulmonary dysplasia in a population-based cohort. JAMA Pediatr 2015;169(2):e143676.
16. Fawke J, Lum S, Kirkby J, et al. Lung function and respiratory symptoms at 11 years in children born extremely preterm: the EPICure study. Am J Respir Crit Care Med Jul 15 2010;182(2):237–45.

17. DeMauro SB. Neurodevelopmental outcomes of infants with bronchopulmonary dysplasia. Pediatr Pulmonol 2021;56(11):3509–17.
18. Aschner JL, Bancalari EH, McEvoy CT. Can we prevent bronchopulmonary dysplasia? J Pediatr 2017;189:26–30.
19. Jensen EA, Dysart K, Gantz MG, et al. The diagnosis of bronchopulmonary dysplasia in very preterm infants. An evidence-based approach. Am J Respir Crit Care Med 2019;200(6):751–9.
20. Provost LP, Murray SK. The health care data guide: learning from data for improvement. 1st edition. San Francisco, CA: Jossey-Boss; 2011.
21. Vincent C, Burnett S, Carthey J. Safety measurement and monitoring in healthcare: a framework to guide clinical teams and healthcare organisations in maintaining safety. BMJ Qual Saf Aug 2014;23(8):670–7.
22. Jaworski M, Janvier A, Bourque CJ, et al. Parental perspective on important health outcomes of extremely preterm infants. Arch Dis Child Fetal Neonatal Ed 2022 Sep;107(5):495–500.
23. Dylag AM, Kopin HG, O'Reilly MA, et al. Early neonatal oxygen exposure predicts pulmonary morbidity and functional deficits at 1 year. J Pediatr 2020;223:20–28 e2.
24. Bapat R, Nelin L, Shepherd E, et al. A multidisciplinary quality improvement effort to reduce bronchopulmonary dysplasia incidence. J Perinatol 2020;40(4):681–7.
25. Hatch LD, Sala C, Araya W, et al. Increasing volume-targeted ventilation use in the NICU. Pediatrics 2021;147(5).
26. Hatch LD, Scott TA, Rivard M, et al. Building the driver Diagram: a mixed-methods approach to identify causes of unplanned extubations in a large neonatal ICU. Jt Comm J Qual Patient Saf 2019;45(1):40–6.
27. Watkins PL, Dagle JM, Bell EF, et al. Outcomes at 18 to 22 Months of corrected age for infants born at 22 to 25 Weeks of gestation in a center practicing active management. J Pediatr 2020;217:52–8.e1.
28. Morley CJ, Davis PG, Doyle LW, et al. Nasal CPAP or intubation at birth for very preterm infants. N Engl J Med 2008;358(7):700–8.
29. Foglia EE, Jensen EA, Kirpalani H. Delivery room interventions to prevent bronchopulmonary dysplasia in extremely preterm infants. J Perinatol 2017;37(11):1171–9.
30. Schmölzer GM, Kumar M, Pichler G, et al. Non-invasive versus invasive respiratory support in preterm infants at birth: systematic review and meta-analysis. BMJ 2013;347:f5980.
31. Perlman JM, Wyllie J, Kattwinkel J, et al. Part 7: neonatal resuscitation: 2015 international consensus on cardiopulmonary resuscitation and emergency cardiovascular care science with treatment recommendations. Circulation Oct 20 2015;132(16 Suppl 1):S204–41.
32. Oei JL, Vento M, Rabi Y, et al. Higher or lower oxygen for delivery room resuscitation of preterm infants below 28 completed weeks gestation: a meta-analysis. Arch Dis Child Fetal Neonatal Ed 2017;102(1):F24–30.
33. Bahadue FL, Soll R. Early versus delayed selective surfactant treatment for neonatal respiratory distress syndrome. Cochrane Database Syst Rev 2012;11:CD001456.
34. Isayama T, Iwami H, McDonald S, et al. Association of noninvasive ventilation strategies with mortality and bronchopulmonary dysplasia among preterm infants: a systematic review and meta-analysis. JAMA 2016;316(6):611–24.
35. Ashmeade TL, Haubner L, Collins S, et al. Outcomes of a neonatal golden hour implementation project. Am J Med Qual 2016;31(1):73–80.

36. Peleg B, Globus O, Granot M, et al. Golden Hour" quality improvement intervention and short-term outcome among preterm infants. J Perinatol 2019;39(3): 387–92.
37. Mola SJ, Annibale DJ, Wagner CL, et al. NICU bedside caregivers sustain process improvement and decrease incidence of bronchopulmonary dysplasia in infants < 30 weeks gestation. Respiratory care 2015;60(3):309–20.
38. Waskosky A, Huey TK. Quality improvement project: implementing guidelines supporting noninvasive respiratory management for premature infants. Neonatal Netw 2014;33(5):245–53.
39. Davidson LM, Berkelhamer SK. Bronchopulmonary dysplasia: chronic lung disease of infancy and long-term pulmonary outcomes. J Clin Med Jan 6 2017;6(1).
40. Dunn MS, Kaempf J, de Klerk A, et al. Randomized trial comparing 3 approaches to the initial respiratory management of preterm neonates. Pediatrics 2011; 128(5):e1069–76.
41. Finer NN, Carlo WA, Walsh MC, et al. Early CPAP versus surfactant in extremely preterm infants. N Engl J Med May 27 2010;362(21):1970–9.
42. AAP Committee on Fetus, Newborn. Respiratory support in preterm infants at birth. Pediatrics 2014;133(1):171–4.
43. Boel L, Hixson T, Brown L, et al. Non-invasive respiratory support in preterm infants. Paediatr Respir Rev 2022;43:53–9.
44. Levesque BM, Burnham L, Cardoza N, et al. Improving respiratory support practices to reduce chronic lung disease in premature infants. Pediatr Qual Saf Jul-Aug 2019;4(4):e193.
45. Bamat NA, Zhang H, McKenna KJ, et al. The clinical evaluation of severe bronchopulmonary dysplasia. Neoreviews 2020;21(7):e442–53.
46. Hatch LD, Clark RH, Carlo WA, et al. Changes in use of respiratory support for preterm infants in the US, 2008-2018. JAMA Pediatr Oct 1 2021;175(10):1017–24.
47. Kakkilaya VB, Weydig HM, Smithhart WE, et al. Decreasing continuous positive airway pressure failure in preterm infants. Pediatrics Oct 2021;148(4).
48. Kakkilaya V, Jubran I, Mashruwala V, et al. Quality improvement project to decrease delivery room intubations in preterm infants. *Pediatrics*. Feb 2019; 143(2).
49. Jensen EA, DeMauro SB, Kornhauser M, et al. Effects of multiple ventilation courses and duration of mechanical ventilation on respiratory outcomes in extremely low-birth-weight infants. JAMA Pediatr 2015;169(11):1011–7.
50. Klingenberg C, Wheeler KI, McCallion N, et al. Volume-targeted versus pressure-limited ventilation in neonates. Cochrane Database Syst Rev Oct 17 2017;10: CD003666.
51. Klingenberg C, Wheeler KI, Davis PG, et al. A practical guide to neonatal volume guarantee ventilation. J Perinatol 2011;31(9):575–85.
52. Peng W, Zhu H, Shi H, et al. Volume-targeted ventilation is more suitable than pressure-limited ventilation for preterm infants: a systematic review and meta-analysis. Arch Dis Child Fetal Neonatal Ed 2014;99(2):F158–65.
53. Gupta A, Keszler M. Survey of ventilation practices in the neonatal intensive care units of the United States and Canada: use of volume-targeted ventilation and barriers to its use. Am J Perinatol 2019;36(5):484–9.
54. Kaempf JW, Campbell B, Sklar RS, et al. Implementing potentially better practices to improve neonatal outcomes after reducing postnatal dexamethasone use in infants born between 501 and 1250 grams. Pediatrics 2003;111(4 Pt 2): e534–41.

55. Birenbaum HJ, Pfoh ER, Helou S, et al. Chronic lung disease in very low birth weight infants: persistence and improvement of a quality improvement process in a tertiary level neonatal intensive care unit. J Neonatal Perinat Med 2016; 9(2):187–94.

56. Hermeto F, Bottino MN, Vaillancourt K, et al. Implementation of a respiratory therapist-driven protocol for neonatal ventilation: impact on the premature population. Pediatrics 2009;123(5):e907–16.

57. Ely EW, Meade MO, Haponik EF, et al. Mechanical ventilator weaning protocols driven by nonphysician health-care professionals: evidence-based clinical practice guidelines. Chest 2001;120(6 Suppl):454S–63S.

58. Shalish W, Anna GM. The use of mechanical ventilation protocols in Canadian neonatal intensive care units. Paediatr Child Health 2015;20(4):e13–9.

59. Courtney SE, Durand DJ, Asselin JM, et al. High-frequency oscillatory ventilation versus conventional mechanical ventilation for very-low-birth-weight infants. N Engl J Med Aug 29 2002;347(9):643–52.

60. Cools F, Offringa M, Askie LM. Elective high frequency oscillatory ventilation versus conventional ventilation for acute pulmonary dysfunction in preterm infants. Cochrane Database Syst Rev 2015;3:CD000104.

61. Clark RH, Gerstmann DR, Null DM Jr, et al. Prospective randomized comparison of high-frequency oscillatory and conventional ventilation in respiratory distress syndrome. Pediatrics 1992;89(1):5–12.

62. Hatch LD 3rd, Scott TA, Slaughter JC, et al. Outcomes, resource use, and financial costs of unplanned extubations in preterm infants. Pediatrics 2020;145(6).

63. Merkel L, Beers K, Lewis MM, et al. Reducing unplanned extubations in the NICU. Pediatrics 2014;133(5):e1367–72.

64. Klugman D, Melton K, Maynord PO, et al. Assessment of an unplanned extubation bundle to reduce unplanned extubations in critically ill neonates, infants, and children. JAMA Pediatr 2020;174(6):e200268.

65. Schmidt B, Roberts RS, Davis P, et al. Caffeine therapy for apnea of prematurity. N Engl J Med 2006;354(20):2112–21.

66. Tyson JE, Wright LL, Oh W, et al. Vitamin A supplementation for extremely-low-birth-weight infants. National institute of child health and human development neonatal research Network. N Engl J Med 1999;340(25):1962–8.

67. Abdel-Latif ME, Davis PG, Wheeler KI, et al. Surfactant therapy via thin catheter in preterm infants with or at risk of respiratory distress syndrome. Cochrane Database Syst Rev 2021;5:CD011672.

68. Payne NR, LaCorte M, Karna P, et al. Reduction of bronchopulmonary dysplasia after participation in the breathsavers group of the Vermont Oxford Network neonatal intensive care quality improvement collaborative. Pediatrics 2006; 118(Suppl 2):S73–7.

69. Stark A, Smith PB, Hornik CP, et al. Medication use in the neonatal intensive care unit and changes from 2010 to 2018. J Pediatr. Jan 2022;240:66–71 e4.

70. Pakvasa MA, Saroha V, Patel RM. Optimizing caffeine use and risk of bronchopulmonary dysplasia in preterm infants: a systematic review, meta-analysis, and application of grading of recommendations assessment, development, and evaluation methodology. Clin Perinatol 2018;45(2):273–91.

71. Tolia VN, Murthy K, McKinley PS, et al. The effect of the national shortage of vitamin A on death or chronic lung disease in extremely low-birth-weight infants. JAMA Pediatr 2014;168(11):1039–44.

72. Ramaswamy VV, Bandyopadhyay T, Nanda D, et al. Assessment of postnatal corticosteroids for the prevention of bronchopulmonary dysplasia in preterm

neonates: a systematic review and Network meta-analysis. JAMA Pediatr 2021; 175(6):e206826.

73. Barrington KJ. The adverse neuro-developmental effects of postnatal steroids in the preterm infant: a systematic review of RCTs. BMC Pediatr 2001;1:1.

74. Puia-Dumitrescu M, Wood TR, Comstock BA, et al. Dexamethasone, prednisolone, and methylprednisolone use and 2-year neurodevelopmental outcomes in extremely preterm infants. JAMA Netw Open 2022;5(3):e221947.

75. Network NNR. Neonatal BPD outcome estimator. Available at: https://neonatal.rti. org/index.cfm. Accessed July 30, 2022.

76. Hansen TP, Oschman A, E KP, et al. Using quality improvement to implement consensus guidelines for postnatal steroid treatment of preterm infants with developing bronchopulmonary dysplasia. J Perinatol. Apr 2021;41(4):891-7.

77. Berneau P, Nguyen Phuc Thu T, Pladys P, et al. Impact of surfactant administration through a thin catheter in the delivery room: a quality control chart analysis coupled with a propensity score matched cohort study in preterm infants. PLoS One 2018;13(12):e0208252.

78. De Martino L, Yousef N, Ben-Ammar R, et al. Lung ultrasound score predicts surfactant need in extremely preterm neonates. Pediatrics 2018;142(3).

79. Lau CSM, Chamberlain RS, Sun S. Less invasive surfactant administration reduces the need for mechanical ventilation in preterm infants: a meta-analysis. Glob Pediatr Health 2017;4. 2333794X17696683.

80. Conlon SM, Osborne A, Bodie J, et al. Introducing less-invasive surfactant administration into a level IV NICU: a quality improvement initiative. Children Jul 7 2021;8(7).

81. Poindexter BB, Martin CR. Impact of nutrition on bronchopulmonary dysplasia. Clin Perinatol 2015;42(4):797-806.

82. Patel AL, Johnson TJ, Robin B, et al. Influence of own mother's milk on bronchopulmonary dysplasia and costs. Arch Dis Child Fetal Neonatal Ed 2017;102(3): F256-61.

83. Hartnoll G, Betremieux P, Modi N. Randomised controlled trial of postnatal sodium supplementation on oxygen dependency and body weight in 25-30 week gestational age infants. Arch Dis Child Fetal Neonatal Ed 2000;82(1):F19-23.

84. Lapcharoensap W, Kan P, Powers RJ, et al. The relationship of nosocomial infection reduction to changes in neonatal intensive care unit rates of bronchopulmonary dysplasia. J Pediatr 2017;180:105-109 e1.

85. Razak A, Alshehri N. Azithromycin for preventing bronchopulmonary dysplasia in preterm infants: a systematic review and meta-analysis. Pediatr Pulmonol 2021; 56(5):957-66.

86. Thebaud B, Goss KN, Laughon M, et al. Bronchopulmonary dysplasia. Nat Rev Dis Primers 2019;5(1):78.

87. Abman SH, Collaco JM, Shepherd EG, et al. Interdisciplinary care of children with severe bronchopulmonary dysplasia. J Pediatr 2017;181:12-28.e1.

88. Sabnis A, Hagen E, Tarn DM, et al. Increasing timely family meetings in neonatal intensive care: a quality improvement project. Hospital Pediatrics 2018;8(11): 679-85.

89. Malloy KW, Austin ED. Pulmonary hypertension in the child with bronchopulmonary dysplasia. Pediatr Pulmonol 2021 Nov;56(11):3546-56.

90. Swier NL, Richards B, Cua CL, et al. Pulmonary vein stenosis in neonates with severe bronchopulmonary dysplasia. Am J Perinatol 2016;33(7):671-7.

91. Krishnan U, Feinstein JA, Adatia I, et al. Evaluation and management of pulmonary hypertension in children with bronchopulmonary dysplasia. J Pediatr 2017;188:24–34.e1.
92. Abman SH, Hansmann G, Archer SL, et al. Pediatric pulmonary hypertension: guidelines from the American heart association and American thoracic society. Circulation 2015;132(21):2037–99.
93. Levesque BM, Kalish LA, LaPierre J, et al. Impact of implementing 5 potentially better respiratory practices on neonatal outcomes and costs. Pediatrics Jul 2011;128(1):e218–26.
94. Bizzarro MJ, Li FY, Katz K, et al. Temporal quantification of oxygen saturation ranges: an effort to reduce hyperoxia in the neonatal intensive care unit. J Perinatol 2014;34(1):33–8.
95. Chu SS, White HO, Rindone SL, et al. An initiative to reduce preterm infants pre-discharge growth failure through time-specific feeding volume increase. Pediatr Qual Saf 2021;6(1):e366.

Next Steps for Health Care-Associated Infections in the Neonatal Intensive Care Unit

Sandhya S. Brachio, MD[a],*, Wendi Gu, MD[a],
Lisa Saiman, MD, MPH[b,c]

KEYWORDS

- NICU • HAI • Infection prevention • Stewardship • Quality improvement

KEY POINTS

- Infection prevention and control (IP&C) strategies can reduce health care-associated infections (HAIs) in the neonatal intensive care unit caused by *Staphylococcus aureus*, multidrug-resistant gram-negative organisms, Candida, and respiratory viruses.
- IP&C strategies for HAIs include optimizing hand hygiene, active surveillance programs for selected pathogens, use of isolation precautions, and cohorting infected and colonized infants.
- Implementing evidence-based bundle strategies to prevent central-line-associated bloodstream infections and surgical site infections requires multidisciplinary quality improvement (QI) initiatives.
- Engagement with multidisciplinary teams, parents, and families; data transparency and detailed case review; accountability; and participation in collaborative efforts are effective QI strategies that can reduce HAIs.

INTRODUCTION

Infection prevention and control (IP&C) strategies in the neonatal intensive care unit (NICU) are essential to protecting neonates, who are uniquely susceptible to health care-associated infections (HAIs) due to immature host immune defenses, invasive devices that breach skin and mucosal surfaces, frequent use of antibiotics that disrupt the microbiome, and need for prolonged hospitalization which increases their risk of

[a] Division of Neonatology, Department of Pediatrics, Columbia University Vagelos College of Physicians and Surgeons, 622 West 168th Street, PH17, New York, NY 10032, USA; [b] Division of Pediatric Infectious Diseases, Department of Pediatrics, Columbia University Vagelos College of Physicians and Surgeons, 622 West 168th Street, PH1-470, New York, NY 10032, USA; [c] Department of Infection Prevention and Control, NewYork-Presbyterian Hospital, New York, NY, USA
* Corresponding author.
E-mail address: ss4016@cumc.columbia.edu
Twitter: @SBrachio (S.S.B.)

Clin Perinatol 50 (2023) 381–397
https://doi.org/10.1016/j.clp.2023.02.001
0095-5108/23/© 2023 Elsevier Inc. All rights reserved.
perinatology.theclinics.com

exposure to potential pathogens.[1,2] Neonates with HAIs have increased risk of mortality, adverse neurodevelopmental outcomes, and have associated increased health care costs.[3,4] Numerous institutions and structured collaboratives have successfully reduced HAIs using quality improvement (QI) methodologies.[5–7] QI methods to promote strategies like hand hygiene and use of aseptic techniques have been instrumental in IP&C in low-resourced units and high-resourced units.[8,9]

In this review, we provide context for QI and IP&C in the NICU as related to the burden of selected pathogens that cause late-onset sepsis (LOS), including methicillin-susceptible and methicillin-resistant *Staphylococcus aureus* (MSSA/MRSA), multi-drug resistant gram-negative bacteria (GNB), *Candida* species, and respiratory viruses. We also describe the burden of central-line-associated bloodstream infections (CLABSIs) and surgical site infections (SSIs). We highlight approaches that have been successful in mitigating LOS risk in NICUs and suggest potential next steps to improve IP&C.[10,11] Although there are interventions that can impact early-onset infection risk, those are mostly obstetric-based, and therefore, not included in this review. Finally, we conclude with general considerations for QI and IP&C, including family involvement, engagement of the multidisciplinary team, and participation in larger collaborative efforts.

SPECIFIC PATHOGENS
Methicillin-Susceptible and Methicillin-Resistant Staphylococcus aureus

Both MSSA and MRSA can colonize the anterior nares and skin of hospitalized infants, their families, and health care workers, and can contaminate surrounding surfaces and equipment in the NICU. MSSA and MRSA colonization occurs less commonly from perinatal transmission from mothers' anogenital tract.[12] The overall rate of *S aureus* infections, including MSSA and MRSA, in the NICU has ranged from 0.4% to 3.7% with an incidence ranging from 44.8 to 300 infections per 10,000 infants.[13–15] Although the rate of MSSA infections is approximately three-fold to four-fold higher than the rate of MRSA infections, the incidence of MRSA infections has increased.[16,17]

In addition to lower birthweight, prematurity, and invasive devices, colonization with *S. aureus* is an important risk factor for infection. Compared with uncolonized infants, colonized infants had 24.2 times the relative risk of developing MRSA infections.[18] As further evidence, bloodstream isolates from bacteremia were genetically identical to either the MSSA or MRSA isolates colonizing the nasal mucosa.[19]

S. aureus causes bloodstream infections (BSI), CLABSIs, skin and soft tissue infections, SSIs, and bone and joint infections. Such infections are associated with increased mortality, increased length of hospitalization, the potential need for debridement, disseminated infections, and long-term complications.[14,20,21]

Multidrug-resistant gram-negative bacteria

GNB cause life-threatening LOS in neonates.[22,23] GNB are becoming increasingly multidrug-resistant (MDR), resulting in fewer therapeutic options and higher mortality rates. In fact, lower rates of microbiological cure are reported in infants with MDR-GNB sepsis compared with infants with non-MDR-GNB sepsis.[24] In tertiary care NICUs in India, GNB accounted for 60% of LOS episodes, of which 45% were resistant to carbapenems.[25]

Although antimicrobial susceptibility profiles of GNB may vary regionally and nationally, there is much concern about the increasing burden of MDR-GNB infections in NICUs worldwide, particularly in lower- and middle-income countries. Thus, there is a focus on decreasing risk by avoiding prolonged use of empiric, broad-spectrum antibiotics as such treatment alters the microbiome and increases selective pressure on endogenous flora, creating antimicrobial resistance and increasing the risk of necrotizing enterocolitis.[26–28]

Candida species
The highest incidence of invasive candidiasis occurs in extremely preterm infants <1000 g in birthweight or <27 weeks gestation. Disseminated candidiasis in term infants is more common in those treated with systemic steroids or born with congenital anomalies requiring abdominal or neurosurgical surgery.[29] Prolonged hospitalization and interventions needed in intensive care are risk factors for invasive fungal infections, most commonly caused by C albicans (~75%).[30] Less common non-albicans species include C tropicalis, C parapsilosis, C glabrata, and C lusitaniae.

Candida species are normal gastrointestinal (GI) flora. Use of broad-spectrum antibiotics can result in unopposed proliferation of Candida, resulting in translocation across GI mucosa and invasive infections.[22,31] In addition, indwelling central venous catheters (CVC) provide a portal of entry for fungi which can thrive in dextrose-containing and intralipid solutions.[22,31]

Candida spp. can cause BSI, urinary tract infections, endocarditis, meningitis, and renal or skeletal abscesses. Candidal infections can also present as non-invasive, mucocutaneous infections which can recur, but typically do not result in disseminated candidiasis.

Respiratory viruses
The availability of multiplex reverse transcriptase polymerase chain reaction (PCR) assays has increased the appreciation of health care-associated respiratory viral infections (HA-RVIs). NICU outbreaks of respiratory syncytial virus (RSV), influenza, human coronaviruses, parainfluenza, adenovirus, and rhinovirus/enteroviruses have been reported.[32–36] Severe acute respiratory syndrome coronavirus 2 (SARS-CoV-2) has also been reported in NICUs, albeit at lower rates than other populations.[37] Risk factors for sporadic cases of HA-RVIs include longer length of stay and contact with ill staff or visitors.[38] The incidence of HA-RVIs is somewhat difficult to ascertain due to variability in study designs, but has ranged from 6% to 30% in symptomatic infants and from 6.6% to 8% in infants evaluated for LOS.[38,39]

Infants with HA-RVIs may present with symptoms mimicking common manifestations of prematurity. However, we and others found that some infants with HA-RVI can be, somewhat surprisingly, asymptomatic.[40] In an active surveillance study of HA-RVI, 52% (26/50) infants <33 weeks gestation tested positive for one or more HA-RVI, some of whom were sequentially positive. These infections were not clinically suspected by treating providers. We found that 17% (15/83) of infants with HA-RVIs remained asymptomatic, which included unchanged oxygen saturation during continuous bedside monitoring.[41]

Adverse outcomes of HA-RVIs may include a longer hospitalization, unnecessary antibiotics, increased nutritional and respiratory support, risk of bronchopulmonary dysplasia, and home oxygen use on discharge.[40–42] The pooled worldwide case fatality rate is estimated to be 13%.[43]

Specific Health Care-Associated Infections

Central-line associated bloodstream infections
CLABSIs are viewed as preventable HAIs that should be prioritized in NICU QI and safety protocols due to adverse neurodevelopmental and growth outcomes in early childhood, increased mortality rates, and increased health care costs.[44–46] Preterm infants are most susceptible to developing CLABSIs due to immunologic immaturity,

poor skin and mucous membrane integrity, the need for prolonged use of central lines, and prolonged hospitalizations.

The CDC's National Healthcare Safety Network (NHSN) uses standardized infection ratio (SIR) as a summary measure to track HAIs over time; a SIR less than 1.0 indicates that fewer HAIs were observed than predicted.[47] Thanks to evidence-based prevention strategies described below, the national CLABSI SIR was 0.662 (CI$_{95}$ 0.625–0.700) in pediatric hospital units, pediatric ICUs, and NICUs in 2020—the first year these data were reported for this subpopulation.[48]

Surgical site infections

The neonatal surgical population is increasing as NICU admissions increase, and as neonatal surgical care is advancing for congenital and acquired conditions. In addition to the association of SSIs with increased mortality, health care costs, and length of hospitalization, neonates with SSIs are significantly more likely to have pneumonia or sepsis, and require reintubation, re-operation, and readmission.[49]

Risk factors for SSIs in infants include modifiable and non-modifiable risk factors (**Fig. 1**). Increased SSI rates have been associated with wound class; clean, clean/contaminated, contaminated, and dirty/infected wounds had SSI rates of 1.8%, 2.7%. 3.9%, and 4.4%, respectively (P =.002). Length of surgery was also a risk factor; cases ≤1 hour had an SSI rate of 2.1% whereas those >1 hour had an SSI rate of 31% (P =.01).[49] MRSA colonization, blood loss requiring transfusion, higher postoperative glucose, lower gestational age, younger chronologic age, and prolonged hospitalization before surgery are SSI risk factors.[50–53]

Rates of SSIs are higher in neonates when compared with older children. In a single center study, SSI rates after cardiac surgery in infants <30 days was 6.8% compared with 3.4% in infants <1 year of age.[51] The American College of Surgeons National Surgical Improvement Program Pediatric (NSQIP-P) reported an SSI rate of 3% in neonatal surgical cases compared with 1.8% in all pediatric cases; higher SSI rates in neonates were most notable after general surgery and neurosurgery.[54] In the NSQIP-P database of 7,379 neonatal surgical procedures, most SSIs (70.5%) were deemed superficial whereas 8.3% were deep incisional and 18.7% were organ space infections.[49]

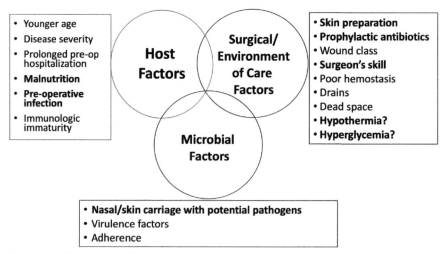

Fig. 1. Sample key driver diagram for MSSA and MRSA IP&C in the NICU.

Specific Quality Improvement Opportunities and Approaches

Hand hygiene
Hand hygiene, particularly the use of alcohol-based hand rub, is the standard of care globally and considered the most important evidence-based IP&C measure to prevent HAIs.[55,56] A volume of 2 to 3 mL of alcohol-based hand rub used for 20 to 30 seconds to cover all surfaces, between fingers and fingertips is adequate, but a larger volume may be needed for larger hands to ensure whole hand coverage.[57,58] Quality of hand hygiene can improve with return demonstrations of hand hygiene practices performed by staff and families.

Artificial nails and rings with stones can be contaminated with *S aureus*, GNB, or *Candida* species, and the presence of watches, rings, and artificial nails can impede effective hand hygiene. Long sleeves from clothes and white coats can become contaminated and lead to patient-to-patient transmission. Thus, some studies suggest that Bare Below the Elbows practices (**Box 1**) can reduce infection risk. Unlike hand hygiene, Bare Below the Elbows is not currently a universal standard practice, but may be useful in some settings.[59–65]

Box 1
Bare Below the Elbows practices for the NICU —sample policy

Rationale for Bare Below the Elbows
- Hand hygiene remains one of the most effective IP&C strategies to protect patients, families, and staff.
  - Alcohol-based hand sanitizers are highly active against gram-positive and gram-negative organisms and majority of viruses and fungi.
- Bare Below the Elbows can improve effectiveness of hand hygiene and reduce transmission of pathogens to patients.

Elements of Bare Below the Elbows
- Hand hygiene
- $< \frac{1}{4}$ inch long, clean, well-manicured nails
- No jewelry on hands or wrists except smooth ring without stones
- Sleeves above the elbows
- No white coats in the NICU

Hand hygiene effectiveness increases when:
- Skin is intact.
  - Dermatitis or cuts can harbor potential pathogens that are not effectively removed by hand hygiene.
  - Using moisturizers and protecting hands from irritation, for example, wearing gloves while using cleaning products outside of work, can maintain good skin condition.
- Artificial nails are not permitted.
  - Artificial nails can become heavily contaminated with gram-negative, gram-positive, and fungal organisms that can be transferred to patients and result in invasive infections.
- Hands and wrists are free of jewelry except for a smooth ring without stones
  - Wearing rings is associated with increased number of organisms on hands.
  - Rings can become contaminated with *S aureus*, gram-negative bacilli, and/or fungi.
  - Risk of contamination increases with more rings worn.
  - Jewelry can impede effective hand hygiene.
- Sleeves are above the elbow.
  - Long sleeves can be contaminated with pathogens.
  - Long sleeves can impede effective hand hygiene.
- White coats are removed before entering the NICU.
  - White coats can be contaminated, particularly with *S aureus*, including MRSA. Contamination of white coats can result in patient-to-patient transmission of *S aureus*.

Methicillin-susceptible and methicillin-resistant Staphylococcus aureus infection prevention and control strategies

Efforts to monitor the incidence and prevalence of MSSA and MRSA and implement strategies to reduce patient-to-patient transmission are increasingly common (**Fig. 2**). Successful strategies include geographic cohorting of infants colonized with MRSA and limiting the number of health care workers in direct contact with them.[66–68]

The CDC recommends active surveillance for *S aureus* when there is ongoing health care-associated transmission, higher rates of infections, and/or outbreaks. Guidelines also suggest surveillance at "regular intervals" based on local epidemiology and resources.[69] Many NICUs have implemented active surveillance for both MRSA and MSSA due to the higher prevalence of MSSA colonization and infections.[14,70,71] Data support targeting out-born infants for surveillance as the prevalence of colonization is as much as 29-fold higher than among inborn neonates. The proportion of out-born infants colonized with MRSA increases with older age at the time of transfer.[18]

Surveillance sites include the anterior nares, which are most likely to be colonized, and sometimes the umbilicus, perineum, and axillae.[18] Although PCR technologies have increased sensitivity compared with traditional cultures, disadvantages include lower specificity for MRSA detection and lack of isolates to undergo strain typing, which may be helpful during clusters and outbreaks.[72–74]

Some NICUs have implemented decolonization strategies for MRSA and/or MSSA routinely or in response to an outbreak to prevent infection in colonized infants and prevent transmission. The most used topical agents have been mupirocin applied to the anterior nares and chlorhexidine gluconate (CHG) baths. However, time and resources are needed to identify colonized patients and depending on the type of screening used, there may be false negative results. A NICU described their universal decolonization

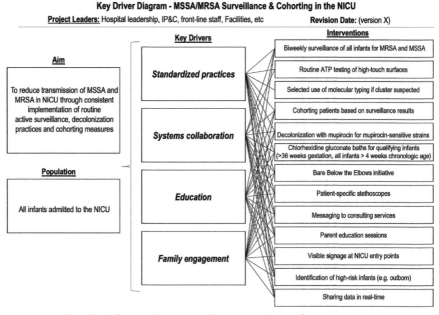

Fig. 2. *Examples of risk factors for SSIs in infants.* Host factors, factors related to the surgical environment of care, and microbial factors are associated with SSIs in infants. Risk factors that are potentially modifiable are bolded.

strategy with mupirocin which successfully decreased S aureus infection rates over 5 years, but this strategy has been studied primarily in adult ICU settings.[75,76]

Long-term efficacy and safety profiles of mupirocin and CHG remain of concern, especially in preterm neonates and young infants. There is potential for skin irritation and systemic absorption of CHG in premature infants, although infants with detectable serum levels did not exhibit harmful effects. The emergence of mupirocin resistance has been described, but not associated with adverse outcomes.[77] Rates of recolonization after decolonization measures have not been well studied in the NICU population, particularly because mupirocin is only directed to S aureus in the nares.

Strategies for multidrug-resistant gram-negative bacteria
NICUs can implement active surveillance for MDR-GNB, routinely update and disseminate their antimicrobial resistance patterns, and provide antimicrobial stewardship education for health care personnel.[78,79] Clinical pathways for antibiotic use, including shorter treatment durations when feasible, pre-approval of restricted broad-spectrum antimicrobials, and post-prescription review of these agents may slow the emergence of MDR-GNB.[80,81] Use of contact precautions for infants colonized or infected with MDR-GNB may reduce patient-to-patient transmission.[82]

Strategies for Candida
The stewardship strategies described above are also relevant for prevention of invasive candidiasis (IC). Additionally, antifungal prophylaxis with fluconazole has been studied for decades.[83] The incidence of IC varies among NICUs, and while fluconazole prophylaxis for very low birthweight infants did reduce fungal infection in NICUs with higher rates of IC, prophylaxis did not decrease mortality. Therefore, targeted use of fluconazole prophylaxis has been studied in infants deemed at high risk, such as those colonized with Candida, with a CVC, or receiving third generation cephalosporin agents or broad-spectrum antibiotics. Similarly, targeted fluconazole prophylaxis demonstrated a reduced incidence of IC, but did not impact overall mortality rates.[84–86] Further refining our understanding of high-risk populations and developing rapid, sensitive diagnostic methods for IC could improve the use of fluconazole prophylaxis.

Strategies for health care-associated respiratory viral infections
IP&C strategies for HA-RVI include optimizing hand hygiene for staff and visitors, restriction of visitors <12 year, rapid diagnosis and screening of exposed infants, use of transmission precautions, and cohorting of infected infants.[41,87,88] Other strategies include screening visitors for symptoms of viral infections and not permitting symptomatic visitors in the NICU. Policies that support staff not to work when ill, and that optimize vaccination of visitors and staff for vaccine-preventable illnesses, can prevent HA-RVIs.

IP&C related to SARS-CoV-2 exposure was a new frontier in the NICU. In addition to the aforementioned strategies, tactics for SARS-CoV-2 included admitting infected or exposed infants to single rooms on droplet and contact precautions, and airborne precautions, when available, for those requiring aerosol-generating procedures, such as intubation or open-line suctioning.[89]

Central line-associated bloodstream infections prevention strategies
The core tenets of national, regional, and local initiatives surrounding CLABSI reduction and prevention focus on standardized definitions, interdisciplinary collaboration, shared accountability, use of insertion and maintenance checklists and bundles, and routine surveillance with data transparency (**Table 1**).

Table 1 Core tenets of central line-associated bloodstream infections prevention	
Standardized Definitions	*Central line: an arterial or venous intravascular catheter that terminates at or close to the heart or one of the great vessels, and is used for infusion, withdrawal of blood, or hemodynamic monitoring* *CLABSI: laboratory-confirmed primary bloodstream infection that develops in a patient with a central line in place within the 48-h period before onset of the bloodstream infection that is not related to infection at another site* *CLABSI rate: number of bloodstream infections attributable to central line per 1000-catheter days*
Interdisciplinary and hospital-wide collaboration	Nurses, advanced practice providers, resident physicians, neonatologists, hospital epidemiologists, hospital administrators, pharmacists, parents/family members
Shared accountability	Family engagement and empowerment related to hand hygiene and line care Unit-specific and role-specific champions Data transparency Shared mental model that CLABSIs are preventable infections
Checklists & bundles	Insertion bundles • Hand hygiene • Maximal sterile barrier precautions • Skin antisepsis with povidone-iodine, CHG, or alcohol • Stop procedure immediately if sterility compromised Maintenance bundles • Daily assessment of catheter need • Assessment of dressing integrity and line site cleanliness • Sterile dressing change procedures • Closed line system for infusion, blood draws, or medication administration
Routine surveillance	Patient safety rounds Tracking local rates in real time Comparison to national benchmarks Collaborative root cause analyses

The CDC's NHSN comprehensive standard definitions are used to classify a BSI as a CLABSI.[90] These definitions must be shared with patient-facing NICU staff to accurately identify the CLABSI rates and to gain the necessary buy-in required to consistently implement successful CLABSI reduction strategies. Creating a culture of responsibility among all health care providers, accurate data reporting, transparency surrounding central-line insertions and related complications, and a shared mental model that CLABSIs are preventable infections are crucial.[91]

The Agency for Healthcare Research and Quality created a neonatal CLABSI reduction project in 2011 with 100 NICUs across nine states.[92] This collaborative and several other published QI reports have demonstrated the success of bundle strategies, which are a set of evidence-based practices implemented together that result in better outcomes than each measure alone, especially related to line insertion and line maintenance.[93,94]

Strategies for surgical site infection

SSI prevention strategies include adequate pre-operative skin disinfection, appropriate timing of perioperative antibiotics, and maintenance of perioperative euthermia. Using the Research and Development Corporation and the University of California Los Angeles appropriateness method, a multidisciplinary consensus panel evaluated 20 clinical scenarios and provided expert guidance for implementing non-pharmacologic prevention strategies.[95] Monitoring adherence to pre-operative, intra-operative, and post-operative preventive strategies can reduce SSIs (**Table 2**).[95]

Next Steps for Infection Improvement

Although CLABSI rates are declining, less is known about the preventive strategies for BSIs that are not considered CLABSIs.[79,80] As such, the CDC NHSN plans to conduct surveillance for all hospital-onset bacteremia in qualifying NICUs. Retrospective data from our NICU from 2010 to 2019 demonstrated a higher rate of non-CLABSI BSIs than BSIs, as well as higher risk of total BSIs and CLABSIs in infants <33 weeks gestation in comparison to term neonates ≥38 weeks gestation.[96] Prevention strategies for non-CLABSIs are less well defined as these are likely to have multiple etiologies.

General Considerations for Quality Improvement and Infection Prevention and Control

Quality improvement approaches

Effective QI initiatives include tangible tests of change, measurable outcomes and balancing measures, and an understanding of systems issues that could impact success. These approaches can be useful in IP&C. For example, management strategies for MSSA and MRSA could involve regular screening and tracking of colonization and decolonization through the use of standard guidelines for surveillance. This may result in potentially negative consequences, such as development of mupirocin resistance with decolonization, and they can be expensive, so it is imperative to track and share these outcomes in real time. The need for cohorting based on surveillance results involves consideration of systems issues, such as NICU census, staffing, and geography. **Table 3** highlights specific QI opportunities related to IP&C in the NICU.

Engaging the multidisciplinary team

The QI work requires a team approach with key stakeholders including NICU front-line staff, hospital epidemiology, hospital administration, and families, who share a mental model regarding desired outcomes, real-time data transparency, and iterative feedback about successes and failures. Collaboration and communication at multiple levels are key—within the NICU among multidisciplinary providers and families, within the hospital among all units, within regional centers, and within national/international organizations. Interventions must move beyond education alone, which can at most achieve 80% to 90% success; teams must analyze how change processes can be embedded into the workflow. Data sharing and non-punitive open-forum review of cases to identify learning opportunities provide accountability so teams can be consistently successful.[97]

Family involvement in infection prevention and control

Family partnerships can and should be leveraged to promote IP&C. Several frameworks exist for family engagement, ranging from ad hoc focus groups to family advisory councils to families co-leading improvement initiatives.[98] One example of family involvement in CLABSI prevention was holding "germ school" to actively engage families with their own and provider compliance with hand hygiene and line care.[94]

Table 2
Pre-operative, intra-operative, and post-operative preventive strategies for surgical site infections

Timing	Example of Prevention Strategies	Comments
Pre-operative	Screening of anterior nares for *S. aureus* and decolonization with mupirocin	Consider for infants undergoing surgical procedures high rates of *S aureus* SSIs
	Bath with non-antiseptic or antiseptic soap on the day of or the day before surgery	Limited evidence that chlorhexidine gluconate antiseptic soap reduces SSIs compared with non-antiseptic soap
Intra-operative	Clean skin around incision site with dual-agent skin preparation containing alcohol	Alcohol-containing products are active against gram-negative and gram-positive bacteria, including multidrug-resistant organisms, and yeast.
		Risk of skin irritation in preterm infants
	Use appropriate perioperative antibiotic prophylaxis based on surgery type	Parameters should include choice of agent, timing before incision, dose, intra-operative redosing, if needed, and discontinuation
		No available data on children
	Maintain normothermia	Infants at increased risk of hypothermia due to less thermoregulatory capacity, less subcutaneous fat, and increased heat loss from larger head and surface area-to-body ratio
Post-operative	Standardize wound care	Consider use for high-risk wounds with negative pressure wound therapy that removes exudate and promotes wound healing
	Standardize wound dressing	
	Perform SSI surveillance using standard case definitions	Centers for Disease Control and Prevention National Health Care Surveillance case definitions applicable to infants

Table 3
Specific quality improvement opportunities and measures

Topic	QI Initiative	Measurable Outcomes	Balancing Measure	Tests of Change	Systems Issues
Hand hygiene	Hand hygiene practices and awareness	% HCW with appropriate hand hygiene practices	HCW dermatitis	Bare Below the Elbows	Supply chain issues
MSSA/MRSA	Active surveillance for MRSA/MSSA	% infants with surveillance cultures sent % with positive cultures % successfully decolonized % reduction in invasive infections	Mupirocin resistance CHG intolerance Cost of testing	Standard guidelines and timeline for surveillance	Cohorting Decolonization practices
CLABSI prevention	Practices surrounding central line care	% CLABSI reduction % device round audits Central line days Time to full feeds	Need for immediate line reinsertion Dermatitis	Insertion and prevention bundles	Staffing Clinical acuity
SSI prevention	Practices surrounding surgical site care	% MRSA/MSSA screening % appropriate peri-operative antibiotics % euthermic intraoperatively % euglycemic postoperatively	Cost of screening Antibiotic overuse	Standardizing perioperative antibiotics Optimizing nutrition	Coordinating with surgical and anesthesia teams

Engagement in larger collaborative efforts
Collaborative efforts and data sharing networks created by the NHSN, Children's Hospital's SPS, Vermont Oxford Network, Children's Hospitals Neonatal Consortium, and various state and regional perinatal quality collaboratives demonstrate similar strategies that can be utilized by every NICU to reduce the burden of HAIs. Collaborative networks should be easily accessible to all types of NICUs so that best practices can be shared among small and larger units alike.

SUMMARY

Neonates are uniquely susceptible to HAIs due to their immunologic immaturity and need for prolonged hospitalization. Pathogens like *S aureus*, MDR-GNB, *Candida,* and respiratory viruses can cause severe illness in this vulnerable population. CLABSIs and SSIs are prevalent in the NICU due to the need for long-term CVCs and a growing number of neonatal surgical admissions. IP&C strategies include universal hand hygiene, surveillance, cohorting, and care bundles. QI methodology, with its focus on involving the multidisciplinary team, actively engaging family partners, and providing real-time data transparently, has been successful in various IP&C initiatives. Participation in larger collaboratives can provide a forum to gauge local successes with national benchmarks and for bidirectional learning to improve care.

DISCLOSURE

The authors have nothing to disclose.

REFERENCES

1. Johnson J, Akinboyo IC, Schaffzin JK. Infection prevention in the neonatal intensive care unit. Clin Perinatol 2021;48(2):413–29.
2. Fleiss N, Tarun S, Polin RA. Infection prevention for extremely low birth weight infants in the NICU. Semin Fetal Neonatal Med 2022;27(3):101345.
3. Stoll BJ, Hansen NI, Adams-Chapman I, et al. Neurodevelopmental and growth impairment among extremely-low-birth-weight infants with neonatal infection. JAMA 2004;292(19):2357–65.
4. Donovan EF, Sparling K, Lake MR, et al. The investment case for preventing NICU-associated infections. Am J Perinatol 2013;30(3):179–84.
5. Schulman J, Wirtschafter DD, Kurtin P. Neonatal intensive care unit collaboration to decrease hospital-acquired bloodstream infections: from comparative performance reports to improvement networks. Pediatr Clin North Am 2009;56(4): 865–92.
6. Schaffzin JK, Harte L, Marquette S, et al. Surgical site infection reduction by the solutions for patient safety hospital engagement network. Pediatrics 2015;136(5): e1353–60.
7. Foster CB, Ackerman K, Hupertz V, et al. Catheter-associated urinary tract infection reduction in a pediatric safety engagement network. Pediatrics 2020;146(4): e20192057.
8. Kibira J, Kihungi L, Ndinda M, et al. Improving hand hygiene practices in two regional hospitals in Kenya using a continuous quality improvement (CQI) approach. Antimicrob Resist Infect Control 2022;11(1):56.
9. Johnson J, Akinboyo IC, Curless MS, et al. Saving neonatal lives by improving infection prevention in low-resource units: tools are needed. J Glob Health 2019;9(1):010319.

10. Cortese F, Scicchitano P, Gesualdo M, et al. Early and late infections in newborns: where do we stand? A review. Pediatr Neonatol 2016;57(4):265–73.
11. Downey LC, Smith PB, Benjamin DK. Risk factors and prevention of late onset sepsis in premature infants. Early Hum Dev 2010;86(Suppl 1):7–12.
12. Jimenez-Truque N, Tedeschi S, Saye EJ, et al. Relationship between maternal and neonatal Staphylococcus aureus colonization. Pediatrics 2012;129(5): e1252–9.
13. Shane AL, Hansen NI, Stoll BJ, et al. Methicillin-resistant and susceptible Staphylococcus aureus bacteremia and meningitis in preterm infants. Pediatrics 2012; 129(4):e914–22.
14. Ericson JE, Popoola VO, Smith PB, et al. Burden of invasive Staphylococcus aureus infections in hospitalized infants. JAMA Pediatr 2015;169(12):1105–11.
15. Carey AJ, Duchon J, Della-Latta P, et al. The epidemiology of methicillin-susceptible and methicillin-resistant Staphylococcus aureus in a neonatal intensive care unit, 2000-2007. J Perinatol 2010;30(2):135–9.
16. Popoola VO, Colantuoni E, Suwantarat N, et al. Active surveillance cultures and decolonization to reduce Staphylococcus aureus infections in the neonatal intensive care unit. Infect Control Hosp Epidemiol 2016;37(4):381–7.
17. Lessa FC, Edwards JR, Fridkin SK, et al. Trends in incidence of late-onset methicillin-resistant Staphylococcus aureus infection in neonatal intensive care units: data from the National Nosocomial Infections Surveillance System, 1995-2004. Pediatr Infect Dis J 2009;28(7):577–81.
18. Zervou FN, Zacharioudakis IM, Ziakas PD, et al. MRSA colonization and risk of infection in the neonatal and pediatric ICU: a meta-analysis. Pediatrics 2014; 133(4):e1015–23.
19. von Eiff C, Becker K, Machka K, et al. Nasal carriage as a source of Staphylococcus aureus bacteremia. Study Group. N Engl J Med 2001;344(1):11–6.
20. Nelson MU, Gallagher PG. Methicillin-resistant Staphylococcus aureus in the neonatal intensive care unit. Semin Perinatol 2012;36(6):424–30.
21. Song X, Perencevich E, Campos J, et al. Clinical and economic impact of methicillin-resistant Staphylococcus aureus colonization or infection on neonates in intensive care units. Infect Control Hosp Epidemiol 2010;31(2):177–82.
22. Benjamin DK, DeLong E, Cotten CM, et al. Mortality following blood culture in premature infants: increased with Gram-negative bacteremia and candidemia, but not Gram-positive bacteremia. J Perinatol 2004;24(3):175–80.
23. Cohen-Wolkowiez M, Moran C, Benjamin DK, et al. Early and late onset sepsis in late preterm infants. Pediatr Infect Dis J 2009;28(12):1052–6.
24. Thatrimontrichai A, Premprat N, Janjindamai W, et al. Risk factors for 30-day mortality in neonatal gram-negative bacilli sepsis. Am J Perinatol 2020;37(7):689–94.
25. Johnson J, Robinson ML, Rajput UC, et al. High burden of bloodstream infections associated with antimicrobial resistance and mortality in the neonatal intensive care unit in pune, India. Clin Infect Dis 2021;73(2):271–80.
26. Alexander VN, Northrup V, Bizzarro MJ. Antibiotic exposure in the newborn intensive care unit and the risk of necrotizing enterocolitis. J Pediatr 2011;159(3): 392–7.
27. Kuppala VS, Meinzen-Derr J, Morrow AL, et al. Prolonged initial empirical antibiotic treatment is associated with adverse outcomes in premature infants. J Pediatr 2011;159(5):720–5.
28. Cotten CM, Taylor S, Stoll B, et al. Prolonged duration of initial empirical antibiotic treatment is associated with increased rates of necrotizing enterocolitis and death for extremely low birth weight infants. Pediatrics 2009;123(1):58–66.

29. Baley JE. Neonatal candidiasis: the current challenge. Clin Perinatol 1991;18(2): 263–80.

30. Lee JH, Hornik CP, Benjamin DK, et al. Risk factors for invasive candidiasis in infants >1500 g birth weight. Pediatr Infect Dis J 2013;32(3):222–6.

31. Zaoutis TE, Heydon K, Localio R, et al. Outcomes attributable to neonatal candidiasis. Clin Infect Dis 2007;44(9):1187–93.

32. Gagneur A, Sizun J, Vallet S, et al. Coronavirus-related nosocomial viral respiratory infections in a neonatal and paediatric intensive care unit: a prospective study. J Hosp Infect 2002;51(1):59–64.

33. Cunney RJ, Bialachowski A, Thornley D, et al. An outbreak of influenza A in a neonatal intensive care unit. Infect Control Hosp Epidemiol 2000;21(7):449–54.

34. Halasa NB, Williams JV, Wilson GJ, et al. Medical and economic impact of a respiratory syncytial virus outbreak in a neonatal intensive care unit. Pediatr Infect Dis J 2005;24(12):1040–4.

35. Faden H, Wynn RJ, Campagna L, et al. Outbreak of adenovirus type 30 in a neonatal intensive care unit. J Pediatr 2005;146(4):523–7.

36. Hall CB, Kopelman AE, Douglas RG, et al. Neonatal respiratory syncytial virus infection. N Engl J Med 1979;300(8):393–6.

37. Machado de Miranda Costa M, Guedes AR, Nogueira MDSP, et al. Nationwide surveillance system to evaluate hospital-acquired COVID-19 in Brazilian hospitals. J Hosp Infect 2022;123:23–6.

38. Ronchi A, Michelow IC, Chapin KC, et al. Viral respiratory tract infections in the neonatal intensive care unit: the VIRIoN-I study. J Pediatr 2014;165(4):690–6.

39. Pichler K, Assadian O, Berger A. Viral respiratory infections in the neonatal intensive care unit—a review. Front Microbiol 2018;9:2484.

40. Bennett NJ, Tabarani CM, Bartholoma NM, et al. Unrecognized viral respiratory tract infections in premature infants during their birth hospitalization: a prospective surveillance study in two neonatal intensive care units. J Pediatr 2012;161(5): 814–8.

41. Shui JE, Messina M, Hill-Ricciuti AC, et al. Impact of respiratory viruses in the neonatal intensive care unit. J Perinatol 2018;38(11):1556–65.

42. Poole CL, Camins BC, Prichard MN, et al. Hospital-acquired viral respiratory infections in neonates hospitalized since birth in a tertiary neonatal intensive care unit. J Perinatol 2019;39(5):683–9.

43. Civardi E, Tzialla C, Baldanti F, et al. Viral outbreaks in neonatal intensive care units: what we do not know. Am J Infect Control 2013;41(10):854–6.

44. Karagiannidou S, Zaoutis T, Maniadakis N, et al. Attributable length of stay and cost for pediatric and neonatal central line-associated bloodstream infections in Greece. J Infect Public Health 2019;12(3):372–9.

45. Karagiannidou S, Triantafyllou C, Zaoutis TE, et al. Length of stay, cost, and mortality of healthcare-acquired bloodstream infections in children and neonates: a systematic review and meta-analysis. Infect Control Hosp Epidemiol 2020; 41(3):342–54.

46. Stoll BJ, Hansen N, Fanaroff AA, et al. Late-onset sepsis in very low birth weight neonates: the experience of the NICHD Neonatal Research Network. Pediatrics 2002;110(2 Pt 1):285–91.

47. The NHSN standardized infection ratio (SIR): a guide to the SIR (updated april 2022). Available at: https://www.cdc.gov/nhsn/pdfs/ps-analysis-resources/nhsn-sir-guide.pdf. Accessed January 24, 2023.

48. Central line-associated bloodstream infections | A.R. & patient safety portal. Available at: https://arpsp.cdc.gov/profile/nhsn/clabsi. Accessed October 24, 2022.

49. Gilje EA, Hossain MJ, Vinocur CD, et al. Surgical site infections in neonates are independently associated with longer hospitalizations. J Perinatol 2017;37(10): 1130–4.

50. Inoue M, Uchida K, Ichikawa T, et al. Contaminated or dirty wound operations and methicillin-resistant Staphylococcus aureus (MRSA) colonization during hospitalization may be risk factors for surgical site infection in neonatal surgical patients. Pediatr Surg Int 2018;34(11):1209–14.

51. Murray MT, Krishnamurthy G, Corda R, et al. Surgical site infections and bloodstream infections in infants after cardiac surgery. J Thorac Cardiovasc Surg 2014;148(1):259–65.

52. Prasad PA, Wong-McLoughlin J, Patel S, et al. Surgical site infections in a longitudinal cohort of neonatal intensive care unit patients. J Perinatol 2016;36(4): 300–5.

53. Lejus C, Dumont R, Gall CL, et al. A preoperative stay in an intensive care unit is associated with an increased risk of surgical site infection in neonates. J Pediatr Surg 2013;48(7):1503–8.

54. Bruny JL, Hall BL, Barnhart DC, et al. American College of Surgeons national surgical quality improvement program pediatric: a beta phase report. J Pediatr Surg 2013;48(1):74–80.

55. Lotfinejad N, Peters A, Tartari E, et al. Hand hygiene in health care: 20 years of ongoing advances and perspectives. Lancet Infect Dis 2021;21(8):e209–21.

56. Lam BCC, Lee J, Lau YL. Hand hygiene practices in a neonatal intensive care unit: a multimodal intervention and impact on nosocomial infection. Pediatrics 2004;114(5):e565–71.

57. Consensus recommendations. World Health Organization. 2009. Available at: https://www.ncbi.nlm.nih.gov/books/NBK144035/. Accessed October 25, 2022.

58. Bellissimo-Rodrigues F, Soule H, Gayet-Ageron A, et al. Should alcohol-based handrub use Be customized to healthcare workers' hand size? Infect Control Hosp Epidemiol 2016;37(2):219–21.

59. Bearman G, Bryant K, Leekha S, et al. Expert guidance: healthcare personnel attire in non-operating room settings. Infect Control Hosp Epidemiol 2014;35(2): 107–21.

60. John A, Alhmidi H, Gonzalez-Orta M, et al. Bare below the elbows: a randomized trial to determine whether wearing short-sleeved coats reduces the risk for pathogen transmission. Open Forum Infect Dis 2017;4(Suppl 1):S34.

61. Yildirim I, Ceyhan M, Cengiz AB, et al. A prospective comparative study of the relationship between different types of ring and microbial hand colonization among pediatric intensive care unit nurses. Int J Nurs Stud 2008;45(11):1572–6.

62. Trick WE, Vernon MO, Hayes RA, et al. Impact of ring wearing on hand contamination and comparison of hand hygiene agents in a hospital. Clin Infect Dis 2003; 36(11):1383–90.

63. Treakle AM, Thom KA, Furuno JP, et al. Bacterial contamination of health care workers' white coats. Am J Infect Control 2009;37(2):101–5.

64. Munoz-Price LS, Arheart KL, Mills JP, et al. Associations between bacterial contamination of health care workers' hands and contamination of white coats and scrubs. Am J Infect Control 2012;40(9):e245–8.

65. Lena P, Ishak A, Karageorgos SA, et al. Presence of methicillin-resistant Staphylococcus aureus (MRSA) on healthcare workers' attire: a systematic review. Trop Med Infect Dis 2021;6(2):42.

66. Milstone AM, Budd A, Shepard JW, et al. Role of decolonization in a comprehensive strategy to reduce methicillin-resistant Staphylococcus aureus infections in the neonatal intensive care unit: an observational cohort study. Infect Control Hosp Epidemiol 2010;31(5):558–60.

67. Kaushik A, Kest H, Zauk A, et al. Impact of routine methicillin-resistant Staphylococcus aureus (MRSA) surveillance and cohorting on MRSA-related bloodstream infection in neonatal intensive care unit. Am J Perinatol 2015;32(6):531–6.

68. Geva A, Wright SB, Baldini LM, et al. Spread of methicillin-resistant Staphylococcus aureus in a large tertiary NICU: network analysis. Pediatrics 2011; 128(5):e1173–80.

69. Recommendation summary | NICU: S. aureus guidelines | infection control | CDC. 2022. Available at: https://www.cdc.gov/infectioncontrol/guidelines/nicu-saureus/recommendations.html. Accessed October 24, 2022.

70. Nurjadi D, Eichel VM, Tabatabai P, et al. Surveillance for colonization, transmission, and infection with methicillin-susceptible Staphylococcus aureus in a neonatal intensive care unit. JAMA Netw Open 2021;4(9):e2124938.

71. Wisgrill L, Zizka J, Unterasinger L, et al. Active surveillance cultures and targeted decolonization are associated with reduced methicillin-susceptible Staphylococcus aureus infections in VLBW infants. Neonatology 2017;112(3):267–73.

72. Sarda V, Molloy A, Kadkol S, et al. Active surveillance for methicillin-resistant Staphylococcus aureus in the neonatal intensive care unit. Infect Control Hosp Epidemiol 2009;30(9):854–60.

73. Francis ST, Rawal S, Roberts H, et al. Detection of meticillin-resistant staphylococcus aureus (MRSA) colonization in newborn infants using real-time polymerase chain reaction (PCR). Acta Paediatr 2010;99(11):1691–4.

74. Paule SM, Pasquariello AC, Hacek DM, et al. Direct detection of Staphylococcus aureus from adult and neonate nasal swab specimens using real-time polymerase chain reaction. J Mol Diagn JMD 2004;6(3):191–6.

75. Huang SS, Septimus E, Kleinman K, et al. Targeted versus universal decolonization to prevent ICU infection. N Engl J Med 2013;368(24):2255–65.

76. Delaney HM, Wang E, Melish M. Comprehensive strategy including prophylactic mupirocin to reduce Staphylococcus aureus colonization and infection in high-risk neonates. J Perinatol 2013;33(4):313–8.

77. Grohs E, Hill-Ricciuti A, Kelly N, et al. Spa typing of Staphylococcus aureus in a neonatal intensive care unit during routine surveillance. J Pediatr Infect Dis Soc 2021;10(7):766–73.

78. Saporito L, Graziano G, Mescolo F, et al. Efficacy of a coordinated strategy for containment of multidrug-resistant Gram-negative bacteria carriage in a Neonatal Intensive Care Unit in the context of an active surveillance program. Antimicrob Resist Infect Control 2021;10(1):30.

79. Cantey JB, Sreeramoju P, Jaleel M, et al. Prompt control of an outbreak caused by extended-spectrum β-lactamase-producing Klebsiella pneumoniae in a neonatal intensive care unit. J Pediatr 2013;163(3):672–9, e1-3.

80. de Man P, Verhoeven BA, Verbrugh HA, et al. An antibiotic policy to prevent emergence of resistant bacilli. Lancet Lond Engl 2000;355(9208):973–8.

81. Calil R, Marba ST, von Nowakonski A, et al. Reduction in colonization and nosocomial infection by multiresistant bacteria in a neonatal unit after institution of

educational measures and restriction in the use of cephalosporins. Am J Infect Control 2001;29(3):133–8.

82. Goldmann DA, Weinstein RA, Wenzel RP, et al. Strategies to prevent and control the emergence and spread of antimicrobial-resistant microorganisms in hospitals. A challenge to hospital leadership. JAMA 1996;275(3):234–40.

83. Kaufman DA. Challenging issues in neonatal candidiasis. Curr Med Res Opin 2010;26(7):1769–78.

84. Kaufman D, Boyle R, Hazen KC, et al. Fluconazole prophylaxis against fungal colonization and infection in preterm infants. N Engl J Med 2001;345(23):1660–6.

85. Kicklighter SD, Springer SC, Cox T, et al. Fluconazole for prophylaxis against candidal rectal colonization in the very low birth weight infant. Pediatrics 2001;107(2):293–8.

86. Manzoni P, Stolfi I, Pugni L, et al. A multicenter, randomized trial of prophylactic fluconazole in preterm neonates. N Engl J Med 2007;356(24):2483–95.

87. Peluso AM, Harnish BA, Miller NS, et al. Effect of young sibling visitation on respiratory syncytial virus activity in a NICU. J Perinatol 2015;35(8):627–30.

88. Groothuis J, Bauman J, Malinoski F, et al. Strategies for prevention of RSV nosocomial infection. J Perinatol 2008;28(5):319–23.

89. Saiman L, Acker KP, Dumitru D, et al. Infection prevention and control for labor and delivery, well baby nurseries, and neonatal intensive care units. Semin Perinatol 2020;44(7):151320.

90. National Healthcare Safety Network. Bloodstream Infection Event (Central Line-Associated Bloodstream Infection and Non-central Line Associated Bloodstream Infection). Available at: https://www.cdc.gov/nhsn/pdfs/pscmanual/4psc_clabs current.pdf. Accessed January 2023.

91. Mobley RE, Bizzarro MJ. Central line-associated bloodstream infections in the NICU: successes and controversies in the quest for zero. Semin Perinatol 2017;41(3):166–74.

92. Eliminating clabsi, A national patient safety imperative: neonatal clabsi prevention. Available at: https://www.ahrq.gov/hai/cusp/clabsi-neonatal/index.html. Accessed October 24, 2022.

93. Fisher D, Cochran KM, Provost LP, et al. Reducing central line-associated bloodstream infections in North Carolina NICUs. Pediatrics 2013;132(6):e1664–71.

94. Neill S, Haithcock S, Smith PB, et al. Sustained reduction in bloodstream infections in infants at a large tertiary care neonatal intensive care unit. Adv Neonatal Care 2016;16(1):52–9.

95. Meoli A, Ciavola L, Rahman S, et al. Prevention of surgical site infections in neonates and children: non-pharmacological measures of prevention. Antibiot Basel Switz 2022;11(7):863.

96. Manickam S, Paul A, Frantzis I, et al. Association of gestational age with central line and non-central line-associated bloodstream infections in the neonatal ICU. Presented at: 2022 American academy of pediatrics national conference exhibition; 2022; Anaheim, CA.

97. 08_ReliabilityWhitePaper2004revJune06.pdf. Available at: https://www.ihi.org/education/IHIOpenSchool/Courses/Documents/CourseraDocuments/08_ReliabilityWhite Paper2004revJune06.pdf. Accessed October 26, 2022.

98. Celenza JF, Zayack D, Buus-Frank ME, et al. Family involvement in quality improvement. Clin Perinatol 2017;44(3):553–66.

All Care is Brain Care

Neuro-Focused Quality Improvement in the Neonatal Intensive Care Unit

Melissa Liebowitz, MD[a], Katelin P. Kramer, MS, MD[b,c,*],
Elizabeth E. Rogers, MD[b,c]

KEYWORDS

- Quality improvement • Neonatology • Neurodevelopment • Neuroprotection
- Neonatal brain care

KEY POINTS

- Infants requiring intensive care at birth are at high risk of brain injury and long-term neuro-developmental impairment.
- There are 3 pillars of neonatal neuroprotective care: prevention of acquired injury, protection of normal maturation, and promotion of a positive environment.
- Limitations in measuring long-term neurologic outcomes have made neuro-focused quality improvement historically challenging to implement and measure.
- There are ample opportunities for improvement in consistent implementation of best and potentially better neuro-focused practices.
- Many centers have shown success with quality improvement strategies targeting brain health.

INTRODUCTION

Over the past 10 years, quality improvement (QI) initiatives in the Neonatal Intensive Care Unit (NICU), far more than novel therapies, have been responsible for the observed improvement in neonatal morbidity and mortality.[1–4] During this time, neonatal and perinatal teams have implemented initiatives to consistently deliver proven therapies, such as consistent use of antenatal steroids and magnesium sulfate, improvement in thermoregulation, infection prevention, and avoidance of hypocarbia

[a] Envision Physician Services, St. Francis Hospital, 6001 East Woodmen Road, Colorado Springs, CO 80923, USA; [b] Department of Pediatrics, University of California, 550 16th Avenue, 5th Floor, San Francisco, CA 94143, USA; [c] University of California, Benioff Children's Hospital, 550 16th Avenue, 5th Floor, San Francisco, CA 94143, USA
* Corresponding author. Department of Pediatrics, University of California, 550 16th Avenue, 5th Floor, San Francisco, CA 94143.
E-mail address: katelin.kramer@ucsf.edu
Twitter: @kpkrame (K.P.K.); @eerogersmd (E.E.R.)

Clin Perinatol 50 (2023) 399–420
https://doi.org/10.1016/j.clp.2023.01.004   perinatology.theclinics.com

and hyperoxia. These interventions have had both direct and indirect effects on brain injury prevention in neonates.[5–8] Unfortunately, these efforts have not resulted in significant improvements in survival without neurodevelopmental impairment (NDI) for preterm infants.[9,10] Decreased mortality without reported improvements in survival without NDI has also been observed in other populations of critically ill newborns, such as those with congenital heart disease and congenital diaphragmatic hernia.[11,12]

The gap between decreased mortality and stagnant rates of NDI across the spectrum of neonates requiring intensive care may be explained by the critical period of brain development that coincides with NICU hospitalization. From 20 weeks gestation into early postnatal life, a complex milieu of cellular events establishes the anatomic organization of the human brain and lays the foundation for future cognitive, motor, and sociobehavioral function. The cerebral cortex of neonates born during this critical period of brain development is particularly susceptible to injury and deviations and/or interruptions of the normal developmental program.[13,14] Furthermore, the environment in which these infants undergo this vulnerable period of brain development may also trigger further disruptions in these complex developmental processes. Many infants who require neonatal intensive care are at high risk of abnormal cognitive, sensory, and motor development, both related to and independent of acquired brain injury.[9,15–19]

Many, if not all, of the circumstances that occur in the NICU can affect brain development and therefore ND outcomes (**Fig. 1**). Multiple QI initiatives have targeted processes occurring around the time or shortly after birth with the goal of preventing acquired brain injury in neonates. Yet, preventing injury may only be a part of what is needed to achieve improvements in ND outcome. Recently, more QI work has concentrated on protecting normal maturation and promoting a positive and nurturing environment during this particularly vulnerable developmental stage. In this review, the authors highlight QI efforts focused on prevention of acquired injury, protection of normal maturation, and promotion of a positive environment.

Defining and Measuring Neurodevelopmental Impairment

Before reviewing specific QI successes and potentially better practices in this area, we must consider limitations in how brain development is currently measured in NICUs.

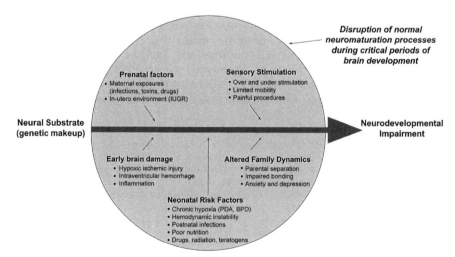

Fig. 1. Perinatal and postnatal factors that have an impact on neurodevelopmental impairment.

The gold standard is long-term neurodevelopmental and behavioral functioning, in later childhood, adolescence, or even as an adult. NDI, as frequently defined in the neonatal literature, is a composite outcome that includes cognitive, sensory, motor, and behavioral developmental components. NDI measured at 18 to 24 months is commonly used by researchers and neonatologists as the primary outcome for brain function; however, its use has many limitations. Even when patients do undergo developmental assessment between 18 and 24 months of age, it is unclear if cognitive and motor outcomes measured at this age predict school-aged, or later, performance. The authors defer a more extensive discussion of the challenges with NDI measurement to other published reviews.[19–21]

Because the long-term nature of assessing ND does not allow for the immediate feedback that is necessary to inform QI initiatives, NICU teams embarking on initiatives focused on brain care should not only consider NDI as an outcome (despite its challenges) but also be prepared to identify intermediate markers of improvements in brain-centered care. For example, many units have used early radiographic evidence of brain injury, such as the presence of intraventricular hemorrhage (IVH) or white matter injury, and intermediate neurologic outcomes. There is also evolving evidence about the predictive ability of the neurologic examination at sequential time points to predict longer-term outcome,[22] making these assessments potentially attractive measures for QI initiatives. Specifically, the General Movements Assessment (GMAs),[23–25] the Assessment of Preterm Infants' Behavior (APIB),[26,27] and others could be used as process measures that can provide earlier evidence of improvement over time. In addition, measures of parental confidence or competence at discharge have been shown to correlate with access to early developmental support services and therefore might also serve as QI targets. Finally, ND is influenced by many postnatal factors that may explain why early assessment may not be predictive of school age function. Some of the most consistently associated postnatal factors include the environment of racism and privilege, socioeconomic status, maternal education, and access to early intervention; therefore, identifying and directly addressing these social determinants of health are also key targets for improvement.[28–30] The challenging lack of real-time ND metrics and complexity of ND has slowed neurologic-focused QI efforts, but consideration of the many correlates of long-term outcome as process/outcome measures can help accelerate this critical area of focus.

PREVENTION OF ACQUIRED INJURY

Critically ill neonates are susceptible to acquired injury for a variety of reasons. The cells of the developing brain are vulnerable to hypoxic, ischemic, and inflammatory insults in the prenatal, perinatal, and postnatal periods.[13] There are a number of strategies that have been shown to prevent acquired injury of the newborn brain (**Table 1**). The authors detail the evidence and examples of QI initiatives to increase the implementation of that evidence later in this article.

Antenatal Corticosteroids

Antenatal steroids have been associated with a decrease in the incidence of severe IVH in multiple meta-analyses.[31–33] **Fig. 2** shows the slow increase in antenatal steroid administration over the past 3 decades annotated by major publications on the topic. Consensus statements from American College of Obstetrics and Gynecology (ACOG) as well as National Institute of Health (NIH) were released in 1995 in support of antenatal steroids. The process of translating this recommendation into consistent

Table 1	
Prevention of Acquired Injury	
Best Practices	**Potentially Better Practices**
Antenatal steroids for IVH prevention	IVH prevention bundle
Magnesium sulfate for neuroprotection	Golden hour bundle
Delayed cord clamping	Expedited treatment of seizures
Timely recognition of candidates for therapeutic hypothermia	
Active therapeutic hypothermia on transport	

Best practices: interventions and/or treatments supported by many well-designed randomized controlled trials. *Potentially better practices*: interventions and/or treatments rooted in physiology, common sense, and/or supported by observational studies, but lack well-designed randomized control trials as these would not be ethical or feasible.

practice took almost 5 years. Within the Neonatal Research Network, antenatal steroid administration improved dramatically from 20% to 60% from 1993 to 1996 and then plateaued at 80% in 2000, and the current reported rate is 88% (from 2013–2018).[2,10] In California, the CPQCC recognized the opportunity for improvement in the delivery of antenatal steroids and initiated a state-wide QI cycle in 1998 that included dissemination of recommended interventions using member-developed educational materials and presentations to California neonatologists. Through these efforts they were able to increase the rate of antenatal steroid use from 76% in 1998 to 86% in 2001.[34] The collaborative has observed continued improvements in antenatal steroid exposure, most recently published rates of 90% in 2016,[35] but this demonstrates how long implementation of evidence-based practice can take to achieve.

Antenatal Magnesium

Antenatal magnesium is thought to reduce cerebral palsy (CP) by decreasing apoptosis and inflammation.[36] Several randomized controlled trials (RCTs) and

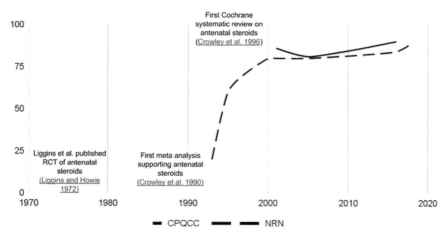

Fig. 2. Key antenatal steroid publications and rates of antenatal steroid use in large US cohorts. CPQCC, California Perinatal Quality Care Collaborative; NRN, Neonatal Research Network.

meta-analyses support the use of magnesium sulfate in mothers with threatened pre-term delivery before 32 weeks gestation, and [37–40] by 2010 to 2011 its use was widely recommended.[41,42] Despite this, uptake was quite low in the United Kingdom. In response, a regional collaborative was formed to expedite the consistent use of antenatal magnesium sulfate.[43] The PReventing Cerebral palsy in PreTerm labor (PRe-CePT) was a well-designed implementation science project that used evidence-based codesign in partnership with parents with lived experiences of preterm birth along with midwife project champions. Their codesigned materials were distributed to participant centers and meant to be adapted to local environments. They improved the use of magnesium sulfate from 12% in 2014 to 100% by 2015 and sustained this rate for 1 year. In contrast to the slow uptake of antenatal steroids, which required almost 10 years to improve rates to 90%, the PReCept group showed that a well-designed, structured implementation initiative can accelerate the translation of new evidence-based practices into clinical settings.

Delayed Cord Clamping

Postnatally, the transition to extrauterine life requires swift, complex, coordinated changes in blood flow and vascular resistance to meet metabolic demands. Delayed cord clamping (DCC), specifically until after the initiation of ventilation, as opposed to immediate cord clamping (ICC) before commencement of ventilation, is thought to improve the resilience of preterm infants to this transition by preventing dramatic changes to heart rate, blood pressures, and blood flow.[44] Systematic meta-analyses of RCTs have supported this hypothesis. Preterm infants who receive DCC are at lower risk of death and any grade IVH compared with preterm infants who receive ICC.[45] In 2012, the American College of Obstetrics and Gynecology (ACOG) released an opinion recommending DCC for premature infants that was endorsed by the American Academy of Pediatrics.[46,47] Despite this, DCC was slowly adopted into clinical practice for preterm births mainly because of concerns for delayed resuscitation.[48] Several groups have published their experience with implementation of this practice in their local settings, summarized in **Table 2**.[49–52] Some key interventions that have been successful in increasing rates of DCC include engagement of a multi-disciplinary team, dissemination of educational materials, standardization of the DCC procedure (which includes prespecified contraindications), and regular data review. Other select interventions included as part of QI initiatives to increase DCC include (1) having an experienced provider assessing infants during DCC, (2) inclusion of DCC in the operating room time out, and (3) creation of a "preterm pause" for vaginal deliveries of preterm infants where plans for DCC are discussed.[53] One area of controversy is providing DCC to infants who require resuscitation, for example, those who may have apnea or low heart rate after the initial steps of the National Resuscitation Program (NRP). Currently, the AAP does not recommend providing DCC to infants requiring resuscitation,[54] but this is an active area of research and innovation. If RCTs show that resuscitation during DCC is effective and safe, implementing this may be an opportunity for future QI initiatives.

Therapeutic Hypothermia

Therapeutic hypothermia (TH) is the gold-standard treatment of infants with presumed moderate-to-severe neonatal hypoxic ischemic encephalopathy (HIE) and is supported by multiple RCTs and meta-analyses.[55] One observational study has suggested that infants who achieve the target temperature sooner have improved outcomes.[56] Therefore, consistent and timely identification of candidates for TH as well as initiation of therapy to achieve goal temperature within 6 hours has been the

Table 2
Summary of quality improvement initiatives to improve rates of delayed cord clamping

Study Author and Publication Year	Setting	Types of Interventions	Baseline Rate	Postintervention Rate
Aziz et al,[51] 2012	Teaching Hospital	Multidisciplinary team Education efforts Clarified contraindications Staged introduction (older babies first)	50%	68%
Bolstridge et al,[49] 2016	Community	Multidisciplinary team Clarified contraindications Standardized procedure	<1%	73%
Pantoja et al,[50] 2018	Teaching Hospital	Standardized procedure Education Quality incentive Weekly & monthly data review	20%	85%
Pauley et al,[52] 2021	Teaching Hospital	Multidisciplinary team EMR changes Timers Weekly data review	12%	96%
UCSF cohort[53]	Teaching Hospital	Quality incentive Multidisciplinary team Clarified contraindications Modification to delivery workflows Experienced provider assessing baby during DCC Timers Monthly data review	56%	86%

Teaching hospital defined by having residents regularly rotate through Obstetrics or Neonatal units.
Abbreviation: EMR, electronic medical record.

focus of several QI initiatives. Select Vermont Oxford Network (VON) centers partici-pated in a QI collaborative program to increase timely identification of at-risk infants who were eligible for TH, standardize the referral and TH cooling processes, and ensure standard neurodevelopmental follow-up of infants with HIE.[57] TH during trans-port is another area for QI. Once the decision is made to provide TH, the goal is for infants to achieve the target temperature by 6 hours of life; this can be a challenge particularly for infants who require transport to a center that provides TH. In one notable QI study, a regional referral center was successful in reducing the time from birth to initiation of TH as well as the percentage of infants achieving goal temperature by 6 hours of life. Their interventions included combining device cooling during trans-port with high visibility "cheat sheets" outlining criteria for TH at birth centers, support reference guidelines for providing passive TH at the referring center while awaiting transport, and regional birth center educational events.[58]

Intraventricular Hemorrhage and Golden Hour Bundles

Bundles of care have been effective in a range of QI efforts across multiple patient populations.[59–61] Care bundles generally contain 3 to 5 evidence-based elements that are relatively independent of each other but together achieve a shared goal. "Golden Hour" and IVH prevention bundles have been developed by QI teams as part of initiatives to prevent acquired brain injury in preterm infants. The "Golden Hour" is a term that refers to the time period immediately after delivery when the NICU team is focused on stabilization of the preterm. Care practice bundles focused on optimizing care during this critical timeframe often include conducting a team pre-briefing to establish clear roles and responsibilities along with interventions targeted at maintaining normothermia, establishing effective ventilation, avoiding hypocapnia, titrating oxygen, and timely initiation of parenteral nutrition.[62,63] Several groups have shown that implementation of golden hour bundles has improved outcomes (**Table 3**). Similarly, neuroprotection bundles have also been effective in decreasing the rates of IVH (**Table 4**).[64–66] IVH bundles generally target care practices within the first 72 hours of life and specifically focus on preventing dramatic shifts in cerebral blood flow. Administration of antenatal magnesium and corticosteroids, delayed cord clamping, avoidance of hypocapnia, utilization of gentle ventilation,[67] slow blood draws and intravenous (IV) boluses,[68] mild elevation of the head of the infant's bed,[69] and midline positioning[70] are some of the care practices that are typically included in IVH bundles.

Seizure Management

Seizures have the greatest incidence of the lifespan during the neonatal period, affecting 1 to 3.5 neonates per 1000 live births.[71,72] Evidence from animal models sug-gests seizures themselves may cause further injury to the immature brain[73–75] and in humans, seizure burden has been independently associated with poor neurodevelop-mental outcomes.[76] Therefore, expedited treatment of seizures is recommended[77] but delays can be common.[78] To address delays in antiepileptic administration, one cen-ter developed a process that used in-room technology to dispatch pharmacy to the patient's bedside in order to quickly dispense antiepileptic medications.[79] Using QI methodology, Kramer and colleagues implemented this novel seizure rescue process in the NICU to decrease average time to treatment from 27 minutes to 14 minutes.[80] Timely recognition of seizures and expedited treatment has the potential to decrease risk of prolonged seizures and further brain injury, and these are important areas for neuroprotective QI efforts in the NICU.

Table 3
Summary of studies on implementation of golden hour bundles

Study Author and Publication Year	Types of Interventions	Results				
		Improved Admit Temperature	Decreased Time to IV Access/IV Nutrition	Decreased Time to Antibiotic Initiation	Decreased Time to Surfactant Delivery	Decreased IVH
Castrodale & Rhinehart,[114] 2014	Evidence-based guideline	✓	✓	NS	NS	NS
Reuter et al,[115] 2014	Evidence-based guideline	x	✓	NS	NS	✓
Lambeth et al,[116] 2016	Evidence-based guideline Golden hour checklist	x	✓	✓	x	NS
Harriman et al,[117] 2018[a]	Evidence-based guideline Roles chart NICU admit worksheet Charge nurse training	✓	✓	✓	x	NS
Peleg et al,[118] 2019	Evidence-based guideline Simulation Prebriefing checklist	✓	NS	NS	NS	x

Key: improvement (✓), no improvement (x), not studied, (NS).
[a] Note: Harriman study was a small study and improvements did not achieve statistical significance.

Table 4
Summary of studies on implementation of intraventricular hemorrhage bundles

Author	Types of Interventions	Summary of Results
De Bijl-Marcus et al,[64] 2020	Midline head positioning x 72 h Elevated head position Avoid head down position, leg elevation Avoid rapid boluses and blood draws	Decreased IVH, cystic PVL, and/or mortality (aOR 0.42, 95% CI 0.27–0.65) Decreased IVH, cystic PVL (aOR 0.54, 95% CI 0.33–0.91)
Murthy et al,[65] 2020	Minimal handling Midline head position x 72 h Delayed cord clamping Protocolization of hemodynamic and respiratory management	Decreased death or severe brain injury (aOR 0.34; 95% CI 0.2–0.59) Decreased sIVH, severe posthemorrhagic ventricular dilation, or cystic PVL (aOR 0.31; 95% CI 0.17–0.58)
Kramer et al,[66] 2022	Minimize stimuli and handling Midline head positioning x 72 h Avoid rapid boluses and blood draws Delayed cord clamping Protocolization of hemodynamic and respiratory management Positive touch (skin-to-skin within 72 h, 2 person cares) Risk based indomethacin prophylaxis Rescue betamethasone when eligible	Decreased sIVH from 14% to 1.2% (sustained x 2 y) Mortality decreased by 50%

Abbreviations: aOR, adjusted odds ratio; sIVH, severe IVH (grade 3 or 4 IVH).

PROTECTION OF NORMAL MATURATION

The NICU environment is fraught with barriers to normal maturation, including separation from the birthing parent and family; exposure to noxious stimuli such as bright lighting, loud noises, and painful procedures; and limitations to the infant's normal mobility. Developmental care in the NICU focuses on mitigating the negative or noxious environmental stimulation, supporting normal developmental processes, and fostering relationship building between an infant and her family. Many units around the country have adopted a QI approach to optimize developmental care and protect neuromaturation. Similar to the discussion of strategies to prevent acquired brain injury of the newborn brain, there are a number of interventions designed to protect normal brain maturation in the NICU (**Table 5**). Again, the authors detail the evidence and examples of QI initiatives to protect maturation later.

Minimizing Noxious Interventions

Avoidance of noxious interventions, or limiting procedures such as skin breaks, may be neuroprotective. Steven Miller and his research group have shown that infants who receive more invasive procedures demonstrate more evidence of disrupted development of regions of the thalamus that are involved in somatosensory processing, as well as reduced white matter and cortical gray matter.[81,82] The POKE Program, which stands for "Prevent pain and Organisms from sKin and catheter Entry," was created in 2008 at Dixie Medical Center in the Intermountain Health System in Utah

Table 5 Protection of Normal Maturation	
Best Practices	**Potentially Better Practices**
Skin-to-skin care	Infant-driven feeding
Decreasing opiate use	
Minimizing noxious interventions	

Best practices: interventions and/or treatments supported by many well designed randomized controlled trials. *Potentially better practices:* interventions and/or treatments rooted in physiology, common sense, and/or supported by observational studies but lack well-designed randomized control trials, as these would not be ethical or feasible.

to minimize infections and other consequences of invasive procedures in the NICU. The program reports that since its conception, the hospital has avoided 11,000 "pokes," NICU length of stay has decreased by 21%, and the cost of NICU hospitalization has decreased by 28%. They used QI methodology to implement and sustain the project, which has been replicated by Loma Linda University Health System and others.[83]

Skin-to-Skin Care

Skin-to-skin care (SSC) is an important part of optimal neurodevelopment care in the NICU. It has been shown to improve breastfeeding rates,[84,85] maternal-infant bonding,[84] infant autonomic regulation,[86] and short and long-term neurodevelopmental outcomes[87–89] in addition to decreasing sepsis, nosocomial infection, and mortality.[84] Common barriers to SSC care include nursing comfort, parent availability, personnel resources, and concerns regarding infant clinical instability (eg, low gestational age, presence of umbilical catheters, and invasive respiratory support). Despite these barriers SSC is well tolerated by preterm infants. There has been increased recognition that SSC is not just an adjunct therapy or "nice" option for neonates and parents but is an essential developmental therapy with proven benefits, even for unstable and low-birth-weight infants. Using QI approaches, many units have successfully increased their rates of SSC, even with more unstable infants (**Table 6**).

Infant-Driven Feeding

Attainment of oral feeds is a developmental milestone that is critical for successful transition to home for most infants and is the foundation for further neurodevelopment.[90,91] Infant-driven feeding (IDF) has been suggested as a way to support normal feeding maturation in preterm infants. IDF is an innovative approach originally developed by Ludwig and Waitzman to assess an infant's feeding readiness, quality of oral feeding, and techniques used for feeding.[92] Although there have been no RCTs that have compared IDF with volume-driven feeding, observational studies and QI initiatives have shown that implementation of IDF can lead to decreased length of stay (LOS) and earlier attainment of full oral feedings. In one systematic review of QI initiatives targeting IDF,[93] of the 7 included studies, 5 showed improvement in LOS (decrease by 2–5 days) and 5 showed improvement in attainment of full oral feedings. Similarly, Osman and colleagues conducted a retrospective study comparing provider-driven feeding with IDF and found that infants in the IDF group achieved full oral feedings on average, 3 days earlier than those in the provider-driven group, although this did not translate to difference in LOS.[94] Gentle and colleagues[95] implemented early assessment for oral feeding readiness (before 33 weeks postmenstrual

Table 6
Summary of quality improvement interventions to increase skin-to-skin care

Author	Patient Population	Interventions	Outcome Measure	Results
WHO Immediate KMC Study Group, 2021[119]	1–1.799 kg infants in Ghana	Randomized controlled trial of immediate Kangaroo Care compared vs conventional care in an incubator or a radiant warmer	28 d mortality	Kangaroo Care had lower 28 d mortality RR 0.75 (0.64–0.89) P-value 0.001
Levesque et al,[120] 2021	Neonatal postoperative cardiac and surgical patients	Alternative holds and alternative parent touch methods Patient transfer simulation pretransfer huddles Champion-assisted transfers	# of patients receiving 1 SSC or APT/total patient census for the day	Baseline 20%; postintervention 50%
Nation,[121] 2021	Infants <29 wk first 30 d of life	Updated SSC guideline Education Patient transfer simulation	SSC sessions/SSC eligible days per patient	Baseline 3%–17%; postintervention 30%–35%
Minot et al,[122] 2022	Infants <28 wk and/or <1000 g	SSC readiness checklist Visual aids	% of patients who received SSC within the first 72 h of life	Baseline 7%; postintervention 84%

Abbreviations: APT, alternative parent touch; SSC, skin-to-skin care.

age), cue-based feeding with readiness scores, transition to provider-driven feeding for infants who had not achieved full oral feedings by 36 weeks, and removal of NG tubes after achieving 120 mL/kg/d consistently. After implementation, they observed a reduction in LOS and time to full oral feeding by an average of 7 days.

Managing Pain While Minimizing Opioid Use

Neonatal pain management presents a clinical conundrum. Untreated pain can cause alterations to brain structural development.[81] On the contrary, treatment with opiates has also been associated with poor neurodevelopmental outcomes.[96] Given this uncertainty regarding the effects of neonatal pain and treatment with opiates, a prudent approach has been to use opiates cautiously while at the same time optimizing other nonpharmacologic and pharmacologic approaches. In a QI effort reported by Grabski and colleagues, their team implemented a number of strategies in postoperative patients to decrease opioid use including the following: (1) implementing standing IV acetaminophen as a primary postoperative pain management tool, (2) conducting educational sessions on postoperative pain management for multidisciplinary team members, and (3) standardizing postoperative pain management sign-outs that included anesthesia, surgery, and NICU providers. Using this approach they significantly decreased the use of opiates and benzodiazepines in the postoperative period, without any increases in Neonatal Pain, Agitation, and Sedation Scale (N-PASS) scores. Specifically, they observed a reduction in the number of patients placed on opiate infusions postoperatively (88% preintervention; 14% postintervention) and an increase in the percentage of patients who were managed without opiates postoperatively (10% preintervention; 35% postintervention).[97,98]

PROMOTION OF POSITIVE ENVIRONMENT

It has long been observed that the context of care, including the physical environment of the NICU, affects providers, patients, and families. Researchers are working to better understand the impact of our care context and the right timing and dosage of developmental therapies in the NICU environment.[99] Although no one approach or system of environmental manipulation or optimization has been shown through RCTs to be the one single solution rising above the rest, it is clear that being aware of and intentionally altering the environment to provide positive sensory experiences is impactful for both infants and their families. Again, there are a number of strategies that have been shown to promote positive relationships and create a supportive sensory environment (**Table 7**), which are detailed later.

Table 7 Promotion of a Positive Environment	
Best Practices	**Potentially Better Practices**
Family as partners	SENSE
Referral to early intervention	NIDCAP

Best practices: interventions and/or treatments supported by many well-designed randomized controlled trials. *Potentially better practices:* interventions and/or treatments rooted in physiology, common sense, and/or supported by observational studies but lack well-designed randomized control trials, as these would not be ethical or feasible

Abbreviations: NIDCAP, Newborn Individualized Developmental Care and Assessment Program; SENSE, Supporting and Enhancing NICU Sensory Experiences.

Newborn Individualized Developmental Care and Assessment Program

The Newborn Individualized Developmental Care and Assessment Program (NIDCAP) was designed by Dr Heidelise Als as a standardized approach to assessment of an individual infant's capacity for stimulation and need for developmental support.[26,100–103] NIDCAP is both a philosophy and a practical, ordered observational system that can be used to describe an infant's developmental strengths and also challenges to assist caregivers in designing a precision-based care plan based on both. As a potentially better practice, it has been shown in mostly single-center and observational studies to result in improved short-term neurobehavioral and neurologic outcomes and reduce parental and infant markers of stress,[101] although in RCTs, it has not been shown to result in significantly different long-term neurodevelopmental outcomes than standard care.[100] In a single-center QI initiative, early application of NIDCAP within the first week of life reduced length of stay for preterm infants.[104] The extensive training required for NIDCAP certification is often seen as a barrier for implementation.

Supporting and Enhancing Neonatal Intensive Care Unit Sensory Experiences Program

The supporting and enhancing NICU sensory experiences (SENSE) program, designed by Dr Bobbi Pineda, describes by gestational age the types and doses of positive sensory exposures and stimulation to mitigate the negative sensory experiences of the critical care environment in a way that is beneficial for brain development.[105,106] The SENSE program relies primarily on parental interaction to achieve positive sensory interventions, although medical caregivers are also provided education and play a role in providing promotive sensory experiences. Interventions are designed to address multiple domains of sensory development including auditory, tactile, vestibular, visual, kinesthetic, and olfactory/gustatory. The SENSE program has been implemented in the context of neuro-focused QI initiatives, such as in the CPQCC NEOBrain QI Collaborative focused on neuroprotective for preterm infants, and long-term outcomes continue to be assessed in ongoing clinical trials, such as the Sensory Optimization of the Hospital Environment (SOOTHE) study[107] (**Table 8**).

Families as Partners

Ensuring that families are integrated into the care of their infants as true partners, described by many as family-centered care (FCC), or more recently as family-integrated care, describes an intentional approach to acknowledging parents and families as critical team members and building structures and systems to involve them into an infant's care plan starting from birth and NICU admission.[87] See the article by Franck and colleagues (Improving NICU Quality and Safety with Family-Centered Care) in this issue for a more detailed discussion of FCC care and QI approaches for improving FCC. It is important to emphasize that even beyond FCC within the NICU, the impact of the parent and parenting environment after NICU discharge is likely more important long-term than the NICU environment, given the ongoing brain development that happens after term gestation in the first years of life.[108]

Referral to Early Intervention

It is important to recognize that brain development continues well past the neonatal period when infants have transitioned home and into their communities and that NICU providers have a responsibility not only to provide developmentally focused NICU care throughout the infant's hospitalization but also to ensure a thoughtful and comprehensive transition to home programs and services. Supportive

Table 8
Summary of quality improvement programs to promote positive environment

Author	Program	Types of Interventions	Summary of Results
Vandenburg et al,[26] 2007	NIDCAP	Standardized approach to assess development Identification of developmental needs Formation of developmental care plan	RCT: Early application reduced length of stay (median: NIDCAP: 74 d; control: 84 d; P = .003)[102] Single-center and observational studies: • Improved short-term neurobehavioral outcomes • Reduced parental and infant stress markers
Pineda et al,[105] 2019	SENSE	Recommendation of positive sensory exposures by gestational age Age-appropriate types and doses of experiences Reliance on parental interaction and education	Small RCT: higher communication scores on ages and stages questionnaire at 1 y, lost significance after controlling for medical/social risk[106] Ongoing larger clinical trial: SOOTHE study[107]

Abbreviations: NIDCAP, Newborn Individualized Developmental Care and Assessment Program; SENSE, Supporting and Enhancing NICU Sensory Experiences.

developmental therapies after discharge, such as through Early Intervention (EI) services, can assist with ongoing promotive experiences while starting to also glean any deficits that need to be addressed with focused physical, occupational, or speech/language therapies, for example,[109] EI has been shown to improve long-term outcomes for infants and children who demonstrate high social needs.[110] In general, short-term cognitive gains have been shown with EI, but longer term impact on neurodevelopmental outcome has been inconsistent. It is considered best practice to put developmental supports in place for infants upon transition to home from the NICU, but the types, frequency, and duration of these supports remain potentially better practices and must be adapted to local context and individual child needs.

Robust programs in place such as the CPQCC HIgh Risk Infant Follow Up Program (HRIF) mandate enrollment for high-risk infants and importantly backstops payment for visits. Even with these programs, there are still challenges with referrals and follow-up. For example, the CPQCC HRIF referral rate at hospital discharge was only 80%, and in both the CPQCC and New England Follow up Network (NEFN) follow-up rates were only 53% for the 18- to 24-month visit.[111–113]

SUMMARY

All care provided to critically ill newborns has both the potential to be harmful and the opportunity to be neuroprotective to the developing brain. Adopting best and potentially better practices in the 3 main areas of prevention of acquired injury, protection of normal maturation, and promotion of positive sensory experiences and relationships can mitigate the negative impact of NICU care on long-term outcomes and optimize and reinforce the resilience and strength of infants and families.

DISCLOSURE

The authors have nothing to disclose.

REFERENCES

1. Spitzer AR. Has quality improvement really improved outcomes for babies in the neonatal intensive care unit? Clin Perinatol 2017;44(3):469–83.
2. Stoll BJ, Hansen NI, Bell EF, et al. Trends in care practices, morbidity, and mortality of extremely preterm neonates, 1993-2012. JAMA 2015;314(10):1039–51.
3. Kaempf J, Morris M, Steffen E, et al. Continued improvement in morbidity reduction in extremely premature infants. Arch Dis Child Fetal Neonatal Ed 2021; 106(3):265–70.
4. Pearlman SA. Advancements in neonatology through quality improvement. J Perinatol 2022. https://doi.org/10.1038/s41372-022-01383-9. Published online April 2.
5. Abiramalatha T, Ramaswamy VV, Bandyopadhyay T, et al. Delivery room interventions for hypothermia in preterm neonates: a systematic review and network meta-analysis. JAMA Pediatr 2021;175(9):e210775.
6. Resch B, Neubauer K, Hofer N, et al. Episodes of hypocarbia and early-onset sepsis are risk factors for cystic periventricular leukomalacia in the preterm infant. Early Hum Dev 2012;88(1):27–31.
7. Sewell E, Roberts J, Mukhopadhyay S. Association of infection in neonates and long-term neurodevelopmental outcome. Clin Perinatol 2021;48(2):251–61.
8. Ortgies T, Rullmann M, Ziegelhöfer D, et al. The role of early-onset-sepsis in the neurodevelopment of very low birth weight infants. BMC Pediatr 2021;21(1):289.

9. Adams-Chapman I, Heyne RJ, DeMauro SB, et al. Neurodevelopmental impairment among extremely preterm infants in the neonatal research network. Pediatrics 2018;141(5).

10. Bell EF, Hintz SR, Hansen NI, et al. Mortality, in-hospital morbidity, care practices, and 2-year outcomes for extremely preterm infants in the US, 2013-2018. JAMA 2022;327(3):248–63.

11. Oster ME, Lee KA, Honein MA, et al. Temporal trends in survival among infants with critical congenital heart defects. Pediatrics 2013;131(5):e1502–8.

12. Politis MD, Bermejo-Sánchez E, Canfield MA, et al. Prevalence and mortality in children with congenital diaphragmatic hernia: a multicountry study. Ann Epidemiol 2021;56:61–9.e3.

13. Volpe JJ. Dysmaturation of premature brain: importance, cellular mechanisms, and potential interventions. Pediatr Neurol 2019;95:42–66.

14. Miller SP, Ferriero DM. From selective vulnerability to connectivity: insights from newborn brain imaging. Trends Neurosci 2009;32(9):496–505.

15. Montalva L, Raffler G, Riccio A, et al. Neurodevelopmental impairment in children with congenital diaphragmatic hernia: not an uncommon complication for survivors. J Pediatr Surg 2020;55(4):625–34.

16. Elgendy MM, Puthuraya S, LoPiccolo C, et al. Neonatal stroke: clinical characteristics and neurodevelopmental outcomes. Pediatr Neonatol 2022;63(1):41–7.

17. Finder M, Boylan GB, Twomey D, et al. Two-Year neurodevelopmental outcomes after mild hypoxic ischemic encephalopathy in the era of therapeutic hypothermia. JAMA Pediatr 2020;174(1):48–55.

18. Gaudet I, Paquette N, Bernard C, et al. Neurodevelopmental outcome of children with congenital heart disease: a cohort study from infancy to preschool age. J Pediatr 2021;239:126–35.e5.

19. Rogers EE, Hintz SR. Early neurodevelopmental outcomes of extremely preterm infants. Semin Perinatol 2016;40(8):497–509.

20. Marlow N. Is survival and neurodevelopmental impairment at 2 years of age the gold standard outcome for neonatal studies? Arch Dis Child Fetal Neonatal Ed 2015;100(1):F82–4.

21. Kilbride HW, Aylward GP, Carter B. What are we measuring as outcome? looking beyond neurodevelopmental impairment. Clin Perinatol 2018;45(3):467–84.

22. Huf IU, Baque E, Colditz PB, et al. Neurological examination at 32-weeks postmenstrual age predicts 12-month cognitive outcomes in very preterm-born infants. Pediatr Res 2022. https://doi.org/10.1038/s41390-022-02310-6.

23. Noble Y, Boyd R. Neonatal assessments for the preterm infant up to 4 months corrected age: a systematic review. Dev Med Child Neurol 2012;54(2):129–39.

24. Kwong AKL, Doyle LW, Olsen JE, et al. Early motor repertoire and neurodevelopment at 2 years in infants born extremely preterm or extremely-low-birth-weight. Dev Med Child Neurol 2022;64(7):855–62.

25. Salavati S, Bos AF, Doyle LW, et al. Very preterm early motor repertoire and neurodevelopmental outcomes at 8 years. Pediatrics 2021;(3):148. https://doi.org/10.1542/peds.2020-049572.

26. Vandenberg KA. Individualized developmental care for high risk newborns in the NICU: a practice guideline. Early Hum Dev 2007;83(7):433–42.

27. Als H, Duffy FH, McAnulty GB. Behavioral differences between preterm and full-term newborns as measured with the APIB system scores: I. Infant Behav Dev 1988;11(3):305–18.

28. Ment LR, Vohr B, Allan W, et al. Change in cognitive function over time in very low-birth-weight infants. JAMA 2003;289(6):705–11.

29. Breslau N, Chilcoat HD, Susser ES, et al. Stability and change in children's intelligence quotient scores: a comparison of two socioeconomically disparate communities. Am J Epidemiol 2001;154(8):711–7.
30. Manley BJ, Roberts RS, Doyle LW, et al. Social variables predict gains in cognitive scores across the preschool years in children with birth weights 500 to 1250 grams. J Pediatr 2015;166(4):870–6.e1.
31. Crowley P, Chalmers I, Keirse MJ. The effects of corticosteroid administration before preterm delivery: an overview of the evidence from controlled trials. Br J Obstet Gynaecol 1990;97(1):11–25.
32. Crowley P, Roberts D, Dalziel S, et al. Antenatal corticosteroids to accelerate fetal lung maturation for women at risk of preterm birth. In: The Cochrane Collaboration. In: Cochrane database of systematic reviews: protocols. John Wiley & Sons, Ltd; 1996. https://doi.org/10.1002/14651858.CD004454.
33. McGoldrick E, Stewart F, Parker R, et al. Antenatal corticosteroids for accelerating fetal lung maturation for women at risk of preterm birth. Cochrane Database Syst Rev 2020;12(12):CD004454.
34. Wirtschafter DD, Danielsen BH, Main EK, et al. Promoting antenatal steroid use for fetal maturation: results from the California Perinatal Quality Care Collaborative. J Pediatr 2006;148(5):606–12.
35. Gould JB, Bennett MV, Phibbs CS, et al. Population improvement bias observed in estimates of the impact of antenatal steroids to outcomes in preterm birth. J Pediatr 2021;232:17–22.e2.
36. Brookfield KF, Vinson A. Magnesium sulfate use for fetal neuroprotection. Curr Opin Obstet Gynecol 2019;31(2):110–5.
37. Rouse DJ, Hirtz DG, Thom E, et al. A randomized, controlled trial of magnesium sulfate for the prevention of cerebral palsy. N Engl J Med 2008;359(9):895–905.
38. Magnesium sulphate given before very-preterm birth to protect infant brain: the randomised controlled PREMAG trial. Obstet Anesth Digest 2007;27(4):175–6.
39. Crowther CA, Hiller JE, Doyle LW, et al. Australasian Collaborative Trial of Magnesium Sulphate (ACTOMg SO4) Collaborative Group. Effect of magnesium sulfate given for neuroprotection before preterm birth: a randomized controlled trial. JAMA 2003;290(20):2669–76.
40. Doyle LW, Crowther CA, Middleton P, et al. Magnesium sulphate for women at risk of preterm birth for neuroprotection of the fetus. Cochrane Database Syst Rev 2009;1:CD004661.
41. American College of Obstetricians and Gynecologists Committee on Obstetric Practice. Magnesium sulfate before anticipated preterm birth for neuroprotection: opinion No. 455. Obstet Gynecol 2010;115:669–71.
42. Royal College of Obstetricians and Gynaecologists. Magnesium sulphate to prevent cerebral palsy following preterm birth. Scientific impact paper 2011;29.
43. Burhouse A, Lea C, Ray S, et al. Preventing cerebral palsy in preterm labour: a multiorganisational quality improvement approach to the adoption and spread of magnesium sulphate for neuroprotection. BMJ Open Qual 2017;6(2): e000189.
44. Bhatt S, Alison BJ, Wallace EM, et al. Delaying cord clamping until ventilation onset improves cardiovascular function at birth in preterm lambs. J Physiol (Lond). 2013;591(8):2113–26.
45. Rabe H, Gyte GM, Díaz-Rossello JL, et al. Effect of timing of umbilical cord clamping and other strategies to influence placental transfusion at preterm birth on maternal and infant outcomes. Cochrane Database Syst Rev 2019;9(9): CD003248.

46. The American College of O, Committee opinion no G. 684: delayed umbilical cord clamping after birth. Obstet Gynecol 2017;129(1):1.

47. The American Academy of P. Delayed umbilical cord clamping after birth. Pediatrics 2017;139(6). https://doi.org/10.1542/peds.2017-0957.

48. Jelin AC, Kuppermann M, Erickson K, et al. Obstetricians' attitudes and beliefs regarding umbilical cord clamping. J Matern Fetal Neonatal Med 2014;27(14): 1457–61.

49. Bolstridge J, Bell T, Dean B, et al. A quality improvement initiative for delayed umbilical cord clamping in very low-birthweight infants. BMC Pediatr 2016; 16(1):155.

50. Pantoja AF, Ryan A, Feinberg M, et al. Implementing delayed cord clamping in premature infants. BMJ Open Qual 2018;7(3):e000219.

51. Aziz K, Chinnery H, Lacaze-Masmonteil T. A single-center experience of implementing delayed cord clamping in babies born at less than 33 weeks' gestational age. Adv Neonatal Care 2012;12(6):371–6.

52. Pauley AN, Roy A, Balfaqih Y, et al. A quality improvement project to delay umbilical cord clamping time. Pediatr Qual Saf 2021;6(5):e452.

53. Chan S, Duck M, Frometa K, et al. Improving the rate of delayed cord clamping in preterm infants: a quality improvement project. . Abstract presentation presented at the. Pediatric Academic Society 2021. Virtual.

54. Perlman JM, Wyllie J, Kattwinkel J, et al. Part 7: neonatal resuscitation: 2015 international consensus on cardiopulmonary resuscitation and emergency cardiovascular care science with treatment recommendations (reprint). Pediatrics 2015;136(Suppl 2):S120–66.

55. Jacobs SE, Berg M, Hunt R, et al. Cooling for newborns with hypoxic ischaemic encephalopathy. Cochrane Database Syst Rev 2013;2013(1):CD003311.

56. Thoresen M, Tooley J, Liu X, et al. Time is brain: starting therapeutic hypothermia within three hours after birth improves motor outcome in asphyxiated newborns. Neonatology 2013;104(3):228–33.

57. Olsen SL, Dejonge M, Kline A, et al. Optimizing therapeutic hypothermia for neonatal encephalopathy. Pediatrics 2013;131(2):e591–603.

58. Redpath S, Moore H, Sucha E, et al. Therapeutic hypothermia on transport: the quest for efficiency: results of a quality improvement project. Pediatr Qual Saf 2022;7(3):e556.

59. Ista E, van der Hoven B, Kornelisse RF, et al. Effectiveness of insertion and maintenance bundles to prevent central-line-associated bloodstream infections in critically ill patients of all ages: a systematic review and meta-analysis. Lancet Infect Dis 2016;16(6):724–34.

60. de Neef M, Bakker L, Dijkstra S, et al. Effectiveness of a ventilator care bundle to prevent ventilator-associated pneumonia at the PICU: a systematic review and meta-analysis. Pediatr Crit Care Med 2019;20(5):474–80.

61. Lavallée JF, Gray TA, Dumville J, et al. The effects of care bundles on patient outcomes: a systematic review and meta-analysis. Implement Sci 2017; 12(1):142.

62. Vento M, Cheung P-Y, Aguar M. The first golden minutes of the extremely-low-gestational-age neonate: a gentle approach. Neonatology 2009;95(4):286–98.

63. Wyckoff MH. Initial resuscitation and stabilization of the periviable neonate: the Golden-Hour approach. Semin Perinatol 2014;38(1):12–6.

64. de Bijl-Marcus K, Brouwer AJ, De Vries LS, et al. Neonatal care bundles are associated with a reduction in the incidence of intraventricular haemorrhage

in preterm infants: a multicentre cohort study. Arch Dis Child Fetal Neonatal Ed 2020;105(4):419–24.

65. Murthy P, Zein H, Thomas S, et al. Neuroprotection care bundle implementation to decrease acute brain injury in preterm infants. Pediatr Neurol 2020;110:42–8.

66. Kramer KP, Minot K, Butler C, et al. Reduction of severe intraventricular hemorrhage in preterm infants: a quality improvement project. Pediatrics 2022;149(3). https://doi.org/10.1542/peds.2021-050652.

67. McLendon D, Check J, Carteaux P, et al. Implementation of potentially better practices for the prevention of brain hemorrhage and ischemic brain injury in very low birth weight infants. Pediatrics 2003;111(4 Pt 2):e497–503.

68. Schulz G, Keller E, Haensse D, et al. Slow blood sampling from an umbilical artery catheter prevents a decrease in cerebral oxygenation in the preterm newborn. Pediatrics 2003;111(1):e73–6.

69. Kochan M, Leonardi B, Firestine A, et al. Elevated midline head positioning of extremely low birth weight infants: effects on cardiopulmonary function and the incidence of periventricular-intraventricular hemorrhage. J Perinatol 2019; 39(1):54–62.

70. Malusky S, Donze A. Neutral head positioning in premature infants for intraventricular hemorrhage prevention: an evidence-based review. Neonatal Netw 2011;30(6):381–96.

71. Ronen GM, Penney S, Andrews W. The epidemiology of clinical neonatal seizures in Newfoundland: a population-based study. J Pediatr 1999;134(1):71–5.

72. Glass H, Wu Y. Epidemiology of neonatal seizures. J Pediatr Neurol 2015;07(01): 013–7.

73. Jiang M, Lee CL, Smith KL, et al. Spine loss and other persistent alterations of hippocampal pyramidal cell dendrites in a model of early-onset epilepsy. J Neurosci 1998;18(20):8356–68.

74. McCabe BK, Silveira DC, Cilio MR, et al. Reduced neurogenesis after neonatal seizures. J Neurosci 2001;21(6):2094–103.

75. Ben-Ari Y, Holmes GL. Effects of seizures on developmental processes in the immature brain. Lancet Neurol 2006;5(12):1055–63.

76. McBride MC, Laroia N, Guillet R. Electrographic seizures in neonates correlate with poor neurodevelopmental outcome. Neurology 2000;55(4):506–13.

77. Glass HC, Wirrell E. Controversies in neonatal seizure management. J Child Neurol 2009;24(5):591–9.

78. Sánchez Fernández I, Abend NS, Agadi S, et al. Time from convulsive status epilepticus onset to anticonvulsant administration in children. Neurology 2015; 84(23):2304–11.

79. Pollet S, Bekmezian A, Wilson-Ganz J, et al. Innovative use of in-room technology to expedite treatment of seizures in hospitalized pediatric patients. Pediatr Qual Saf 2019;4(Supplement 2):e143.

80. Kramer K, Bekmezian A, Nash K, et al. Expediting treatment of seizures in the intensive care nursery. Pediatrics 2021;148(3). https://doi.org/10.1542/peds. 2020-013730.

81. Brummelte S, Grunau RE, Chau V, et al. Procedural pain and brain development in premature newborns. Ann Neurol 2012;71(3):385–96.

82. Duerden EG, Grunau RE, Guo T, et al. Early procedural pain is associated with regionally-specific alterations in thalamic development in preterm neonates. J Neurosci 2018;38(4):878–86.

83. McGlothlin JP, Crawford E, Wyatt J, et al. Poke-R - using analytics to reduce patient. In: Proceedings of the 10th international Joint Conference on Biomedical

Engineering systems and Technologies. SCITEPRESS - Science and Technology Publications; 2017. p. 362–9. https://doi.org/10.5220/0006174603620369.

84. Conde-Agudelo A, Díaz-Rossello JL. Kangaroo mother care to reduce morbidity and mortality in low birthweight infants. Cochrane Database Syst Rev 2014;4: CD002771.

85. Hake-Brooks SJ, Anderson GC. Kangaroo care and breastfeeding of mother-preterm infant dyads 0-18 months: a randomized, controlled trial. Neonatal Netw 2008;27(3):151–9.

86. Carbasse A, Kracher S, Hausser M, et al. Safety and effectiveness of skin-to-skin contact in the NICU to support neurodevelopment in vulnerable preterm infants. J Perinat Neonatal Nurs 2013;27(3):255–62.

87. Pineda R, Bender J, Hall B, et al. Parent participation in the neonatal intensive care unit: predictors and relationships to neurobehavior and developmental outcomes. Early Hum Dev 2018;117:32–8.

88. Marvin MM, Gardner FC, Sarsfield KM, et al. Increased frequency of skin-to-skin contact is associated with enhanced vagal tone and improved health outcomes in preterm neonates. Am J Perinatol 2019;36(5):505–10.

89. Schneider C, Charpak N, Ruiz-Peláez JG, et al. Cerebral motor function in very premature-at-birth adolescents: a brain stimulation exploration of kangaroo mother care effects. Acta Paediatr 2012;101(10):1045–53.

90. Pineda RG. Feeding: an important, complex skill that impacts nutritional, social, motor and sensory experiences. Acta Paediatr 2016;105(10):e458.

91. Grabill M, Pineda R, VanRoekel K. Early feeding behaviors in preterm infants and their relationships to neurobehavior. Am J Occup Ther 2019;73(4_Supplement_1). 7311500021p1.

92. Ludwig S.M. and Waitzman K.A., Changing Feeding Documentation to Reflect Infant-Driven Feeding Practice, Newborn Infant Nurs Rev, 7, 2007, 155–160.

93. Fry TJ, Marfurt S, Wengier S. Systematic review of quality improvement initiatives related to cue-based feeding in preterm infants. Nurs Womens Health 2018;22(5):401–10.

94. Osman A, Ibrahim M, Saunders J, et al. Effects of implementation of infant-driven oral feeding guideline on preterm infants' abilities to achieve oral feeding milestones, in a tertiary neonatal intensive care unit. Nutr Clin Pract 2021;36(6): 1262–9.

95. Gentle SJ, Meads C, Ganus S, et al. Improving time to independent oral feeding to expedite hospital discharge in preterm infants. Pediatrics 2022;149(3). https://doi.org/10.1542/peds.2021-052023.

96. de Graaf J, van Lingen RA, Simons SHP, et al. Long-term effects of routine morphine infusion in mechanically ventilated neonates on children's functioning: five-year follow-up of a randomized controlled trial. Pain 2011;152(6):1391–7.

97. Grabski DF, Vavolizza RD, Lepore S, et al. A quality improvement intervention to reduce postoperative opiate use in neonates. Pediatrics 2020;146(6). https://doi.org/10.1542/peds.2019-3861.

98. Grabski DF, Vavolizza RD, Roecker Z, et al. Reduction of post-operative opioid use in neonates following open congenital diaphragmatic hernia repairs: a quality improvement initiative. J Pediatr Surg 2022;57(1):45–51.

99. Øberg GK, Handegård BH, Campbell SK, et al. Two-year motor outcomes associated with the dose of NICU based physical therapy: the Noppi RCT. Early Hum Dev 2022;174:105680.

100. Ohlsson A, Jacobs SE. NIDCAP: a systematic review and meta-analyses of randomized controlled trials. Pediatrics 2013;131(3):e881–93.

101. Aita M, De Clifford Faugère G, Lavallée A, et al. Effectiveness of interventions on early neurodevelopment of preterm infants: a systematic review and meta-analysis. BMC Pediatr 2021;21(1):210.

102. Peters KL, Rosychuk RJ, Hendson L, et al. Improvement of short- and long-term outcomes for very low birth weight infants: edmonton NIDCAP trial. Pediatrics 2009;124(4):1009–20.

103. Wielenga JM, Smit BJ, Merkus MP, et al. Development and growth in very preterm infants in relation to NIDCAP in a Dutch NICU: two years of follow-up. Acta Paediatr 2009;98(2):291–7.

104. Moody C, Callahan TJ, Aldrich H, et al. Early initiation of newborn individualized developmental care and assessment program (NIDCAP) reduces length of stay: a quality improvement project. J Pediatr Nurs 2017;32:59–63.

105. Pineda R, Raney M, Smith J. Supporting and enhancing NICU sensory experiences (SENSE): defining developmentally-appropriate sensory exposures for high-risk infants. Early Hum Dev 2019;133:29–35.

106. Pineda R, Smith J, Roussin J, et al. Randomized clinical trial investigating the effect of consistent, developmentally-appropriate, and evidence-based multisensory exposures in the NICU. J Perinatol 2021;41(10):2449–62.

107. Pineda R. Sensory optimization of the hospital environment (SOOTHE). NCT05230199. 2022. Available at: https://clinicaltrials.gov/ct2/show/NCT05230199. Accessed November 1, 2022.

108. Bhutta ZA, Guerrant RL, Nelson CA. Neurodevelopment, nutrition, and inflammation: the evolving global child health landscape. Pediatrics 2017;139(Suppl 1):S12–22.

109. Anderson PJ, Treyvaud K, Spittle AJ. Early developmental interventions for infants born very preterm - what works? Semin Fetal Neonatal Med 2020;25(3):101119.

110. Fauth RC, Kotake C, Manning SE, et al. Timeliness of early identification and referral of infants with social and environmental risks. Prev Sci 2022. https://doi.org/10.1007/s11121-022-01453-6.

111. Hintz SR, Gould JB, Bennett MV, et al. Referral of very low birth weight infants to high-risk follow-up at neonatal intensive care unit discharge varies widely across California. J Pediatr 2015;166(2):289–95.

112. Litt JS, Edwards EM, Lainwala S, et al. Optimizing high-risk infant follow-up in nonresearch-based paradigms: the new England follow-up network. Pediatr Qual Saf 2020;5(3):e287.

113. Lakshmanan A, Rogers EE, Lu T, et al. Disparities and early engagement associated with the 18-36 month high risk infant follow up visit among very low birthweight infants in California. J Pediatr 2022. https://doi.org/10.1016/j.jpeds.2022.05.026.

114. Castrodale V, Rinehart S. The golden hour: improving the stabilization of the very low birth-weight infant. Adv Neonatal Care 2014;14(1):9–14, quiz 15.

115. Reuter S, Messier S, Steven D. The neonatal Golden Hour–intervention to improve quality of care of the extremely low birth weight infant. S D Med 2014;67(10). 397-403, 405.

116. Lambeth TM, Rojas MA, Holmes AP, et al. First golden hour of life: a quality improvement initiative. Adv Neonatal Care 2016;16(4):264–72.

117. Harriman TL, Carter B, Dail RB, et al. Golden hour protocol for preterm infants: a quality improvement project. Adv Neonatal Care 2018;18(6):462–70.

118. Peleg B, Globus O, Granot M, et al. Golden Hour" quality improvement intervention and short-term outcome among preterm infants. J Perinatol 2019;39(3): 387–92.

119. WHO Immediate KMC Study Group, Arya S, Naburi H, et al. Immediate "kangaroo mother care" and survival of infants with low birth weight. N Engl J Med 2021;384(21):2028–38.

120. Levesque V, Johnson K, McKenzie A, et al. Implementing a skin-to-skin care and parent touch initiative in a tertiary cardiac and surgical neonatal intensive care unit. Adv Neonatal Care 2021;21(2):E24–34.

121. Nation H, Sanlorenzo L, Lebar K, et al. A quality improvement project to increase frequency of skin-to-skin contact for extreme low-birth-weight infants in the neonatal intensive care unit. J Perinat Neonatal Nurs 2021;35(3):247–57.

122. Minot KL, Kramer KP, Butler C, et al. Increasing early skin-to-skin in extremely low birth weight infants. Neonatal Netw 2021;40(4):242–50.

The Evolution of Neonatal Patient Safety

Nicole K. Yamada, MD, MS*, Louis P. Halamek, MD

KEYWORDS

- Neonate • Patient safety • Human factors • Systems engineering • Simulation
- Debriefing

KEY POINTS

- Neonatal patients are particularly vulnerable to medical errors due to their unique fragility and the complexity of their care.
- The synergy between human factors science and patient safety has led to a fundamental shift in health care away from blaming individual health care professionals and instead acknowledging that adverse events occur because of system failures.
- Integrating human factors principles into simulation, debriefing, and quality improvement initiatives will strengthen the quality and resilience of the process improvements and systems changes that are developed.

INTRODUCTION

Patient safety is defined by the Agency for Healthcare Research and Quality as "freedom from accidental or preventable injuries produced by medical care."[1] The modern focus on patient safety was ignited by the 1999 publication "To Err Is Human: Building a Safer Health System" by the Institute of Medicine (IOM).[2] Since then, improving patient safety has become a major goal within all areas of health care, and the integration of patient safety as a component of improving quality in patient care was the focus of the complementary IOM book "Crossing the Quality Chasm: A New Healthy System for the 21st Century."[3] In the decades since these publications, the understanding of patient safety and mechanisms for improvement have evolved under the influence of human factors science and principles, and so these concepts are woven throughout this article. We will review the history of safety frameworks in health care, discuss how simulation and debriefing dovetail with efforts to improve care in the actual clinical environment, and describe the role of recording and analyzing safety data for better-understanding patient safety. Finally, we will look into the future of patient safety as it continues to evolve in the context of neonatal care.

Division of Neonatal and Developmental Medicine, Department of Pediatrics, Stanford University, 453 Quarry Road, MC 5660, Palo Alto, CA 94304, USA
* Corresponding author.
E-mail address: nkyamada@stanford.edu

Clin Perinatol 50 (2023) 421–434
https://doi.org/10.1016/j.clp.2023.01.005   perinatology.theclinics.com

DEFINITIONS AND CONCEPTS

To understand patient safety, we must first define the foundational terms to understand the types of problems that can be detected during clinical care: adverse events, active errors, latent errors, and near misses. *Adverse events* in health care are defined as any injury caused by medical care.[4] An adverse event does not indicate that an error or failure has occurred; it describes only that an undesirable clinical outcome has resulted from some aspect of medical diagnosis or therapy. *Active errors* are actions committed by the health care professionals who directly care for patients, occurring at the point of contact between a human and some component of the health care environment, that leads to an undesirable outcome.[5] *Latent errors* refer to failures that reside in the design of some component of an environment that set the stage for active errors to occur.[6] Latent errors may exist undetected for long periods before the right set of conditions occur that allow them to manifest and result in patient harm. Finally, *near misses* are also known as "close calls" and are defined as events or situations that did not produce patient injury due to the unintentional benefit of chance.[7]

Historically, health care has primarily focused on adverse events (ie, the situations in which patient harm occurred) and active errors, while devoting fewer resources to understanding latent errors or near misses as well.[8] This approach is known as Safety-I. Many health care professionals are familiar with a Safety-I approach through techniques such as root cause analysis or models for error such as the "Swiss Cheese Model," which explains negative outcomes as the result of a combination of active errors and latent errors.[9] In a Safety-I approach, things are presumed to go wrong because of specific and identifiable failures or malfunctions of the equipment, people, procedures, or system in which they operate.[10] In Safety-I, efforts at improving patient safety are focused on understanding why an adverse event occurred and managing those factors to keep adverse event rates as low as possible. Yet the scope of the Safety-I concept is limited, because many adverse patient safety events are relatively uncommon, constraining the overall relevance of the results of such analyses. In addition, the Safety-I tactics as employed in health care tend to focus on the actions of individual health care professionals, failing to consider the multitude of additional contextual factors present in any complex system that potentially influence the delivery of care. This emphasis on linear relationships between human error and patient harm has for the most part failed to produce significant improvements in patient care.

Patient care delivery is not linear; in fact, it is inherently variable from patient to patient and environment to environment. The Safety-I perspective misses a significant opportunity to learn from circumstances in which, despite such variability, humans and systems perform correctly. The Safety-II perspective is based on this principle and emphasizes understanding successful interventions–rather than only individual or system failures–to enable things to go right more often and under varying circumstances.[10] In other words, successful safety management is about understanding how systems effectively respond to stressors and how the system can be configured for best performance, and then actively seeking to design the system to achieve that.[11] By doing so, the Safety-II approach takes a proactive and more comprehensive approach to examining human and system performance.[12,13]

An appreciation for the complexity of health care systems has also led to the development of several models for patient safety in health care. The Systems Engineering Initiative for Patient Safety (SEIPS) model is one of the most commonly used and was developed by Carayon and colleagues[14] out of the understanding that "Most errors and inefficiencies in patient care arise not from the solitary actions of individuals but from conflicting, incomplete, or suboptimal systems of which they are a part and with which they interact." SEIPS 1.0 describes a work system where a person performs tasks using tools and technologies within an environment under certain organizational conditions. The work completed influences clinical processes, and these processes impact patient care. SEIPS 2.0 expands this initial approach by adding the concepts of configuration, engagement, and adaptation as significant influences existing beyond the original (limited) internal environment. It emphasizes outcomes affecting not just patients but also health care professionals and organizations.[15] Most recently, SEIPS 3.0 included patient experience over time as patients move through their health care journey, encountering numerous health care professionals in a multitude of clinical and non-clinical settings.[16] These types of constructs provide a framework against which to assess various aspects of patient safety in the health care ecosystem.

CURRENT STATE

Neonatal patients present unique physiology and are cared for in consistently complex systems that present constant challenges to patient safety. Safety in neonatology spans issues ranging from the identification of a fetus that is compromised in some manner, to resuscitation at birth, to ongoing care in the neonatal intensive care unit (NICU), through discharge home. Neonates have immature organ development, and most neonates in the NICU have superimposed serious illnesses. These infants are likely to be exposed to multiple medications, invasive procedures, and extended hospitalizations.[17] During a NICU hospitalization, there are several critical transitions in care, including admission, discharge, shift-to-shift handoffs between multiple levels of health care professionals, within-hospital transfers, and changes in clinical status. In an audit of 95 NICUs in the Vermont Oxford Network Critical Transitions collaborative, 43% of infants experienced ≥1 critical transition during the week before the audit.[18] The fragility of neonatal patients means they are particularly vulnerable to errors, and even minor errors can lead to devastating short-term and long-term consequences.[17]

As an illustrative example, consider for a moment only those neonates requiring resuscitation at birth. These neonates experience a compromise in their oxygen delivery during labor, may have congenital anomalies, or are born prematurely. Every year in the United States, approximately 1 in 10 of all newborns (400,000 neonates) require resuscitation, a time-pressured activity requiring teams of health care professionals to carry out invasive procedures in a specific sequence of steps in a relatively constrained volume of space (**Fig. 1**).[19] Unfortunately, error rates in excess of 50% during neonatal resuscitation have been reported.[20–23]

One can see that neonatal resuscitation does not involve merely a patient and those health care professionals providing care. Through a human factors lens, neonatal resuscitation is best described as a complex system comprised of multiple complex subsystems. The components of this complex system include but are not limited to the physical environment, medical devices, supplies, patient, family, health care professionals, and hospital culture–and within each exists multiple potential points of intervention for improving patient safety (**Fig. 2**).

As work in patient safety has evolved over the last two decades, one of the most important advancements in the field has been the application of complex system thinking to understanding and addressing patient safety threats. Simulation, debriefing, and continuous collection and review of objective performance measures are key to improving and sustaining patient safety in any field.

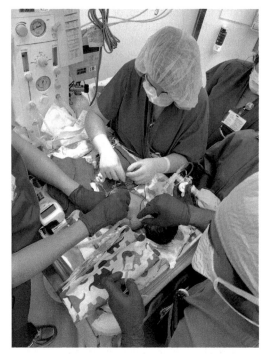

Fig. 1. Neonatal resuscitation in a constrained space.

Simulation

Simulation is an ideal methodology to support the shift from an individual to a systems approach for improving patient safety. The historical model of medical education focuses on education of the individual student or trainee to study and master a body of content knowledge and technical skills. However, individual study is not sufficient to learn or practice the behavioral skills that are necessary to work in a team (including

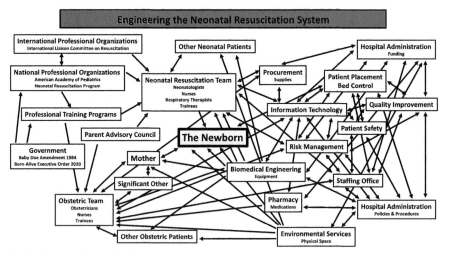

Fig. 2. Neonatal resuscitation system.

communication, task delegation, and leadership) and which are paramount to safe and effective patient care in complex work environments.[24,25]

Simulation-based training is defined as a methodology for learning in which participants are:

1. Immersed in an environment filled with realistic visual, auditory, and tactile cues
2. Required to integrate multiple skill sets while working with colleagues, equipment, and supplies just as in the real world, and
3. Provided the opportunity to reflect on their performance.

The goal of simulation-based training is to evoke the same responses during training as would be elicited in the real environment, thus allowing participants to understand their strengths and how to replicate them as well as their weaknesses and how to avoid them. Simulation-based training is the standard for skill acquisition and maintenance in multiple industries when human or system failure creates a high risk of death or severe injury.[25]

Health care professionals in neonatology are likely most familiar with the use of simulation for neonatal resuscitation training, as simulation has been formally integrated into the Neonatal Resuscitation Program curriculum since 2010.[26] In addition to resuscitation training, however, simulated clinical events conducted in the actual patient care environment (ie, in situ *simulation*) have the additional benefit of the ability to probe elements of that physical environment and the larger system in which care is delivered. The term "simulation" in this context involves more than a simple walkthrough; rather, it represents a true-to-life portrayal of patient care. In situ simulation allows direct observation of work in the real clinical environment, with all component personnel, culture, equipment, supplies, physical features, and care protocols. This type of observation is key to understanding "work as done" (the real everyday challenges and complexities of work) and how, where, and why variations occur from the idealized conception of "work as imagined" (what is expected to happen in ideal circumstances).[27] As such, in situ simulation has been used to probe new NICU environments for latent errors before opening them for the care of actual patients and is a valuable tool for optimizing patient safety.[28,29]

Debriefing

Debriefing is a key tool for analyzing complex systems and improving individual and team performance within them. Debriefing is most associated with its use following simulation for the purposes of enhancing and solidifying the learning that takes place through simulation-based training.[25] However, debriefings can be conducted after any patient care event—whether real or simulated. A debriefing is a discussion about events that have already occurred. In a debriefing, information flows

a. Between the leader(s) of the debriefing and the team being debriefed, as well as
b. Among the members of the team themselves.

The person or persons leading a debriefing may or may not have been involved in the event that is being discussed.

There are essentially two types of debriefings: *technical performance debriefings* that are used to assess human and system performance and *critical incident stress debriefings* conducted to provide emotional or psychological support to humans involved in an event.[22] Technical performance debriefings are used to evaluate human and system performance, and therefore, can provide direct connections to patient safety. The goal of technical performance debriefings is to establish a factual mental model of what occurred during the preceding event, develop a proper understanding of the situation, and determine whether responses during the event were appropriate and executed in accordance with established policies and/or guidelines.[25] The outcome analysis that occurs through technical performance debriefing is a key part of the learning that occurs after both simulated and real clinical events and can contribute to patient safety by identifying performance strengths or gaps in any element of individual, team, or system performance.

A successful debriefing need not rely on complicated and expensive technology nor take excessive time. Critical to a valuable debriefing is the use of a standardized method of addressing what occurred (or did not occur, but should have) during a particular event, with an understanding of the take-home points when considering safe and effective health care.

- Health care is delivered within the context of a complex system comprised of many interrelated subsystems.
- Investigation into patient safety requires examination of both human and system performance.
- It is critically important to understand the circumstances associated with:
  o Weaknesses/errors and develop tactics to avoid those, and
  o Strengths/exemplar performances and develop strategies to replicate those.

These take-home points underlie the debriefing method espoused at the Center for Advanced Pediatric and Perinatal Education at Stanford (**Boxes 1** and **2**).

Recording and Reporting Data

As in all quality improvement efforts, data are needed to provide an understanding of the system. These data can also be used to inform the design of simulations and enhance the context of the debriefings so that these tools can effectively inform changes that may be made to improve patient safety. Process, outcome, and balancing measures to understand how systems impact patient safety can be obtained from multiple data sources that combine both retrospective and prospective data collection including

- Incident reports
- Medical record review
- Morbidity and mortality case review
- Direct observation of clinical activities in real-time
- Analyses of audiovisual recordings of individual and team performance during real clinical events and simulated clinical events

Review of incident reports and medical records are among the most common potential sources of safety data. However, these records are rarely sufficiently comprehensive, detailed, and objective enough to ensure that all important data are present and accurate. *Case reviews* are based on both subjective and objective sources of data but they too have similar limitations. In addition, neither of these data sources allow for a complete understanding of the system dynamics.

More robust sources of data are those that allow detailed analysis of all aspects of clinical care and allow for an understanding of how components of the complex system interact. As described previously, *observation of clinical work in real-time* facilitates an understanding of the differences between "work as imagined" and "work as done." Specific tools can be used to understand sub-components of this work and provide structure and objectivity to recorded data. Examples of such tools include flow disruption analysis and teamwork scales. Flow disruptions are events where a process deviates from the optimal state as identified by a trained observer. They signify instances where the task demands are greater than the ability of the people

> **Box 1**
> **Center for Advanced Pediatric and Perinatal Education guiding principles for debriefing**
>
> Guiding Principles for Effective Human and System Performance Debriefings
> 1. Leaders should set a professional, business-like, matter-of-fact tone for the debriefing and maintain that tone whether the performance of the team members was exemplary or highly flawed.
> 2. The role of the leader in a debriefing is to facilitate, rather than dominate, discussion among team members.
> 3. Debriefings should be focused on:
>   a. The actions of individual team members
>   b. How those actions contributed to the performance of the team
>   c. How team performance influenced patient outcome
>   d. Developing strategies for
>   i. Replicating actions that facilitate successful human and system performance
>   ii. Avoiding actions that are ineffective or harmful

and the system to meet them, often necessitating deviations from planned or accepted procedures.[30] Teamwork scales such as the Oxford Non-Technical Skills (NOTECHS) scale act to assess behavioral skills.[31,32]

Analysis of audiovisual recordings of individual and team performance during actual clinical events limits the negative effects of memory, recall, and hindsight bias that are frequently seen when reviewing notes in the medical record and may negate some of the potential Hawthorne effect that may occur when conducting observations in real-time. It is challenging for health care professionals to possess sufficient situation awareness during patient care to observe all aspects of that care and accurately recall the actions taken and words spoken when they are performed and said. It is even more challenging for them to then accurately document all of their interventions, the time each intervention was initiated and completed, and the patient's response, especially when these actions are carried out during time-pressured care such as resuscitation or intensive care. Many written records of clinical events are limited by time pressure, lack of situation awareness, and/or recall bias, and therefore, cannot be construed to be fully accurate or complete.[33,34] An audiovisual record is the only way to obtain a completely accurate chronology of events.

The use of video to record clinical activities in neonatology is feasible[35–37] and useful in improving performance.[38,39] Some authors have even reviewed recordings of neonatal resuscitations with parents to help them understand what happened to their child and provide them with screenshots or videos as keepsakes, especially in the event of patient death.[40] Before initiating any recording (audio, video, or combined) of real patient care events, neonatologists must review the legal implications of doing so with their hospital risk managers so that they may proceed in a manner that both protects patient and staff confidentiality and provides a mechanism for discussing any deviations from the standard of care with parents and remediating any weaknesses in human and system performance. Similarly, any ethical concerns should be discussed and resolved with coworkers and appropriate bodies (eg, ethics committee).[41–43] Despite real and perceived challenges to recording clinical events in neonatology, we believe that an audiovisual record provides the most accurate account of human and system performance and recommend its use to improve neonatal patient safety in the delivery room and NICU.[44]

NEONATAL PATIENT SAFETY IN EVOLUTION

The future of patient safety will require a continued shift toward thorough integration of human factors science into health care. The fields of human factors and patient safety

---

Box 2
Center for Advanced Pediatric and Perinatal Education specific tactics for debriefing

Specific Tactics for Effective Human and System Performance Debriefings
  Debriefing Basics
  1. Preparing the team: Clearly communicate expectations.
  2. Initiating debriefings: "What happened in 10 words or less?"
  3. Sequencing debriefings: Chronological order is easiest to follow.
  4. Pacing debriefings: Maintain awareness of time remaining for debriefing.
  5. Terminating debriefings: "Any final questions/comments?"
  Facilitating Discussion
  6. Asking questions, avoiding statements: Target a question-to-statement ratio of 3:1.
  7. Using silence: Wait approximately 10–15 s for a response.
  Encouraging Self-Assessment
  8. De-emphasizing debriefer viewpoint: Limit the use of first-person pronouns.
  9. Avoiding qualitative statements: Draw performance assessment from team members.
  10. Minimizing personal anecdotes: Emphasize team member (not debriefer) experiences.
  11. Eschewing hindsight bias: Debrief as if experiencing the event for the first time.
  Asking Questions
  12. Formulating pertinent questions: Create lists of debriefing points from four sources
      a. Primary: expected events during the scenario or learning objectives upon which the
         scenario is based
      b. Secondary: unexpected events during the scenario
      c. Tertiary: concerns raised during the debriefing
      d. Quaternary: hypothetical situations
  13. Listening for "red flags": Recognize phrases that indicate a need to drill down.
  14. Drilling down to root causes: Use a series of four questions
      a. What happened/what did you notice (at that point in the scenario)?
      b. What circumstances led to that?
      c. What happened to the patient as a result?
      d. What can be done to:
          i. Facilitate the recurrence of that positive event?
          ii. Prevent that negative event from happening again?
  Maintaining Focus
  15. Deconstructing defensiveness: Limit use of second-person pronouns.
  16. Dealing with emotion: It is not necessary to assume all team members need to ventilate.
  17. Deciding when to intervene: Interject only when necessary
      a. Inability to recognize performance gaps
      b. Talking over one another
      c. Lack of gravitas
      d. Inappropriate laughter
      e. Harsh criticism
  Special Debriefing Circumstances
  18. Debriefing with video: Scroll to segments of interest and pause playback for discussion.
  19. Debriefing novices and experts: Employ the same strategies regardless of experience.
  20. Debriefing real clinical events: Formal process is required.

---

have both existed since the middle of the twentieth century, but the last two decades have marked the greatest growth and development of synergy between these two fields. Human factors experts know well that the cultural emphasis on the work, knowledge, and individuals that exists in health care fosters a tendency to blame individual persons for adverse events. Only in the last 20 years has health care begun to shift away from this blame-and-retrain approach and toward acknowledging that adverse events instead occur as a result of system failures.[11,45] This has allowed human error to be viewed as a symptom of system failure, and thus turned the focus to building systems and processes that support limitations in human capabilities and prevent errors or mitigate their impact.[46,47]

One example of a future development to improve neonatal patient safety is the creation of a national neonatal safety management system (SMS). Individual NICUs typically have some type of safety committee and system for reporting safety events; many NICUs are also members of a regional and/or national collaborative that shares deidentified safety data among members. A national neonatal SMS would be much more comprehensive in scope than any patient safety system that currently exists in health care. A national neonatal SMS would provide a methodical approach to achieving safety, be modeled after that in use by commercial aviation,[48] and be comprised of four major safety components:

- Policy (organizational methods, processes, and structure)
- Risk management (define and manage acceptable risks)
- Assurance (assess effectiveness of current initiatives)
- Promotion (efforts to create a culture of safety)

A national neonatal SMS would allow NICUs to centrally report safety data as well as view comprehensive reports of that data from NICUs across the country. The neonatal safety database could include frequently measured adverse events from quality improvement work such as medication errors, unplanned extubations, and hospital-acquired infections. It would support the learning around less commonly reported (but critically important) adverse events such as diagnostic errors, detailing both the events and strategies and tactics to reduce the risk of their recurrence.[49] It would also log near misses, which are seldom identified and rarely formally reported. Problems with patient care technologies would be a component of this searchable database, allowing rapid identification of device failures or misguided applications and subsequent recall of said devices or, if necessary, alterations in operating procedures. These data could be reported from events occurring not only during real clinical care but also simulated scenarios. Data could be filtered to allow comparisons between similarly sized, geographically located, or resourced NICUs. It can also allow for the identification and dissemination of the most common problems encountered, similar to what the Federal Aviation Administration tracks in terms of factors that cause aviation accidents (**Box 3**).[50]

Another concept for the future is the development of perinatal operations centers. Tremendous advances in safety, efficiency, and effectiveness have resulted from the development of operations centers in high-risk industries such as mass transit, commercial aviation, aerospace, nuclear power, and the military. Although it is true that "hospital command centers" have come online in various US locations, these

---

Box 3
Aviation accident cause factors

10 Most Frequent Cause Factors for General Aviation Accidents that Involve the Pilot-In-Command
1. Inadequate preflight preparation and/or planning.
2. Failure to obtain and/or maintain flying speed.
3. Failure to maintain direction control.
4. Improper level off.
5. Failure to see and avoid objects or obstructions.
6. Mismanagement of fuel.
7. Improper inflight decisions or planning.
8. Misjudgment of distance and speed.
9. Selection of unsuitable terrain.
10. Improper operation of flight controls.

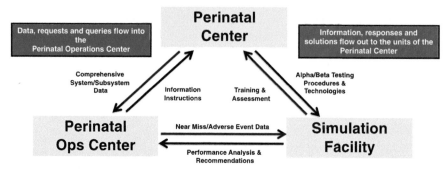

Fig. 3. The perinatal operations center.

centers typically miss their full potential, instead serving only to reinforce existing reactive, inefficient, and unsafe processes while focusing on the function of a single subsystem (typically patient placement and bed management). Current facilities tend to focus on technology (eg, placing multiple computer displays on a desk or a wall) but provide less emphasis on functionality. This outcome can be avoided by re-engineering hospital operations by delineating the components of this complex system, defining the interactions among those components, and crafting performance-based mission rules to guide operations. Because a busy regional perinatal center is a microcosm of a large hospital system, a perinatal operations center could generate unique insights about the interactions between subsystems of these larger health care systems and how those interactions may present opportunities to achieve improvements in the safety, efficiency, and effectiveness of clinical care. Functions of a perinatal operations center could include tracking high-risk pregnancies and maternal and neonatal transports, predicting the probability of delivery and the severity of neonatal disease, simplifying neonatal care coordination within the hospital, supporting local reporting of neonatal patient safety events at the hospital, and facilitating communication between referring physicians in community hospitals and physicians at referral centers. Simulation could be integrated to recreate near misses or adverse events; the lessons learned and system modifications identified during the performance analysis and debriefings of those simulations could be fed back through the operations center to improve the processes through which patient care is delivered (**Fig. 3**).

SUMMARY

The attention on patient safety in health care has been unquestionable for decades, but the mechanisms by which to improve patient safety continue to evolve. Human factors science teaches us that patient safety is not achieved by disciplining or training mistakes out of individual health care professionals, but rather by designing systems, protocols, and work environments that acknowledge human vulnerability and capitalize on the capabilities of the human beings working within them. The integration of human factors principles into patient safety work is increasingly understood to add value to the redesigning of processes, equipment, and systems for safer care. Incorporating human factors knowledge into well-known methodologies such as simulation, debriefing, and quality improvement initiatives based on reported data will strengthen the quality and resilience of the solutions and systems changes that are developed. The future of patient safety in neonatology–and all of health care–will depend on continued efforts to engineer and re-engineer systems that best support the humans who are at the interface of delivering safe patient care.

Best practices

What is the current practice?
- Patient care is comprised of a complex system with numerous components including but not limited to the physical environment, medical devices, supplies, patient, family, health care professionals, and hospital culture.
- Focus on the contribution of an individual health care professional to any adverse event limits the scope of patient safety analyses.

What changes in current practice are likely to improve outcomes?
- Broadening perspectives on patient safety to include the following will enhance the quality of quality improvement efforts:
  - Use objective data from audiovisual recordings of real clinical care and simulated clinical events.
  - Examine the role of system components.
  - Look beyond adverse events. Scrutinize near misses as well as successes in safe patient care.

Major Recommendations:
- Incorporation of human factors science principles will strengthen the quality and resilience of the processes, equipment, and systems implemented for safe patient care.

Bibliographic source(s)
Carayon P, Wooldridge A, Hose BZ, Salwei M, Benneyan J. Challenges And Opportunities For Improving Patient Safety Through Human Factors And Systems Engineering. *Health Aff (Millwood)*. 2018;37(11):1862-1869.
Emanuel L, Berwick D, Conway J, et al. What Exactly Is Patient Safety? In: Henriksen K, Battles JB, Keyes MA, Grady ML, eds. *Advances in Patient Safety: New Directions and Alternative Approaches (Vol. 1: Assessment)*. Advances in Patient Safety. Agency for Healthcare Research and Quality; 2008.
Emanuel L, Berwick D, Conway J, et al. What Exactly Is Patient Safety? In: Henriksen K, Battles JB, Keyes MA, Grady ML, eds. *Advances in Patient Safety: New Directions and Alternative Approaches (Vol. 1: Assessment)*. Advances in Patient Safety. Agency for Healthcare Research and Quality; 2008.

DISCLOSURE

The authors have nothing to disclose.

REFERENCES

1. Agency for healthcare research and quality. Patient safety Network glossary. *Glossary entry for "patient safety.* Available at: https://psnet.ahrq.gov/glossary-0. Accessed October 25, 2022.
2. Institute of medicine (US) committee on quality of Health care in America. To Err is human: building a safer Health system. In: Kohn LT, Corrigan JM, Donaldson MS, editors. National Academies Press (US); 2000. Available at: http://www.ncbi.nlm.nih.gov/books/NBK225182/. Accessed October 24, 2022.
3. Institute of medicine (US) committee on quality of Health care in America. Crossing the quality Chasm: a new Health system for the 21st century. National

Academies Press (US); 2001. Available at: http://www.ncbi.nlm.nih.gov/books/NBK222274/. Accessed October 24, 2022.

4. Agency for healthcare research and quality. Patient safety Network glossary. *Glossary entry for "adverse event.* Available at: https://psnet.ahrq.gov/glossary-0. Accessed October 25, 2022.

5. Agency for healthcare research and quality. Patient safety Network glossary. *Glossary entry for "active error.* Available at: https://psnet.ahrq.gov/glossary-0. Accessed October 25, 2022.

6. Agency for healthcare research and quality. Patient safety Network glossary. *Glossary entry for "latent error.* Available at: https://psnet.ahrq.gov/glossary-0. Accessed October 25, 2022.

7. Agency for healthcare research and quality. Patient safety Network glossary. *Glossary entry for "near miss.* Available at: https://psnet.ahrq.gov/glossary-0. Accessed October 25, 2022.

8. The Joint commission. Human factors analysis in patient safety systems. Joint Comm Source 2015;13(4). Available at: https://www.jointcommission.org/-/media/deprecated-unorganized/imported-assets/tjc/system-folders/assetmanager/humanfactorsthe_sourcepdf.pdf?db=web&hash=085A09275C38FACB50BC3D92CB35450A. Accessed October 24, 2022.

9. Reason J. Human error: models and management. BMJ 2000;320(7237):768–70.

10. Hollnagel E., Wears R.L. and Braithwaite J., From Safety-I to Safety-II: A White Paper, 2015, Resilient Health Care Net: Published simultaneously by the University of Southern Denmark, University of Florida, USA, and Macquarie University, Australia.

11. Yamada NK, Catchpole K, Salas E. The role of human factors in neonatal patient safety. Semin Perinatol 2019;43(8):151174.

12. Patterson M, Deutsch ES. Safety-I, safety-II and resilience engineering. Curr Probl Pediatr Adolesc Health Care 2015;45(12):382–9.

13. Hollnagel E. Safety-I and safety-II: the past and future of safety management. CRC Press; 2017. https://doi.org/10.1201/9781315607511.

14. Carayon P, Schoofs Hundt A, Karsh BT, et al. Work system design for patient safety: the SEIPS model. Qual Saf Health Care 2006;15(Suppl 1):i50–8.

15. Holden RJ, Carayon P, Gurses AP, et al. SEIPS 2.0: a human factors framework for studying and improving the work of healthcare professionals and patients. Ergonomics 2013;56(11):1669–86.

16. Carayon P, Wooldridge A, Hoonakker P, et al. SEIPS 3.0: human-centered design of the patient journey for patient safety. Appl Ergon 2020;84:103033.

17. Raju TNK, Suresh G, Higgins RD. Patient safety in the context of neonatal intensive care: research and educational opportunities. Pediatr Res 2011;70(1):109–15.

18. Kaplan HC, Edwards EM, Soll RF, et al. Variability in the systems of care supporting critical neonatal intensive care unit transitions. J Perinatol 2020;40(10):1546–53.

19. Weiner GM. Textbook of Neonatal Resuscitation. 8th edition. Itasca, IL: American Academy of Pediatrics and American Heart Association; 2021.

20. Yamada NK, Yaeger KA, Halamek LP. Analysis and classification of errors made by teams during neonatal resuscitation. Resuscitation 2015;96:109–13.

21. Yamada NK, Fuerch JH, Halamek LP. Impact of standardized communication techniques on errors during simulated neonatal resuscitation. Am J Perinatol 2016;33(4):385–92.

22. Yamada NK, Kamlin COF, Halamek LP. Optimal human and system performance during neonatal resuscitation. Semin Fetal Neonatal Med 2018;23(5):306–11.
23. Fuerch JH, Yamada NK, Coelho PR, et al. Impact of a novel decision support tool on adherence to Neonatal Resuscitation Program algorithm. Resuscitation 2015; 88:52–6.
24. Halamek LP. Teaching versus learning and the role of simulation-based training in pediatrics. J Pediatr 2007;151(4):329–30.
25. Halamek LP, Cady RAH, Sterling MR. Using briefing, simulation and debriefing to improve human and system performance. Semin Perinatol 2019;43(8):151178.
26. Ades A, Lee HC. Update on simulation for the neonatal resuscitation program. Semin Perinatol 2016;40(7):447–54.
27. Hollnagel E. Why is work-as-imagined different from work-as-done?. In: Resilient health care, 2 London: CRC Press; 2015. p. 249–64.
28. Bender GJ. In situ simulation for systems testing in newly constructed perinatal facilities. Semin Perinatol 2011;35(2):80–3.
29. Krammer T, Kessler L, Aspalter G, et al. Video-recorded in situ simulation before moving to the new combined neonatal/pediatric intensive care facility: an observational study. Pediatr Crit Care Med 2022. https://doi.org/10.1097/PCC.0000000000003080.
30. Cohen TN, Wiegmann DA, Kanji FF, et al. Using flow disruptions to understand healthcare system safety: a systematic review of observational studies. Appl Ergon 2022;98:103559.
31. Robertson ER, Hadi M, Morgan LJ, et al. Oxford NOTECHS II: a modified theatre team non-technical skills scoring system. PLoS One 2014;9(3):e90320.
32. Mishra A, Catchpole K, McCulloch P. The Oxford NOTECHS System: reliability and validity of a tool for measuring teamwork behaviour in the operating theatre. Qual Saf Health Care 2009;18(2):104–8.
33. Avila-Alvarez A, Davis PG, Kamlin COF, et al. Documentation during neonatal resuscitation: a systematic review. Arch Dis Child Fetal Neonatal Ed 2021; 106(4):376–80.
34. Berglund S, Norman M. Neonatal resuscitation assessment: documentation and early paging must be improved. Arch Dis Child Fetal Neonatal Ed 2012;97(3): F204–8.
35. Rüdiger M, Braun N, Gurth H, et al. Preterm resuscitation I: clinical approaches to improve management in delivery room. Early Hum Dev 2011;87(11):749–53.
36. Shivananda S, Twiss J, El-Gouhary E, et al. Video recording of neonatal resuscitation: a feasibility study to inform widespread adoption. World J Clin Pediatr 2017;6(1):69–80.
37. Leone TA. Using video to assess and improve patient safety during simulated and actual neonatal resuscitation. Semin Perinatol 2019;43(8):151179.
38. Gelbart B, Hiscock R, Barfield C. Assessment of neonatal resuscitation performance using video recording in a perinatal centre. J Paediatr Child Health 2010;46(7–8):378–83.
39. den Boer MC, Houtlosser M, Foglia EE, et al. Benefits of recording and reviewing neonatal resuscitation: the providers' perspective. Arch Dis Child Fetal Neonatal Ed 2019;104(5):F528–34.
40. den Boer MC, Houtlosser M, Witlox RSGM, et al. Reviewing recordings of neonatal resuscitation with parents. Arch Dis Child Fetal Neonatal Ed 2021; 106(4):346–51.

41. O'Donnell CPF, Kamlin COF, Davis PG, et al. Ethical and legal aspects of video recording neonatal resuscitation. Arch Dis Child Fetal Neonatal Ed 2008;93(2): F82–4.

42. Gelbart B, Barfield C, Watkins A. Ethical and legal considerations in video recording neonatal resuscitations. J Med Ethics 2009;35(2):120–4.

43. den Boer MC, Houtlosser M, van Zanten HA, et al. Ethical dilemmas of recording and reviewing neonatal resuscitation. Arch Dis Child Fetal Neonatal Ed 2018; 103(3):F280–4.

44. Carbine DN, Finer NN, Knodel E, et al. Video recording as a means of evaluating neonatal resuscitation performance. Pediatrics 2000;106(4):654–8.

45. Emanuel L, Berwick D, Conway J, et al. What exactly is patient safety?. In: Henriksen K, Battles JB, Keyes MA, et al, editors. *Advances in patient safety: new Directions and alternative Approaches (vol. 1: assessment)*. Advances in patient safety. Agency for Healthcare Research and Quality; 2008. Available at: http://www.ncbi.nlm.nih.gov/books/NBK43629/. Accessed October 25, 2022.

46. Carayon P, Wooldridge A, Hose BZ, et al. Challenges and opportunities for improving patient safety through human factors and systems engineering. Health Aff 2018;37(11):1862–9.

47. Dekker S. Patient Safety: A Human Factors Approach. Boca Raton, LA: CRC Press/Taylor & Francis Group; 2011.

48. Federal aviation administration. Safety management system. Available at: https://www.faa.gov/about/initiatives/sms/explained. Accessed January 6, 2023.

49. Shafer G, Singh H, Suresh G. Diagnostic errors in the neonatal intensive care unit: state of the science and new directions. Semin Perinatol 2019;43(8):151175.

50. Federal aviation administration. Safety of flight. In: Aeronautical information manual. United States Department of Transportation; 2022. Available at: https://www.faa.gov/air_traffic/publications/atpubs/aim_html/chap7_section_6.html. Accessed January 6, 2023.

How Design Thinking and Quality Improvement Can Be Integrated into a "Human-Centered Quality Improvement" Approach to Solve Problems in Perinatology

Jessica Gaulton, MD, MPH[a],*, Byron Crowe, MD[b,1],
Jules Sherman, MFA[c,2]

KEYWORDS

- Design thinking • Human-centered design • Innovation • Neonatology
- Perinatology • Neonatal-perinatal

KEY POINTS

- Both design thinking (DT) and quality improvement methodologies have their unique strengths and weaknesses. When integrated together into a "human-centered QI" approach, they can work synergistically to solve complex problems in health care.
- At its core, DT fosters empathy and a deep understanding for how "users" (patients, providers, staff) think, feel, and act when experiencing a problem.
- The Double Diamond model is a DT framework that can be applied to understand a problem from the eyes of the users, develop potential solutions, and test them for viability.
- Although DT has begun to be applied in health care, it has yet to be adopted at scale.

BACKGROUND

In recent decades, health systems have adopted formal methodologies to decrease waste and improve clinical outcomes. Quality improvement (QI) represents one of these methodologies and includes a set of tools adopted from the manufacturing

[a] Department of Neonatology, Beth Israel Deaconess Medical Center, 330 Brookline Avenue, RO-320, Boston, MA 02215, USA; [b] Department of Medicine, Beth Israel Deaconess Medical Center, 330 Brookline Avenue, Boston, MA 02215, USA; [c] Biodesign Program, Children's National Hospital, 111 Michigan Avenue Northwest, Washington, DC 20010, USA
[1] Present address: 93 Beacon Street Apartment #5, Cambridge, MA 02139.
[2] Present address: 905 Forest Avenue, Palo Alto, CA 94301.
* Corresponding author. 330 Brookline Avenue, RO-320, Boston, MA 02215.
E-mail address: jgaulton@bidmc.harvard.edu

Clin Perinatol 50 (2023) 435–448
https://doi.org/10.1016/j.clp.2023.01.006
0095-5108/23/© 2023 Elsevier Inc. All rights reserved.
perinatology.theclinics.com

industry that has permeated health care and made a significant impact on health outcomes.[1,2] However, in some cases, QI methods have led to unintended consequences and criticisms, including burdensome measurement and reporting requirements, perverse financial incentives that have led to gamification of key metrics, and the perception that process improvement deemphasizes the role of individuals and their contributions within complex systems.[3,4] Addressing these challenges with contemporary QI requires a thoughtful reconsideration of the improvement toolkit and an openness to integrating alternative methodologies.

Design thinking (DT), also referred to as "human-centered design," is a structured framework for solving complex problems. Although both DT and QI are improvement methodologies that share common goals, they view the problem-solving process from different perspectives. Conceptually, a simple way to explain the difference is that QI methods apply a process-centered lens when seeking to understand and solve problems, whereas DT applies a human-centered lens.[2]

DT is characterized by an overarching emphasis on solving for unmet human needs as the most important outcome of interest, and its corresponding framework is built to accomplish this task by examining the human experience. Although QI methods excel at deeply examining a process and unmasking drivers of error or opportunities to improve efficiency, DT excels at unmasking how people think, feel, and act when interacting with a product or service. The DT framework also allows us to define the contribution of peoples' emotions and actions within complex health systems and identify opportunities to address unmet human wants and desires through improved systems design.[5] Although DT has been broadly adopted by consumer-facing giants such as Google, General Electric, and Apple to create products and services that delight individuals, health care has yet to adopt DT at scale.[6]

There are many benefits to combining elements of DT alongside contemporary QI, including visibility into how individual actions and behaviors affect processes, as well as increased clarity on how to make tradeoffs between reliable processes and unmet human needs. Earlier study has described how both methods can be used together in a hybrid framework termed *"human-centered QI."*[2] In this article, we provide an overview of DT fundamentals, describe examples of its application in neonatal-perinatal medicine, and recommend next steps for clinicians interested in applying a "human-centered QI" approach to their improvement study.

DESIGN THINKING FRAMEWORK
Double Diamond Model

The Double Diamond (DD) model provides the overarching framework in DT and can be thought of as analogous to the model for improvement in QI.[1] The DD framework (**Fig. 1**) is organized into 4 main phases: discover, define, develop, and deliver. The 2 diamonds represent 2 different, yet equally important stages. The first diamond represents the "problem space" and the second represents the "solution space."[6] The DD model was first developed by the British Design Council in 2004[6] to codify design methods being used widely at the time, and since then, it has achieved broad adoption, providing a nonlinear, interactive path for solving complex problems across diverse industries.

The first diamond captures the "discover" and "define" phases (see **Fig. 1, Table 1**), which help us deeply understand (rather than assume) the problem through the eyes of its users, who may be patients, providers, staff or other individuals. In this stage, designers immerse themselves in learning from the users through *"contextual inquiry,"* which includes interviews, focus groups, and observations of people and processes.[7]

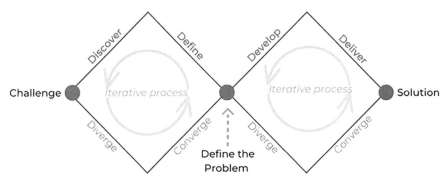

Fig. 1. *DD model.* The DD model is organized into 4 main phases: discover, define, develop, and deliver. The 2 diamonds represent 2 different, equally important stages. The first diamond represents the "problem space" and the second represents the "solution space." Each diamond's shape helps us visualize a key principle in DT: "diverge then converge." In the "diverge" stage of both diamonds, the team explores as many ideas as possible, without judgment, in order to foster creativity and teamwork. After the team has "diverged" on their thinking, they apply their insights and "converge" to either define the problem (*first diamond*) or deliver a solution (*second diamond*). (*Adapted from* Framework for Innovation: Design Council's evolved Double Diamond. Available at: https://www.designcouncil.org.uk/our-work/skills-learning/tools-frameworks/framework-for-innovation-design-councils-evolved-double-diamond/. Accessed Aug 1 2022.)

DT methodology often steers clear of questionnaires as a primary means of collecting data because peoples' actions do not always align with their intentions.[18] Contextual inquiry also helps the team develop *empathy* for the users,[8–10] which is at the core of DT. Investing a significant amount of time and effort in the "discover" phase, often with multiple nonlinear cycles of learning, allows the team to accurately define the problem.

The second diamond represents the "solution space," which includes the "develop" and "deliver" phases (see **Fig. 1**, **Table 1**). During these phases, the design team uses insights gathered from the previous phases to brainstorm potential solutions and test them in the form of low-fidelity *prototypes*. During brainstorming sessions, team members are encouraged to think creatively and collaboratively to collect ideas for potential solutions, which may come in the form of a service, program, device, behavioral change, or technological intervention. In DT, prototypes are tested in *rapid pilots* with small cohorts of users. It is critical to seek feedback from users early and often and to iterate quickly in order to achieve a viable solution that can be studied at a larger scale.

Each diamond's shape helps us visualize a key principle in DT: "diverge then converge" (see **Fig. 1**). In the "diverge" stage of both diamonds, the team explores as many ideas as possible, without judgment, in order to foster creativity and teamwork. "Out-of-the-box" ideas are welcomed in the "diverge" stages of each diamond. After the team has "diverged" on their thinking, they apply their insights and "converge" to either define the problem (first diamond) or deliver a solution (second diamond).[6]

The DT framework also encourages *multidisciplinary collaboration*, often with nonmedical professionals from fields such as anthropology, computer science, business, architecture, among others, to provide unique perspectives and ideas.[19] Design teams often apply the concept of "*codesigning*" with users, who may be patients, providers, staff, or other key stakeholders, who are considered integral members of the

Table 1
Phases of the double diamond model

Phase	Description	Tool
DISCOVER	Discovery is the first phase of the DT process, in which investigators are immersed in learning. This is also called "*contextual inquiry*" and includes the following: conducting interviews, focus groups, and observing people and processes.[7] The goal is to put yourself in the users' shoes in order to foster *empathy* and a deep understanding of the problem you are trying to solve[8-10]	Empathy maps Personas
DEFINE	In the "define" phase, the focus is on defining the unmet need that the users are experiencing. "*How might we…?*" statements[11] are often utilized in the problem definition, which highlight insights synthesized from contextual inquiry. For example, "How might we decrease burnout among nurses in the NICU to decrease job turnover?" Oftentimes, in health care, a problem is defined without input from the users, which can lead to developing interventions that do not ultimately solve the problem at hand	Empathy maps Personas
DEVELOP	*Ideating*, or brainstorming, is a critical component of DT and emphasizes creativity and teamwork. In this phase, it is important to suspend judgment and encourage "out-of-the-box" ideas.[12] One strategy to facilitate communication when brainstorming is to begin a response to a team member's idea with "*Yes, and…*" rather than "No, but…"[13]	Rapid prototyping
DELIVER	Testing is part of an *iterative* process on real users that provides the team with critical feedback. The purpose of testing is to learn what works and what does not in order to iterate quickly. A *prototype* is a low-fidelity, low-cost model of a potential solution that is meant to convey an idea quickly. A prototype can be a sketch,[14] diagram, model, 3D printed representation, skit, or nontangible intervention.[15] Prototypes are tested in *rapid cycles*[16] with small cohorts (as few as 5–10 users) in order to quickly receive feedback and iterate.[17] This type of agile testing allows the team to identify viable solutions that can be studied at a larger scale	Rapid prototyping

design team. The principle of codesign, also called "coproduction," is based on the belief that the user's perspective is essential and should be equally represented throughout the creative process.[20]

DESIGN THINKING TOOLS

Throughout each phase of the DD model, teams can apply tools to generate key insights from user emotions and experiences. Although there are many DT tools,[21–23] the authors have highlighted 4 high-yield tools that are easiest to implement. Each tool is typically applied in specific phases of the DD model outlined below and in **Table 1**.

Empathy Maps

Empathy maps (**Figs. 2** and **3**) allow the design team to visually summarize their learnings from the "contextual inquiry" process in the "discover" phase and are typically fully developed in the "define" phase. An empathy map provides a synthesized overview of the users' experiences and consists of 4 quadrants, which illustrate what the users "said," "did," "thought," and "felt."[24,25] It is usually easier to determine what the users "said" and "did." However, determining what they "thought" and "felt" should be based on real-world observations capturing how they behaved and responded as they experienced the problem being studied. A design team makes inferences and often identifies insights based on their own backgrounds and biases, which is why it is important to have a diverse team analyzing the data.[26] Empathy maps are also helpful as background for constructing personas (see next section).

Personas

A persona (**Fig. 4**) is a visual representation of a composite character profile based on research collected through contextual inquiry. In other words, a persona is a "user archetype," which represents a cohort of individuals with similar characteristics. A persona may include details such as age, gender, occupation, direct quotes, aspirations, hopes, fears, pain points, behaviors, and lifestyle choices.

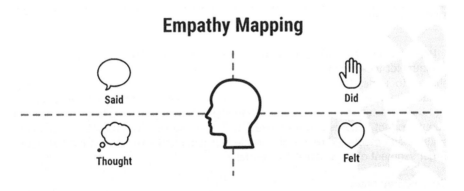

Empathy Mapping

Said

Did

Thought

Felt

Fig. 2. *Empathy Map Template* An empathy map provides a synthesized overview of the users' experiences and consists of 4 quadrants, which illustrate what the users "said," "did," "thought," and "felt."[24,25] The map visually summarizes learnings from the "contextual inquiry" process. (*From* Dam RF, Siang TY. Empathy Map – why and how to use it. The Interaction Design Foundation. Available at: https://www.interaction-design.org/literature/article/empathy-map-why-and-how-to-use-it. Accessed Nov 26 2022.)

Empathy Map

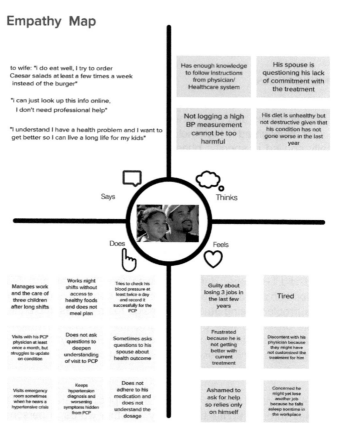

Fig. 3. *Example of Empathy Map.* Empathy map of student work from *Designing Healthcare For Social Justice: Telehealth Design & Access* at Stanford d.school. Qualitative descriptions from patient and spouse interviews as well as direct observations of patient behaviors are shown in each of the 4 quadrants (says, thinks, does and feels). (*Courtesy of* J Sherman, MFA, Washington, DC.)

Personas are typically utilized in the "discover" and "define" phases to build empathy for the users (often patients), so designers can "walk a mile in the person's shoes" to understand their behaviors, motivations, and expectations. Personas replace the need to collect data on the entire community, significantly reducing time and cost. Design teams often develop multiple distinct personas to guide decisions about product features and visual design.[27–30] Personas help us avoid developing a solution that meets the needs of a single individual and ensures that the needs of a larger segment of the population are met.[31]

User Journey Maps

A user journey map (**Fig. 5**) is a visualization of a person's experience interacting with a process. The map includes a timeline of the user's actions, along with their accompanying emotions to create a narrative.[32] The journey map can represent a single individual's experience or the collective journey of a "persona" in order to understand specific trends within a larger group of users. The journey map can be created by the design team, or it can be codeveloped with the user (often the patient), who

Name: Danika

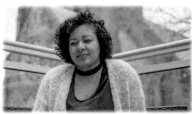

Typical Day:
Danika wakes at 6am, walks to the train .25 miles from her home, walks to her office across the street and begins work at 8am. She sits most of the day, getting up from her chair only to file papers. Food is ordered into the office. She typically eats tacos or burgers for lunch with soda. She leaves work at 5:30pm, grabs a sub sandwich or Chinese food and rushes to get to school by 6:30pm. She stays at school for classes until 9:00pm and takes the train home. At home she has snacks like chips, watches her favorite shows and then goes to bed around at 11:30pm.

Age: 36

Occupation: Paralegal and law student.

Pregnancy History: Pregnant once before, ended in pre-term birth at 22 weeks, baby did not survive.

Health Insurance: Medicaid (through PPACA or "Obamacare").

Lifestyle: Works full time, law school part time at night and weekends.

Diet: Mostly fast food, and packaged food.

Exercise: Walks from home to train station 5 days a week (.5 mile total distance).

Habits: Alcohol consumption every weekend, drinks soda and coffee daily.

Psychological Profile: Has struggled with anxiety on and off during her life. After the death of her baby, she did not receive any therapy and did not seek therapy. Peer support wasn't offered at the hospital.

Home Relationships: Lives with partner who shares similar lifestyle traits, and his mother.

Social Life: Has a few close friends and her sister who she regularly sees on weekends.

Personal Goals: Trying to get pregnant with a healthy full-term baby again ever since the death of her first child 11 months ago.

Professional Goals: Wants to become a family attorney within 4 years.

Based on the above persona, Danika may need (inferring here):
1) Information about becoming pregnant after the loss of a pre-term infant.

"I'm too tired to exercise and I'm not a good cook! I know this affects my health, but I don't know where to start to make changes."

2) Support post discharge from clinicians and peers about what she experienced in the NICU.

What else could you infer Danika might need to reach her healthy pregnancy goal?

Fig. 4. *Example of Persona*. This user archetype illustrates the daily habits, characteristics, interests, and behaviors of a mother with unhealthy lifestyle choices who experienced the loss of a preterm infant. She wishes to get pregnant again and is seeking help to achieve healthier lifestyle choices during her next pregnancy.

may draw pictures or symbols to visually represent their own journey (see **Fig. 5**A). The format of a journey map is often a timeline with notes at specific moments or a series of images, or both. Journey maps help design teams build empathy for the users and uncover insights, particularly when comparing journeys between different personas to find common threads or conflicting emotions and behaviors.[33–35]

Rapid Prototyping

Similar to plan-do-study-act cycles in QI, rapid prototyping facilitates agile testing and learning. A prototype is a low-fidelity, low-cost model of a potential solution that is meant to convey an idea quickly. A prototype can be a sketch,[14] diagram, website, 3D-printed representation, skit, behavioral change, service, or other nontangible intervention.[15] Ideas for prototypes are conceptualized and constructed in the "develop" phase, then tested in the "deliver" phase. Prototypes are tested in rapid pilots[16] over the course of days to weeks with small cohorts (as few as 5–10 users) in order to quickly receive feedback and iterate.[17]

The advantage of rapid prototyping is the ability to quickly test ideas and eliminate those that are not viable. Failure is expected (and welcomed) and allows the team to move on from nonviable prototypes quickly, without significant time or money lost. It is essential to seek feedback from the users early and often during the rapid prototyping process in order to determine which potential solutions show promise and quickly improve those prototypes for subsequent testing. Rapid prototyping allows the team to identify viable solutions that can be studied at a larger scale.

EXAMPLES OF DESIGN THINKING IN NEONATAL-PERINATAL MEDICINE

With the growing popularity of DT in health care, there have been some published examples of successful projects within neonatal-perinatal medicine that have used DT methods. We have chosen to highlight 3 examples and examine the phases of the

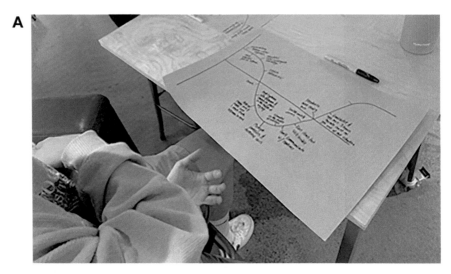

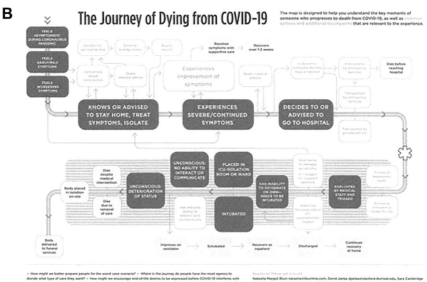

Fig. 5. *Examples of Journey Maps.* (*A*) Journey map from student work from *Designing Healthcare For Social Justice*, at Stanford's design school. This picture illustrates the principle of "codesign," which engages users as active participants in the "journey mapping" process. An important feature of a journey map is the user's emotions that are associated with each step of the journey. Positive experiences are drawn above the x-axis and negative ones below it. (*B*) Journey map from *Project End of Life*, Emergency Design Collective. This map depicts a linear representation of key moments of patients who progress to death from COVID-19 at one hospital. Note that the patient's emotional experiences are not included in this map. David Janka (master architect), Alana Ippolito, Natasha Margot Blum, Sara Cambridge, Scott Witthoft, Leila Roumani, Ben Seligman. ([*A*] *Courtesy of* J Sherman, MFA, Washington, DC.)

DD model (see **Fig. 1**) that were applied in each article. Although no project fully described all phases of the DD model, these examples illustrate the expected progression through the framework, which is often nonlinear and requires exploration of multiple phases concurrently.

Example 1: Using Design Thinking to Assess Environmental Factors and Their Contribution to Childbirth

In this article, the authors applied DT methods to improve patient safety and clinician workflows across 10 labor and delivery (L&D) units in California.[36] The multidisciplinary team included physicians, nurses, engineers, designers, and human factors experts.

Discover phase
Qualitative data, collected through "*contextual inquiry*," were gathered from in-person interviews with clinicians and stakeholders with knowledge of hospital design, observations from site visits, photographs, and sketches. The in-person interviews were intentionally unstructured and open-ended, which is a design tactic that helps facilitate storytelling about how the user feels, behaves, and acts when experiencing a problem.

Define phase
In the "define phase," the DT team identified 3 main insights across the 10 hospitals and offered concrete recommendations that had the potential to (and ultimately did) improve patient safety outcomes.

First, there was a delay in blood availability during emergent cases of postpartum hemorrhage. The team observed that at some hospitals, blood was stored in a different building, sometimes far away, which contributed to significant delays. Based on these key learnings, a set of recommendations for the hospitals were developed that included storage of blood products on the L&D floor, ideally outside of the operating room if possible.

Second, delivery rooms lacked appropriate spaces for neonatal resuscitation, resulting in resuscitation in cramped locations in the corner of the room and often with other equipment blocking the resuscitation space. The team recommended an easily accessible, dedicated space where 3 or more clinicians would be able to comfortably perform the resuscitation.

Third, inefficient and inconsistent restocking of supply rooms on the L&D floors resulted in restocking errors. The team found that what made the biggest difference at one hospital was tied to a basic human motivation. When the patient's primary nurse, rather than a technician who was not involved in patient care, took ownership of restocking the supply room, the responsibility became personal and tied to their patient's outcome, which resulted in fewer restocking errors.

Example 2: Using Design Thinking to Identify Opportunities for Reducing Inequity in Perinatal Care Delivery

The authors applied human-centered design principles to understand the unmet needs of Medicaid-insured pregnant people in San Francisco, California.[37]

Discover phase
In the "discover" phase, the team conducted qualitative, semistructured interviews with pregnant women, as well as focus groups with key stakeholders.

Define phase
The team synthesized the qualitative data and identified several key "*insight statements*," which are short sentences that capture an unmet human need.[38] For

example, one of the insight statements that emerged from this study was as follows: "Marginalized people are not welcomed as equal, trusted partners in their care."

Develop and deliver phases

The design team then translated these insight statements into actionable opportunities to drive the "develop" and "deliver" phases of the DD model, at which time the team developed low-fidelity prototypes of potential solutions that were presented to patients for feedback. One prototype that received enthusiastic feedback from patients visually depicted a "Support Sister," or a peer with similar lived experiences who would be incorporated into the patient's care team and would be the patient's advocate during and after pregnancy. The team "*codesigned*" several prototypes with pregnant women and based on their feedback, came to a consensus about which potential solutions to develop and test.

Example 3: Using Design to Overcome Social Disadvantage in the Neonatal Intensive Care Unit

In this article, the DT team developed an app called "PretermConnect," in order to decrease socioeconomic barriers in neonatal intensive care units (NICUs).[39] The goal of the app is to educate and empower women at risk of preterm birth.

Develop and deliver phases

The authors "*codesigned*" with end users (pregnant women), who were core members of the team. The article described 3 codesign cycles, during which they sought feedback from women from diverse ethnic, economic, and cultural backgrounds in different settings. Three main insights that emerged from the user feedback included the following: (1) pregnant women struggled with social isolation, (2) they felt a lack of social connection, and (3) mothers had similar challenges when caring for their preterm infants. The team integrated these insights when developing the app, which led to features such as facilitating connections between mothers and local community organizations. In order to continuously iterate, the team integrated a feature that allowed the app to collect feedback from users at regular intervals to meet the unmet needs of their users.

RECOMMENDATION FOR USING A "HUMAN-CENTERED QUALITY IMPROVEMENT" APPROACH

Practitioners of QI will likely see many similarities between DT and QI, both offering a codified approach to solving problems at a systems level. The main difference between these 2 frameworks lies in the lens through which the 2 methods view the world; QI sees the world through a process-centered lens and DT through a human-centered lens. We have found that combining both worldviews leads to deeper insights and more effective solutions than using one framework in isolation, as both methods have their strengths and weaknesses that complement each other. Improvement efforts in neonatal-perinatal medicine, and in fact, across all clinical specialties, can be enhanced by integrating DT methods and tools alongside those of contemporary QI. We previously described how these tools can work synergistically as part of a hybrid model of "*human-centered QI*" in a real-world example that improved the breastfeeding experience of mothers in the neonatal intensive care unit.[2]

A common pitfall that clinicians experience when starting an improvement project comes from having a preconceived notion about the solution before fully

Table 2	
Recommendations for implementing a 'human-centered QI' approach within an organization	
Strategy	**Tactics**
Be able to articulate the fundamental value proposition of DT to key stakeholders	Articulate that DT is not a new or experimental method but rather already used across diverse, world-class industries with demonstrated results
	Describe how the DT approach provides a deeper understanding of users' wants, needs, and behaviors
	Describe how DT identifies unmet needs among patients, providers, and staff, and allows for developing solutions that fuel the organization's clinical and financial missions
Gain a working knowledge of fundamental tools and methods of DT	Key staff should be trained in DT methods through widely available courses taught by commercial or academic organizations.
	Identify individuals who can be local advocates and superusers of DT
	Begin small-scale experiments implementing DT tools into current QI projects
Build organizational capacity by partnering with professional designers and their organizations	Avoid "DIY" mentality and instead invest in professionally-supported design work for high-priority projects
	Build effective people, processes, and systems for conducting DT work as part of active improvement projects

understanding the problem. To avoid falling into this trap, we recommend investing a significant amount of time interviewing the users—which may include patients, providers, and staff—to fully understand the problem at hand from *their* perspective. Clinicians should attempt to eliminate any biases that they have about the problem or potential solution in order to avoid implementing a solution that will not ultimately solve the unmet needs of the users. The goal of these interviewers is to draw out the user's stories and accompanying emotions because they experience the problem at hand. For those wishing to implement this new hybrid approach in their organization, we offer the following recommendations in **Table 2**.

SUMMARY

For the past several decades, the field of QI has revolutionized health care's approach to patient safety and quality measures. Similarly, DT methods are foundational to how businesses design products and services. By combining these methodologies and drawing from their strengths, we have the opportunity to rethink how we solve complex problems in health care, by focusing on both the gaps in processes as well as the unmet needs of patients, providers, leaders, and staff.

Similar to QI, DT requires expertise from researchers and practitioners with deep experience in the field. Although basic design methods are approachable and can be self-taught, investing in consultants and organizations with expertise can help accelerate learning across health systems. Whether applied to problems at an individual or enterprise-wide level, DT offers an opportunity to create human-centered solutions that improve care within neonatal-perinatal medicine and beyond.

Best practices

What is the current practice for QI in Perinatology?
Utilizing traditional QI methods to address complex problems in health care.[1]

What changes in current practice are likely to improve outcomes? Is there a clinical algorithm?
The DD model provides an overarching framework in DT and can be thought of as analogous to the Model for Improvement in QI.[6]

Pearls/pitfalls at the point-of-care:
Both DT and QI methodologies have their unique strengths and weaknesses. When integrated together into a "human-centered QI" approach, they can work synergistically to solve complex problems in health care.[2]

Major recommendations:
By integrating QI and DT frameworks, we have a unique opportunity to rethink how we solve problems in health care by elevating the human experience and putting empathy back at the center of medicine.

DECLARATION OF INTERESTS

The authors have nothing to disclose.

REFERENCES

1. The improvement guide: a practical approach to enhancing organizational performance. Qual Manag J 1997;4(4):85–6.
2. Crowe B, Gaulton JS, Minor N, et al. To improve quality, leverage design. BMJ Qual Saf 2022;31(1):70–4.
3. Rosenbaum L. Reassessing quality assessment - the flawed system for fixing a flawed system. N Engl J Med 2022;386(17):1663–7.
4. Berwick DM. Era 3 for medicine and health care. JAMA 2016;315(13):1329–30.
5. Norman D. *The design of everyday things: Revised and expanded edition*. Basic books, 2013. Available at: https://doi.org/10.15358/9783800648108. Accessed March 17, 2023.
6. Framework for innovation: design council's evolved double diamond. Available at: https://www.designcouncil.org.uk/our-work/skills-learning/tools-frameworks/framework-for-innovation-design-councils-evolved-double-diamond/. Accessed August 1, 2022.
7. Beyer H, Holtzblatt K. Contextual design. Interactions 1999;6(1):32–42.
8. Dam RF, Siang TY. What is empathy and why is it so important in design thinking? The Interaction Design Foundation. 2016. Available at: https://www.interaction-design.org/literature/article/design-thinking-getting-started-with-empathy. Accessed November 26, 2022.
9. Oxley JC, Julinna CO. "Conclusion: Implications for Feminist Ethics." The Moral Dimensions of Empathy: Limits and Applications in Ethical Theory and Practice (2011): 151-161. Available at: https://link.springer.com/chapter/10.1057/9780230347809_8. Accessed March 17, 2023.
10. Design kit. Available at: https://www.designkit.org/mindsets/4. Accessed November 26, 2022.
11. Design kit. Available at: https://www.designkit.org/methods/3. Accessed November 26, 2022.

12. What is brainstorming? 10 effective techniques you can use. The Interaction Design Foundation. Available at: https://www.interaction-design.org/literature/topics/brainstorming. Accessed November 26, 2022.

13. Ramirez DM. The 'yes, and' ethos also emphasizes the open-minded and collaborative feature of the design thinking process. Available at: https://sites.duke.edu/opendesignplus/2020/07/27/the-yes-and-ethos-also-emphasizes-the-open-minded-and-collaborative-feature-of-the-design-thinking-process/. Accessed November 26, 2022.

14. Make your ideas tangible through prototypes. IDEO U. 2020. https://www.ideou.com/blogs/page/make-your-ideas-tangible-through-prototypes. Accessed November 26, 2022.

15. Dam RF, Siang TY. Design thinking: get started with prototyping. The Interaction Design Foundation. 2016. Available at: https://www.interaction-design.org/literature/article/design-thinking-get-started-with-prototyping. Accessed November 26, 2022.

16. Design kit. Available at: https://www.designkit.org/methods/rapid-prototyping. Accessed November 26, 2022.

17. Design kit. Available at: https://www.designkit.org/methods/integrate-feedback-and-iterate. Accessed November 26, 2022.

18. What is UX research & what does a UX researcher do? The interaction design foundation. Available at: https://www.interaction-design.org/literature/topics/user-research. Accessed November 26, 2022.

19. Plattner H, Meinel C, Leifer L. Design thinking: understand – Improve – Apply, 2010, Springer Science & Business Media. Available at: https://books.google.com/books?hl=en&lr=&id=LAblwOwHz1MC&oi=fnd&pg=PR3&dq=Plattner+H.,+Meinel+C.+and+Leifer+L.,+Design+thinking:+understand+–+Improve+–+Apply,+2010,+Springer+Science+%26+Business+Media.&ots=2OmdpD3RsN&sig=vUCyiF2eQuMR8eAprIxIpFB5xu0#v=onepage&q=Plattner%20H.%2C%20Meinel%20C.%20and%20Leifer%20L.%2C%20Design%20thinking%3A%20understand%20–%20Improve%20–%20Apply%2C%202010%2C%20Springer%20Science%20%26%20Business%20Media.&f=false. Accessed March 17, 2023.

20. Batalden M, Batalden P, Margolis P, et al. Coproduction of healthcare service. BMJ Qual Saf 2016;25(7):509–17.

21. Design kit. Available at: https://www.designkit.org/methods. Accessed November 26, 2022.

22. Klein J. Using Research Tools in your design practice: negotiating to actually use them. Available at: https://bocoup.com/blog/using-research-tools-in-your-design-practice-negotiating-to-actually-use-them. Accessed November 26, 2022.

23. Chasanidou D, Gasparini AA and Lee E. (2015). Design thinking methods and tools for innovation. In Design, User Experience, and Usability: Design Discourse: 4th International Conference, DUXU 2015, Held as Part of HCI International 2015, Los Angeles, CA, USA, August 2–7, 2015, Proceedings, Part I (pp. 12-23). Springer International Publishing, Chicago.

24. Dam RF, Siang TY. Empathy map – why and how to use it. The interaction design foundation. 2016. Available at: https://www.interaction-design.org/literature/article/empathy-map-why-and-how-to-use-it. Accessed November 26, 2022.

25. Build your creative confidence: empathy maps. Available at: https://www.ideo.com/blog/build-your-creative-confidence-empathy-maps. Accessed November 26, 2022.

26. Polart G. The importance of diversity in the Design Thinking process. Medium. 2019. Available at: https://medium.com/@gaelle.polart/the-importance-of-

diversity-in-the-design-thinking-process-76a40b7ffcce. Accessed November 26, 2022.

27. Dam RF, Siang TY. Personas – a simple introduction. The interaction design foundation. 2016. Available at: https://www.interaction-design.org/literature/article/personas-why-and-how-you-should-use-them. Accessed November 26, 2022.

28. Open design kit. Available at: http://opendesignkit.org/methods/personas/. Accessed November 26, 2022.

29. Perfecting your personas. UX Articles by UIE. 2005. Available at: https://articles.uie.com/perfecting_personas/. Accessed November 26, 2022.

30. Adlin T, Pruitt J. The essential persona lifecycle: Your guide to building and using personas. Morgan Kaufmann; 2010.

31. Binkowska E. UX design: how user personas help build better products. Gorrion Software House. 2022. Available at: https://gorrion.io/blog/ux-design-how-user-personas-help-build-better-products/. Accessed November 28, 2022.

32. Gibbons S. Journey mapping 101. Nielsen norman group. Available at: https://www.nngroup.com/articles/journey-mapping-101/. Accessed November 28, 2022.

33. Design kit. Available at: https://www.designkit.org/methods/journey-map. Accessed November 26, 2022.

34. Customer journey map: definition & process. The interaction design foundation. Available at: https://www.interaction-design.org/literature/topics/customer-journey-map. Accessed November 26, 2022.

35. Quinn C. Use customer journey maps to uncover innovation opportunities. IDEO U. 2016. Available at: https://www.ideou.com/blogs/inspiration/use-customer-journey-maps-to-uncover-innovation-opportunities. Accessed November 26, 2022.

36. Sherman JP, Hedli LC, Kristensen-Cabrera AI, et al. Understanding the heterogeneity of labor and delivery units: using design thinking methodology to assess environmental factors that contribute to safety in childbirth. Am J Perinatol 2020;37(6):638–46, 5.

37. Nijagal MA, Patel D, Lyles C, et al. Using human centered design to identify opportunities for reducing inequities in perinatal care. BMC Health Serv Res 2021; 21:714.

38. What is insight? The 5 principles of insight definition. Thrive. 2016. Available at: https://thrivethinking.com/2016/03/28/what-is-insight-definition/. Accessed November 27, 2022.

39. Jani SG, Nguyen AD, Abraham Z, et al. PretermConnect: leveraging mobile technology to mitigate social disadvantage in the NICU and beyond. Semin Perinatol 2021;45(4):151413, 6.

Improving Neonatal Intensive Care Unit Quality and Safety with Family-Centered Care

Linda S. Franck, RN, PhD, FRCPCH, FAAN[a],*, Anna Axelin, RN, PhD[b],
Nicole R. Van Veenendaal, MD, MPH[c], Fabiana Bacchini, MSc, BJ[d]

KEYWORDS

- Family-centered care • Quality improvement • Neonatal intensive care unit
- Parent participation

KEY POINTS

- There is now strong evidence for family-centered interventions and models of care.
- The family-centered care (FCC) research-to-practice gap can be addressed with quality improvement (QI) approaches.
- Families are essential partners in QI.
- FCC QI measures and strategies are available, and there is opportunity for future innovation.

"I was only 25 weeks gestation when one of my twins died in utero... My surviving twin was rushed into the NICU, where he stayed for 146 days. The first time I saw him, I did not see a baby. I saw the wires; the monitors and I was very scared. I asked myself, how can he survive, how can an entire life be contained in only 900 grams? The nurse asked me if I would like to hold him. I was still recovering from the C-section, sitting on a wheelchair. I got transferred to another chair, and he was placed on my chest. He was so small, it felt like a worm, I held my breath as I didn't want to hurt him.

[a] Department of Family Health Care Nursing, University of California San Francisco, 2 Koret Way, N411F, Box 0606, San Francisco, CA 94143, USA; [b] Department of Nursing Science, University of Turku, 20014 University of Turku, Finland; [c] Department of Pediatrics, Emma Children's Hospital, Amsterdam UMC Location University of Amsterdam, Meibergdreef 9, Amsterdam, the Netherlands; [d] Canadian Premature Babies Foundation, 4225-B Dundas Street West, Etobicoke, ON M8X 1Y3, Canada
* Corresponding author.
E-mail address: linda.franck@ucsf.edu
Twitter: @AnnaAxelin (A.A.); @nicolevan_vee (N.R.V.V.); @fabianabacchini (F.B.)

Clin Perinatol 50 (2023) 449–472
https://doi.org/10.1016/j.clp.2023.01.007
0095-5108/23/© 2023 Elsevier Inc. All rights reserved.
perinatology.theclinics.com

We had two primary nurses who taught me how to change his diaper, take his temperature. As I gained physical strength, I stayed more hours by his bedside and once he got off the ventilator, I was invited to participate in the study of Family Integrated Care. It sounded like a great idea to be able to go to education classes every day so I could learn more about prematurity and what it could mean for him. I was invited to present him at rounds, which was intimidating in the beginning. It was a multidisciplinary team with about ten people, but every day I felt more confident to talk about my son and ask questions. As the days went by, the alarms didn't scare me as much and I learn to identify if my son was breathing well without looking at the monitors. Doctors would always come by the bedside to share information and discuss treatments and involved me in the decision-making. I was welcomed as part of my son's care team. I had access to the hospital 24/7 and it felt like my home away from home.

When I look back…, I realize that I was being prepared for the long road ahead as prematurity does not end when the baby gets discharged. My son came home on oxygen and during the first year of his life we had several trips to the emergency room because of respiratory distress. The first month post-discharge, he got very sick and was admitted in our local hospital. He turned blue while I was breastfeeding him and even after screaming for help, no one came. I ended up doing CPR on him and I saved his life. This monumental day made me realize how important being involved in the care in the NICU is. I learned not only life skills but also the confidence to advocate for my son. My preemie is now 10 years old. He has cerebral palsy and the advocacy never ended, but I'm much more prepared to face the challenges and celebrate the victories. Thanks to the amazing team who care for him and taught me how to be a parent of a child born preterm."

(Excerpt adapted from: Bachinni F. From Surviving to Thriving – A Mother's Journey through Infertility, Loss and Miracles, Toronto: Burman Books, Inc, 2017.)

INTRODUCTION

The essential role of parents (or other primary caregivers) to the survival and optimal development of small and sick newborns has been well documented across the world for more than 60 years. There is now strong evidence that outcomes are improved for infants and families when families are involved in their hospitalized infant's care.[1] The neonatal intensive care unit (NICU) team cannot fully meet the infant's physical and developmental needs during hospitalization or adequately prepare families to care for infants after discharge without strong family engagement as described so powerfully by the mother reflecting on her preterm infant's NICU journey [see Sidebar]. Moreover, the rights of children (including newborns) to fully and continuously be supported by their parents/primary caregivers are codified in the UN Rights of the Child.[2] Therefore, separation of infants from their parents in healthcare settings can be considered a violation of their human rights. Building on this, the European Foundation for the Care of Newborn Infants (EFCNI) states in their *Rights of Parents and Newborns*: "all families have the right to be considered as a unit [..], all parents have the right to receive appropriate education and be actively involved in their baby's care giving in an effective and sensitive manner."[3] The EFCNI also states that "all parents and newborns have the right to family-centered care (FCC) and to stay together while the child receives healthcare."[3,4]

The importance of patient-centered and family-centered healthcare services and the contribution of patients and families in the design and delivery of health care that are safe and high-quality are not unique to the NICU and have been recognized for many years, across all healthcare settings, age groups, and conditions. Patient-centered care and FCC lead to better health outcomes, improved patient and family experience of care, better clinician and staff satisfaction, and wiser allocation of resources when families are fully integrated into the care delivery system and treated as essential and irreplaceable partners in all aspects of healthcare delivery, from the bedside to the health system boardroom.[5–7] Nevertheless, healthcare services remain stubbornly professional-centric and institutional-centric, contributing to underperformance in attainment of quality and safety goals and adverse/suboptimal patient and family outcomes.[8,9]

As illustrated in the mother's personal reflection above, FCC requires intentional and coordinated effort from the healthcare team to overcome emotional, physical, and institutional barriers to achieve the level of parental partnership in care necessary to achieve optimal outcomes for infants and families. The quality improvement (QI) principle of improving reliability[10] applies equally to family partnership in caregiving as it does to other routine QI activities such as infection control. Greater investment in FCC QI to assure maximal family partnership both in caregiving and work undertaken to improve systems and processes of care is essential to optimizing infant and family outcomes during NICU stay, at NICU discharge and for long-term health, development and well-being.

In this review, we describe the principles and main constructs of family-centered neonatal care; discuss the state of the science and practice of FCC in the neonatal intensive care setting; and provide recommendations for assessment, development of practice standards and evaluation of FCC in the NICU setting. In keeping with the principles of family partnership and family-centeredness, a NICU parent advocacy organization leader served as a key partner in this review from the inception and is a coauthor (FB). Throughout we provide commentary from different parents, recognizing the imperfect level of partnership in the current healthcare quality and safety enterprise. We seek to further strengthen the voices and essential contributions of parents and caregivers of neonatal patients.

FAMILY-CENTERED CARE PRINCIPLES, CONSTRUCTS, AND CONCEPTS

FCC terminology and definitions vary by setting, discipline, and geography. The term person-centered care may be used to denote the holistic focus on the needs and strengths of the person that extend beyond health care to all societal systems.[11] In patient-centered care and FCC, the focus is on patients and families receiving healthcare services. Patients and their primary caregivers define their "family" and determine how they will participate in care and decision-making.[12] For neonates (or any other individuals who are unable to express their personal agency), parents or other primary caregivers act on behalf of the patient; hence, the use of the term FCC rather than patient and FCC.

Most models of FCC share the core principles of respect and dignity, information sharing, negotiation, participation, and collaboration (**Fig. 1**, **Table 1**).[12–14] FCC is rooted in the belief that partnerships among healthcare providers, patients, and families are mutually beneficial and lead to higher quality and safer health care. For a health system to be patient-centered and family-centered, there must be collaboration among all stakeholders, including healthcare professionals, administrators, funders, patients, family and community at all levels of care, in all healthcare settings and health systems operations, and health professional education.

Underlying the core principles of FCC are the foundational constructs of mutual trust and power-sharing (see **Fig. 1**). For FCC to occur, the healthcare practitioners must trust in the capabilities, knowledge and worth of the family, and families must trust in the capabilities and intentions of the healthcare team. Healthcare practitioners

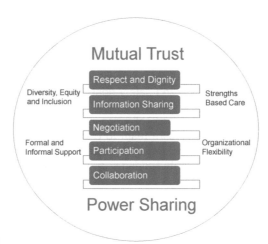

Fig. 1. Family-Centered Care (FCC) ecosystem.[1] The figure depicts the foundational constructs (*large type*), core principles of FCC (*boxes*), and corollary concepts (*regular type*) that comprise the FCC ecosystem. All elements must be addressed for optimal FCC to occur. (*Adapted from* Sigurdson K, Profit J, Dhurjati R, et al. Former NICU Families Describe Gaps in Family-Centered Care. Qual Health Res. 2020;30(12):1861-1875.)

must also be willing to share power and empower families to participate as equal partners in patient care.[15]

Corollary concepts in FCC that are also relevant to quality and safety include the following: strengths-based care; diversity, equity, and inclusion (DEI); formal and informal support; and organizational flexibility. Strengths-based approaches to health care recognize the family as the constant in a child's life and focus first on the positive attributes, capacities, and resources of the infant, family, and community, rather than solely focusing on deficits and needs.[16] DEI are similarly critical concepts, recognizing the preventable yet persistent harmful disparities in health care related to race, ethnicity, gender, and other social identities.[17] Incorporating a DEI focus in delivery of FCC and in FCC QI includes striving for a diverse workforce representative of the population served and training in DEI practices. DEI also pertains to NICU policies that ensure equity in access and delivery of all treatments and services. Formal and informal support refers to the recognition of the importance of providing both formal and structured support to enable FCC as well as encouraging informal peer support among families and with community. Finally, organizational flexibility refers to the concept of adaptable, learning, healthcare systems that can support the tailoring of FCC services to align with the strengths and needs of individual families.[11] FCC approaches that actively incorporate the core principles and corollary concepts create a supportive ecosystem, which then leads to improved quality, safety, and patient/ family experience and outcomes of neonatal care (see **Fig. 1**).

FAMILY-CENTERED CARE MODELS AND INTERVENTIONS

Having defined the principles, constructs, and concepts of FCC, the next step in assuring quality and safety is to evaluate the evidence for the various FCC models and intervention bundles. Adoption of evidence-based models of care has the potential to change not only care delivery but also hospital culture.[18] There are several family-centered and parent partnered-care models for the NICU setting supported by research evidence.[19] The models vary in emphasis but all share common elements:

Table 1
Core principles, constructs, and corollary concepts of patient-centered care and family-centered care[11-13]

Foundational Constructs	Mutual trust	Healthcare practitioners need to trust in the capabilities and worth of the family, and families need to trust in the capabilities and intentions of the healthcare practitioners
	Power sharing	Healthcare practitioners must be willing to share power and empower families to participate as equal partners in patient care and decision-making
Core Principles	Respect and dignity	Healthcare practitioners listen to and honor patient and family perspectives and choices. Patient and family knowledge, values, beliefs, and cultural backgrounds are incorporated into the planning and delivery of care
	Information sharing	Healthcare practitioners communicate and share complete and unbiased information with patients and families in ways that are affirming and useful. Patients and families receive timely, complete, and accurate information in order to effectively participate in care and decision-making
	Negotiation	Healthcare practitioners seek to gain an understanding of the patient and family's perspective, honor the family's right to advocate, explore, rather than explain, differences in perspective so everyone feels heard and validated, promote mutual trust and negotiate differences, which requires flexibility, responsiveness, and compromise
	Participation	Patients and families are encouraged and supported in participating in care and decision-making at the level they choose
	Collaboration	Patients, families, healthcare practitioners, and healthcare leaders collaborate in policy and program development, implementation, and evaluation; in facility design; in professional education; and in research; as well as in the delivery of care
Corollary Concepts	Strengths-based approaches	Healthcare practitioners and health systems recognize the family as the constant in a child's life and focus first on the positive attributes, capacities, and resources of the infant, family and community, rather than solely focusing on deficits and needs
	Diversity, Equity and Inclusion	Healthcare practitioners and health systems recognize the preventable yet persistent harmful disparities in health care related to race, ethnicity, gender, and other social identities
	Formal and informal support	Healthcare providers and health systems provide families with access to formal practical, educational, and emotional support, and encourage informal peer support among families and with community to enable families to participate fully as partners in health care
	Institutional flexibility	The health system works is an adaptable, learning, health systems that can support the tailoring of FCC services to align with the strengths and needs of individual families

providing a supportive environment, clearly defined and collaborative roles and responsibilities for parents, training, and parent-delivered interventions. In addition, there are numerous evidence-based parent-focused and parent-delivered interventions that support or enable FCC. The taxonomy in **Fig. 2** depicts the hierarchy of evidence-based parent support and parent-delivered interventions and the evidence-based parent-partnered care models for NICU FCC.

Family-Centered Models of Care

Many of the models of care, such as Kangaroo Mother Care, Care by Parent and Primary Nursing, have been around for decades and have a solid evidence base, yet have proven difficult to implement sustainably in many settings. Therefore, for the purposes of this review, we will focus on the 2 most recent models, Family Integrated Care (FICare)[20] and Close Collaboration with Parents,[21] which have been designed to address some of the implementation challenges of the prior models while maintaining fidelity to the principles of FCC. These models are briefly described below and in the state of the science and practice in the following section.

Family Integrated Care

In the FICare model (see **Fig. 2**, **Table 2**), parents are welcomed as part of the healthcare team and medical and nursing staff to promote parent involvement toward a level in which parents are supported as primary caregivers. Important to the implementation of FICare is the inclusion and partnership of veteran NICU parents in the core steering group to plan, implement, and sustain the FICare model on the unit. The FICare model has a comprehensive framework of interventions with 4 main pillars: environment; NICU team education and support; parent education/psychological support; and active parent participation/partnership. In this model, the environment is designed or adapted to support 24-hour parental presence/participation. The healthcare team receives training and ongoing support in FCC principles and skills and special needs of NICU families.[22,23] The healthcare team then receives recurring education on the needs of families and provides coaching, education, and mentorship to support parents. Parents are provided group educational sessions as well as individualized bedside teaching. Parents also receive psychosocial support from

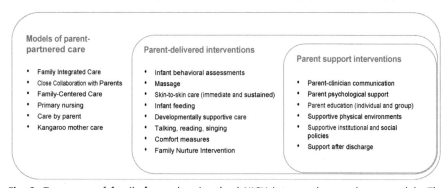

Fig. 2. Taxonomy of family-focused or involved NICU interventions and care models. The taxonomy depicts the hierarchy of evidence-based parent support and parent-delivered interventions and the evidence-based parent-partnered care models for NICU FCC. (*Adapted from* Franck LS, O'Brien K. The evolution of family-centered care: From supporting parent-delivered interventions to a model of family integrated care. Birth Defects Res. 2019;111(15):1044-1059.)

Table 2
Family Integrated Care (FICare) pillars (essential and recommended components)

Environment	NICU Team Education and Support	Parent Education/Psychological Support	Active Parent Participation/Partnership
Essential			
FICare steering committee comprising parent and multidisciplinary NICU team members			
• Comfortable, semireclining chairs at bedside to support prolonged parent presence and skin-to-skin contact	• NICU leadership support	• Regularly scheduled parent group classes	• Parent participation in baby's direct caregiving
• Dedicated parent room for respite away from but nearby NICU	• FICare nurse champions	• Individual teaching and skills building at bedside	• Parent active involvement in medical rounds and daily care planning
• Food storage and preparation area for parents	• Education on FICare for all team members	• Opportunities for peer-peer support with parent mentors	• Parent tracking progress (baby, their own)
• Place for parents to store coats and personal belongings	• Additional education for nurses emphasizing their role as teacher and coach with parents		
• 24-h NICU open access for parents to be with their babies	• FICare education included in orientation and annual skills updates		
• NICU and hospital policies and services that welcome and support parents			
Suggested			

• Dedicated space for families in patient care area	• Enhanced education on:
	  o Developmentally supportive care
	  o Trauma-informed care
	  o Communication skills
		• Parent classes offered evenings and weekends	• Technology support for remote participation in rounds and care planning

(continued on next page)

Table 2
(continued)

Environment	NICU Team Education and Support	Parent Education/Psychological Support	Active Parent Participation/ Partnership
• Single family room NICU	• Parent teaching, coaching, and communication included in NICU team core competencies and performance reviews	• NICU Family Advisory Council	• Technology support for tracking
• Discounted or subsidized food, parking, and transportation between home and hospital		• Stipends or other honoraria for parent mentors	
• Onsite childcare		• Paid parent liaison position	
• Extended paid parental leave for parents of NICU infants		• Technology support for parent education	

Adapted from Franck LS, Waddington C, O'Brien K. Family Integrated Care for Preterm Infants. Crit Care Nurs Clin North Am. 2020;32(2):149-165.

professionals and peer support from former NICU parents. Finally, parents are included on daily rounds and shared decision-making, and they are asked to actively participate in the care for their infant.

Studies have shown that the FICare model in level 2 and level 3 neonatal units across the world is adaptable and associated with improved infant and parent outcomes compared with generic or unstructured FCC implementation.[23] Improved infant outcomes at NICU discharge include higher rates of exclusive breastfeeding; increased weight gain; shorter lengths of stay; and lower infection rates.[24–30] In follow-up studies, preterm infants who were exposed to the FICare model during their NICU stay had more robust self-regulation, fewer challenges with sleep, eating, or communication, and less negative emotionality compared with infants who received NICU FCC.[31–33] Improved parent outcomes for FICare compared with FCC include less stress and improved mental health for mothers and fathers.[34–38] QI and evaluations of FICare indicate that improved infant, parent, and hospital-level outcomes shown in studies are sustained in real-world implementation.[39–42]

Close Collaboration with Parents

The Close Collaboration with Parents model (see **Fig. 2**, **Table 3**) provides education for the whole healthcare team of a neonatal or obstetric unit. By reaching each staff member of the unit, the intervention aims to change the unit's culture to become more family centered. The intervention provides skills for healthcare staff to collaborate with parents and support parenting during the hospital stay. After preparation with the unit leadership, the duration of the training and implementation phase is approximately 1.5 years. The training content includes the following: (1) observations and communication of infant behavior, (2) joint observations of infants with parents, (3) listening to parents' stories about how they become parents for this baby and providing individualized support, and (4) integrating shared decision-making regarding care and discharge planning. The training is integrated into daily practices and supported by reflective discussions. The main implementation strategy is mentoring. The implementation is planned collaboratively with the unit mentors and leaders and adapted to the context.[21]

Close Collaboration with Parents has been shown to improve FCC practices in diverse neonatal units.[43] Nurses reported better mutual trust with parents, better active listening, and shared decision-making skills and emotional support.[44,45] The intervention increased parental presence in the unit and duration of skin-to-skin care.[46] Infant growth was improved in the units that had implemented the Close Collaboration with Parents intervention compared with the units before or without the implementation.[47] Maternal depressive symptoms were decreased at 6 and 24 months after infant's due date.[48,49] The implementation of Close Collaboration with Parents has been more successful in neonatal units that dedicated sufficient time for the training, considered the timing carefully, and had strong support from the leadership and physicians involved.[50]

Family-Centered Care Interventions

Supportive interventions
Within the parent-partnered neonatal care models, or implemented individually, numerous interventions can be provided by NICUs to support FCC. The foundational or most basic of these are the family support interventions (see **Fig. 2**, right panel). These interventions provide the basic and essential services and processes of care to enable FCC to occur. Without these interventions, FCC cannot be implemented with fidelity, and there is risk of bias in access to FCC services, leading to disparities

Table 3
Core elements and implementation process of Close Collaboration with Parents

	Preparation	Training for Unit Leaders and Mentors	Staff Training and Implementation	Sustainability
Target population	Unit leadership	Unit leadership and unit mentors	Whole healthcare team of the unit	Whole healthcare team of the unit
Provider	Training team	Training team	Unit mentors and leadership Support by the training team	Unit staff and leaders Training team
Duration	6–12 mo	18 d per mentor within 3 mo	5 workdays for each staff member within 12–18 mo	Years
Content	Introducing the training program and its outcomes	Education including theory of 4 training phases, bedside practices, and reflective discussions Training about mentoring as facilitation method and reflective practices	E-learning course or manual about the theoretic background, bedside practices related to the content of each phase, and reflections on the practice experiences	E-learning course or manual about the theoretic background, bedside practices related to the content of each phase, and reflections on the practice experiences
Strategies	Negotiating about the commitment to the implementation Visit to the NICU in the training hospital to familiarize with the FCC culture Meetings	Lectures Bedside practices with experienced mentors Reflections with expert mentors	E-learning course or manual including theory, description, and demonstrations of the practices, and reflective questions Bedside practices with unit mentors Reflective discussions with unit mentors about experiences, innovations, and future needs for practice changes	Unit specific strategies for example, planning how to integrate the intervention in staff orientation Yearly seminars for networking organized by the training team

Evaluation	Reviewing unit plan	Reflections with the whole staff of the unit and leadership
		Monitoring by the leadership
		Following the fidelity by documentation of the realization of practices
		Following e-learning use by user statistics
		Reviewing the adherence of practice content
		The unit reports their implementation process and innovated practice changes

in service access, quality, and outcomes.[51] Without these foundational interventions, the other FCC interventions or models will not be effective or sustained.

Parent-Delivered Interventions

Parent-delivered interventions (see **Fig. 2**, middle panel) are specific techniques for NICU care delivery that can be performed with parents, once they have been trained. In many instances, the training can be brief and performed at the bedside. Most of the interventions, such as developmentally supportive care, require staff training and support for ongoing competency for the interventions to be properly implemented with parents.[52] All of the parent-delivered interventions listed in **Fig. 2** have a strong evidence base and should be practiced within any model of FCC.

CURRENT STATE OF FAMILY-STAFF PARTNERSHIP AND FAMILY-CENTERED CARE PRACTICE

Most NICUs purport to provide FCC. However, consistent implementation, ability to meet minimal requirements, and sustained fidelity have proven to be difficult and practice varies greatly among and within units and regions.[51,53–55] For example, in a large European multicenter qualitative study with NICU healthcare professionals, despite implementation of FICare principles in all the units, mother-infant separation was still very common.[55]

Including parents as primary caregivers requires a profound mind shift from professional-centered care and hierarchical hospital culture to ways of working in partnership with parents in all aspects of care, built on mutual trust and power sharing (see **Fig. 1**). The coronavirus disease 2019 (COVID-19)-pandemic has highlighted the relationship between deimplementation of FCC, increased parent-infant separation and disempowerment in infant care, and associated detrimental outcomes for patients and their families.[56,57]

One necessary condition for optimal FCC is unlimited access for parents to their infant. In another large European study, mothers spent approximately 8 hours and fathers 4 hours per day in the unit. Presence varied across units, with parents in some units staying less than an hour, and in others, they were present almost all the time.[58] Design features of NICUs such as single-family rooms, parent bed next to the infant, showers, and cooking facilities encourage and enable family presence.[58–62] However, the cultural and attitudinal environment of FCC are more important than the physical environment, and FCC can be successfully implemented even in crowded NICUs in older facilities if the clinical teams are committed and willing to invest their efforts in developing creative solutions.[55,63]

Another FCC necessity that is frequently lacking is provision of psychological support to parents.[64,65] Despite consensus that postpartum psychosocial care is essential, routine mental health care of primary caregivers in the NICU remains inadequate. In a US national study, less than half of the NICUs surveyed routinely screened for perinatal mental health problems or provided caregivers with psychoeducation about mental health self-care.[65] Neonatal staff are aware of this shortcoming and wish for comprehensive training on how to support parents.

QUALITY IMPROVEMENT STRATEGIES FOR FAMILY-CENTERED CARE

Evidence-based QI methods currently used to improve a wide range of NICU processes and outcomes are also useful for FCC QI. In fact, FCC QI can be accomplished with existing QI infrastructure (eg, roles and responsibilities, tools, communication strategies).[66] Similar to QI efforts targeting other clinical processes and outcomes, successful FCC QI requires building a cohesive team which can make decisions, identifying clear goals and achievable intermediate targets, selecting the appropriate assessments (measurement tools), designing, testing, and implementing interventions to improve performance, and explicitly planning for sustainability.[67] Perhaps, even more important for FCC QI than other NICU QI efforts (where it is also important), NICU families *must* be part of the QI core team and active in all aspects of the QI process, rather than being engaged solely for postimplementation consultation. With respect to measurement, FCC-specific assessments must be selected, adapted, or developed to monitor the agreed priority QI goals. Delivery of family support interventions and parent-delivered interventions must be assessed. Communication with families, support of staff and engagement with parent-led organizations are other areas where the QI focus should be tailored. Below, each of the aspects of FCC QI is discussed in more detail.

Building the Family-Centered Care Quality Improvement Team

Former NICU families should be included in the QI team along with representatives from all the main professional groups and decision-makers involved in providing care to neonates. In preparing this review, we spoke with family representatives involved in NICU QI, and they provided practical tips for engaging and preparing families to serve as NICU QI partners (**Table 4**). There should ideally be more than one parent on the committee so that they are not the "only one" on the committee. It is common to advise parents to reengage in NICU activities once their child has been home for at least a year after discharge. This is because the first year at home with an infant who has spent time in a NICU, with possible subsequent health issues and demands, can be very challenging for families. NICU families need training and ongoing support to prepare and engage in NICU FCC QI.

Useful resources for preparing to engage families in QI work include the Agency for Healthcare Quality evidence-based guidelines toolkit for QI partnership among patients, families, and healthcare professionals.[68] Ultimately, family participation enhances all QI work but for FCC QI, it is essential. The following quotes illustrate the importance of including parents in all NICU QI activities:

"As a parent, I have had the opportunity to collaborate on several QI projects in the NICU where my son was born. I can humbly attest to the value that is brought to the table when the perspective of a parent is shared. In meetings, I have shared my own thoughts and experiences or experiences of other parents on aspects of the project at hand. [I have] come to appreciate that often the ideas, barriers and challenges that I raise, despite best efforts, have not been thought of or realized by the medical team. My participation in QI work is gratifying and rewarding, and I am always thanked by the team for my valued contributions."

Another parent provided a specific example of a practice change resulting from their input:

"We bring a different kind of expertise. I feel valued when I know I've been heard. I've seen my ideas coming to life and this gives me the courage to keep going. For example, my hospital had a check list of practices when the baby was born and the list had a box: 'update the second parent.' I asked about the birthing parent as updating only one parent is not enough. Today, the check list has a box to 'update both parents'."

Assessing Family-Centered Care and Family-Staff Partnership Quality

Measurement and ongoing monitoring are essential components of any QI program. For FCC, (re)assessment must occur at the level of the patient, family, healthcare

Table 4
Tips for engaging and preparing families to serve as neonatal intensive care unit quality improvement partners

Topic	Advice from Parents
Parents' motivation to contribute to QI	"It's been 7 years since I came back to the same NICU where my baby was born. I came back because I was grateful for the care team, but I soon realized that besides being grateful I could advocate and be a voice of the families." "I like QI because you affect change on a policy level, and they happen. The knowledge and connections gained from QI help being an advocate elsewhere." "It's hard work and the pandemic made it harder. I am privileged as I have an emotionally and financially supportive partner, but the possibility of the impact I can make in changing the world is more than the tech job my husband does."
Preparing families and staff for collaborating on NICU QI issues	"Going back to the hospital either as a volunteer or paid position can be very hard for parents who had premature or sick babies admitted in the NICU. Besides the triggers, such as alarms, and the smell of soap, parent-partners learn things that can be emotionally difficult. Helpful framing for this could be: If we knew then what we know now it feels like your story could have changed, but we can't change the past." "The NICU staff need to be aware of the complicated emotions for a parent to have this role. We were not trained for this, parents are allowed to cry, and it doesn't mean that we can't do the job. It just means that we bring out feelings to this professional space. [It helps if] "triggering events" can be announced before they occur (ie, Picture of deceased baby to be shown)." "I was invited to review a new protocol for the NICU where my son was born. I was given a warning that the material could be hard to read as they were changing protocols from the time of birth (the golden hour) to improve outcomes related to the preterm brain. My task was to make sure the language used to inform new families in the NICU was accessible and in lay language. It was emotionally difficult to review and re-word it, but with enough support I got through the document with the QI nurse to create a one-page document that was given to parents informing minimal handling for 72-hours and how they could still participate in the care of their baby."

(continued on next page)

Topic	Advice from Parents
Table 4 ***(continued)***	
	"I felt overwhelmed for first year due to medical jargon. Committees where quite technical and some family participation was really not necessary. Over time found balance to be able to attend when input is valuable and not attend when not needed." *"When you get involved with advocacy there is a learning curve, and as you go from project to project you are more able to step away from your personal experience and allow it to inform your involvement as opposed to it being your involvement."* *"Provide background – explain the purpose of the committee. Language/training would be helpful but doesn't exist – most people don't know what a QI project is."*
Disparities when parents are volunteers and/or only parent and all other participants are paid staff	*"Being the only unpaid person makes speaking up challenging".* *"Need more than the experience from one parent – need other views, experience. In order to create policies or trainings. Diversity of opinions is important to be mindful of, but not possible to be 100% inclusive."* *"I felt dissatisfied with the type of family input in some projects, as it did not reflect the wide range of experiences that many families have. You need a great deal of time and to be of a certain economic status to be able to take 4 days out of your life and donate that time when you have a child with complex health needs."*
Parents as paid members of staff	*"Being a paid member allowed for more collaboration – necessary unless you hold the meetings at 9pm at night or find other ways for the member to become involved – Presence/Access/Respect all need to be in place."*
Parent impact on FCC and QI	*"There were occasions when my own words were used to create the visual flow of needs and presented on posters at conferences. Also was part of a video that was self-scripted and created and is being used. This is the signal that it's not just lip service –[I] felt listened to."*

team, and healthcare organization. Although there are no universally agreed standards or metrics for FCC, there are several useful assessment tools currently available, and more are undergoing testing. The Donabedian Structure-Process-Outcome framework[69,70] is helpful in organizing a comprehensive FCC QI assessment program (**Fig. 3**). Structural assessment includes measures of NICU and hospital-level resources and leadership necessary for FCC to thrive.[71] Process measures include measures of

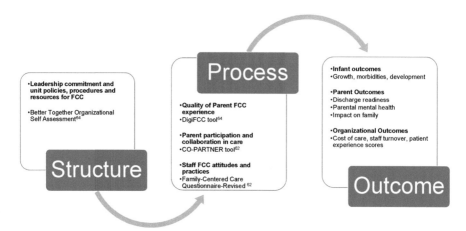

Fig. 3. Potential QI measures for FCC structure, process, and outcomes. This figure shows some potential evidence-informed QI measures for FCC structural elements, processes, and outcomes.

the completion and quality of processes that are essential to FCC implementation, including delivery of family support and parent-delivered interventions; staff knowledge and communication skills competence; interpersonal teamwork and unit culture climate;[72–75] parental presence and participation in caregiving; and shared decision-making, education, and skills.[76] Outcome measures include common infant, family, or organizational outcomes that may be sensitive to FCC interventions. Infant outcomes may include human milk intake, nosocomial infection or other adverse event rates, length of stay, growth, and improved cognitive and motor development or quality of life. Family outcomes may include measures of parental mental health and well-being. Organizational outcomes may include cost of care, adverse event rates, parent experience of care and organizational culture. **Fig. 3** shows some potential QI measures for FCC structural elements, processes, and outcomes. Future study is currently underway in developing core outcome sets and minimal reporting measures for FCC research, which could also be useful for QI in the NICU.[77] Although common metrics are important, the FCC QI team should establish measures that are locally relevant after consultation with all relevant stakeholders to identify and prioritize areas for improvement.

DEI in FCC QI is of particular importance to ensure NICU care quality. Therefore, FCC assessment should include measurement and analysis of structural, interpersonal and intrapersonal barriers to FCC to that specific context and measures should be stratified based on potential inequities. For example, if audits data reveals that parental participation in NICU rounds varies by demographics (eg, race or ethnicity, language spoken at home, education, or employment status), or if there is a difference in the level of parental participation in caregiving related to the concordance between staff role and demographics, then further analysis is warranted to uncover and address the barriers to improve parental participation. These barriers could for instance include the following: unavailability of interpreters or lack of childcare for siblings (structural); unwelcoming verbal or nonverbal communication by NICU staff to families (interpersonal); and extreme parental distress or lack of knowledge about their important role in clinical rounds (intrapersonal).[51] Only by measuring indicators of FCC DEI, can barriers be identified and addressed.

Creating Culture Change

One of the common themes among units that successfully implement and sustain FCC is a nurturing culture.[42,50,55] Culture is described as jointly held characteristics, values, thinking, and behaviors of people in workplaces and organizations. Units that had a comprehensive and sustained FCC approach, commonly included parents as members of hospital or unit boards, directly influencing management and decisions and regarded them as equal partners.[50,55]

Unfortunately, as the following quote illustrates, some units may have to commit to major culture change to transform their current practices to be more family-centered, as illustrated by this quote from a father:

"One nurse told me that when the babies are very sick, parents cannot hold them. I wish I knew what I know today; that I could have asked, that I could have held her, that I could comfort her when she was in pain. I learned years later that parents should be involved and care for their babies while they are in the NICU. This was not my experience and I still feel angry about this."

Changing hospital culture can be very difficult,[70] and approaches to change have been previously proposed,[18] and success stories have been shared.[39–42,50,78] First, attention must be given to how care is delivered at the bedside, listening to parents and staff. Second, all meaningful improvement should be local and tailored to the setting. Standardization and generic strategies are important starting points but may fail when they do not allow for tailoring to individual circumstances. Third, daily successes in the workplace must also be recognized, appreciating how the clinical team successfully handle dynamic situations, highlighting the factors that promote successful delivery of FCC. Successful cases of culture change usually share 4 common characteristics. They always start with the patient at the center of any proposed change; begin with small-scale initiatives and buildup; convert data and information into intelligence shared with appropriate decision makers; and focus on collaboration as the foundation of productive change rather than the lone hero model.[71] Leaders of successful QI focus on helping the team to create a new mental model of their collective work, appreciating the complexity of care systems and understanding that change is always unpredictable and takes time and sustained effort.[18]

Here is a quote on how one NICU medical leader described the culture change:

"Parents are doing this job for a reason. They are unique. They've been through the NICU journey and now they want to give back. We were pioneers here bringing parents voices in the entire QI process. It was a cultural shift so everyone had to become sensitive to the presence of parents. Parents in QI receive peer-to-peer support. They are all very involved in QI and their voices are quite powerful. We would [now] not consider not having a parent in a QI committee. We see them as colleagues."

Supporting Staff to Deliver High-Quality Family-Centered Care

Staff motivation, competence, and multiprofessional collaboration are essential to deliver high-quality FCC. To sustain and implement high-quality FCC with minimal separation between parents and infants, the overarching core values in successful units in Europe were the shared value to promote closeness between parents and their infants and common shared commitment to *collaboration* (between healthcare professionals, management, and parents), *capacities* (physical space, investment in staffing), and *coaching* (education of staff and parents).[55]

When significant professional staff shortages and high turnover, particularly among nurses, are present, hospital leaders have a nonevidence-based tendency to limit family presence as a means of reducing workload. However, as was poignantly learned during the COVID-19 pandemic, curtailing or eliminating family presence and FCC was harmful not only to quality and safety of patient care but also further eroded job satisfaction and caused moral distress for healthcare professionals.[79,80]

Addressing these challenges requires leadership and consistent commitment to daily practice in accordance with the principles of FCC. One US study showed that although FCC practices were overall strongly endorsed; there were indications of lack of knowledge or valuing of several key dimensions of FCC, particularly of family partnership at the organizational level and variability across neonatal units and with years of experience.[51,77] Initial and ongoing training and support of the whole healthcare staff is essential and should be treated with the same dedication and recurrence as advanced life support training. Frontline staff and parents should be consulted as to specific areas that need additional QI efforts. Common staff recommendations for the improvement of FCC included language translation and interpreter services for families; improving communication between staff and families; staffing and workflow; team, culture, and leadership; education; and NICU environment. Previous research has shown the need for greater resources for staffing, education, and environmental supports, as well as team culture and staff–parent communications.[51]

Professional and Parent Organization Engagement

FCC QI efforts can be advanced through engagement of parent-led organizations, which can assist with evaluation of the state of the science, building consensus on minimal standards, quality assessment metrics, and benchmarking. These outcomes in turn can be used to negotiate for necessary resources with healthcare administrators. Parent-led organizations can play a critically important role in providing support for families to fully engage in their infant's care and in NICU FCC QI efforts. Some organizations provide practical support to enable parents to stay in hospital, such as access to transportation, food, or support in finding accommodation near the hospital. Others provide education for families and healthcare professionals, deliver mental health programs, and organize peer support groups and training to hospitals to create peer support groups. Representatives from parent-led organizations can support FCC QI by referring potential parent members who have an interest in serving on a QI committee, providing training for parents and staff and facilitating consultations with former NICU families for the assessment of longer term outcomes.

Partnering with policy makers is a final essential component of FCC QI work to address the systemic barriers to FCC identified through as part of FCC QI initiatives. For example, lack of universal paid parental leave and reliable, quality childcare are 2 policy-level barriers to parental partnership in their infant's NICU care. Creating more equity in NICU FCC will require partnership and advocacy on these issues at local, regional, and national levels.

SUMMARY

Evidence abounds that implementation of FCC is beneficial to the health and safety of infants and families in neonatal care settings. Nevertheless, the systematic uptake of interventions required for high-quality and sustainable FCC remains challenging and suboptimal. Two FCC models with strong research evidence are FICare and Close Collaboration with parents. Well-established QI methodology can be applied to FCC QI and must include authentic partnership with neonatal families in FCC QI planning and activities. To further optimize NICU care, families should be included as essential and irreplaceable team members in all NICU QI activities, not only FCC QI activities.

Greater investment in FCC QI is needed to maximize the promise of FCC and ensure all families have equitable access to the necessary support and partnership with healthcare practitioners, and infants can reach their full health and developmental potential.

BEST PRACTICES

- Include former NICU families in the QI team along with representatives from all the main professional groups and decision-makers involved in providing care to neonates.
- Engage with parent-led organizations to expand support for NICU families and as partners in QI.
- Provide training and support for NICU family QI partners, and training for staff on how to engage families in QI.
- Consider evidence-based FCC models, and NICU culture change that might be needed to improve delivery of FCC.
- Support NICU staff to deliver high-quality FCC.
- Incorporate FCC structure, process and outcome metrics into NICU QI.

DECLARATION OF INTERESTS

The authors have nothing to disclose.

REFERENCES

1. North K, Whelan R, Folger LV, et al. Family involvement in the routine care of hospitalized preterm or low birth weight infants: a systematic review and meta-analysis. Pediatrics 2022;150(Suppl 1). e2022057092O.
2. UN general assembly, convention on the rights of the child, 20 November 1989, united Nations, treaty series, vol. 1577, p. 3. Available at: https://www.refworld.org/docid/3ae6b38f0.html. Accessed 29 October 2022.
3. EFCNI, Pallás-Alonso C, Westrup B, Kuhn P, et al. European standards of care for newborn health: parental involvement. 2022. Available at: https://newborn-health-standards.org/standards/standards-english/infant-family-centred-developmental-care/parental-involvement/. Accessed 29 October 2022.
4. EFCNI, Moen A, Hallberg B, et al. European Standards of Care for Newborn Health: core principles of NICU design to promote family-centred care. 2018. Available at: https://newborn-health-standards.org/standards/standards-english/nicu-design/core-principles-of-nicu-design-to-promote-family-centred-care/. Accessed October 29, 2022.
5. Kokorelias KM, Gignac MAM, Naglie G, et al. Towards a universal model of family centered care: a scoping review. BMC Health Serv Res 2019;19(1):564.
6. Davidson JE, Aslakson RA, Long AC, et al. Guidelines for family-centered care in the neonatal, pediatric, and adult ICU. Crit Care Med 2017;45(1):103–28.
7. Park M, Giap TT, Lee M, et al. Patient- and family-centered care interventions for improving the quality of health care: a review of systematic reviews. Int J Nurs Stud 2018;87:69–83. Epub 2018 Jul 26. PMID: 30056169.
8. Epstein RM, Fiscella K, Lesser CS, et al. Why the nation needs a policy push on patient-centered health care. Health Aff 2010;29(8):1489–95. PMID: 20679652.

9. Kelleher K, Hardy RY. Coming full circle (to hard questions): patient- and family-centered care in the hospital context. Fam Syst Health 2020;38(2):209–11.

10. The Health Foundation. Quality improvement made simple: what everyone should know about health care quality improvement. 2021. Available at: https://doi.org/10.37829/HF-2021-I05. Accessed 29 October 2022.

11. World Health Organization. WHO global strategy on integrated people-centred health services 2016-2026. Sixty-Ninth World Health Assembly, A69/39 Provisional agenda item 16.1. 2016. Available at: https://apps.who.int/gb/ebwha/pdf_files/WHA69/A69_39-en.pdf?ua=1&ua=1. Accessed 29 October 2022.

12. Committee on hospital care and institute for patient and family-centered care; patient- and family-centered care and the pediatrician's role. An Pediatr 2012;129(2):394–404.

13. Johnson BH, Abraham MR. Partnering with patients, residents, and families: a resource for leaders of hospitals, ambulatory care settings, and long-term care communities. (2012). Bethesda, MD: institute for Patient- and Family-Centered Care. Available at: https://ipfcc.org/about/pfcc.html. Accessed 29 October 2022.

14. Kaslow NJ, Dunn SE, Henry T, et al. Collaborative patient- and family-centered care for hospitalized individuals: best practices for hospitalist care teams. Fam Syst Health 2020;38(2):200–8.

15. Sigurdson K, Profit J, Dhurjati R, et al. Former NICU families describe gaps in family-centered care. Qual Health Res 2020;30(12):1861–75.

16. Peyton C, Sukal Moulton T, Carroll AJ, et al. Starting at birth: an integrative, state-of-the-science framework for optimizing infant Neuromotor health. Front Pediatr 2022;9:787196.

17. Parker MG, Hwang SS. Quality improvement approaches to reduce racial/ethnic disparities in the neonatal intensive care unit. Semin Perinatol 2021;45(4):151412.

18. Braithwaite J. Changing how we think about healthcare improvement. BMJ 2018;361:k2014.

19. Franck LS, O'Brien K. The evolution of family-centered care: from supporting parent-delivered interventions to a model of family integrated care. Birth Defects Res 2019;111(15):1044–59.

20. Franck LS, Waddington C, O'Brien K. Family integrated care for preterm infants. Crit Care Nurs Clin 2020;32(2):149–65.

21. Ahlqvist-Björkroth S, Boukydis Z, Axelin AM, et al. Close Collaboration with Parents™ intervention to improve parents' psychological well-being and child development: description of the intervention and study protocol. Behav Brain Res 2017;325(Pt B):303–10.

22. Family integrated care. Available at: http://familyintegratedcare.com. Accessed 29 October 2022.

23. British perinatal association. Family integrated care: a framework for practice. 2021. Available at: https://www.bapm.org/resources/ficare-framework-for-practice.

24. O'Brien K, Bracht M, Macdonell K, et al. A pilot cohort analytic study of Family Integrated Care in a Canadian neonatal intensive care unit. BMC Pregnancy Childbirth 2013;13(Suppl 1):S12.

25. O'Brien K, Robson K, Bracht M, et al. Effectiveness of Family Integrated Care in neonatal intensive care units on infant and parent outcomes: a multicentre, multinational, cluster-randomised controlled trial. Lancet Child Adolesc Health 2018;2(4):245–54 [published correction appears in Lancet Child Adolesc Health. 2018;2(8):e20].

26. Murphy M, Shah V, Benzies K. Effectiveness of alberta family-integrated care on neonatal outcomes: a cluster randomized controlled trial. J Clin Med 2021;10(24):5871.
27. He SW, Xiong YE, Zhu LH, et al. Impact of family integrated care on infants' clinical outcomes in two children's hospitals in China: a pre-post intervention study. Ital J Pediatr 2018;44(1):65.
28. van Veenendaal NR, van der Schoor SRD, Heideman WH, et al. Family integrated care in single family rooms for preterm infants and late-onset sepsis: a retrospective study and mediation analysis. Pediatr Res 2020;88(4):593–600.
29. Chen H, Dong L. The effect of family integrated care on the prognosis of premature infants. BMC Pediatr 2022;22(1):668.
30. Franck LS, Gay CL, Hoffmann TJ, et al. Neonatal outcomes from a quasi-experimental clinical trial of Family Integrated Care versus Family-Centered Care for preterm infants in U.S. NICUs. BMC Pediatr 2022;22(1):674.
31. Synnes AR, Petrie J, Grunau RE, et al. Family integrated care: very preterm neurodevelopmental outcomes at 18 months. Arch Dis Child Fetal Neonatal Ed 2022;107(1):76–81.
32. Church PT, Grunau RE, Mirea L, et al. Family Integrated Care (FICare): positive impact on behavioural outcomes at 18 months. Early Hum Dev 2020;151:105196.
33. Moe AM, Kurilova J, Afzal AR, et al. Effects of alberta family integrated care (FICare) on preterm infant development: two studies at 2 Months and between 6 and 24 Months corrected age. J Clin Med 2022;11(6):1684.
34. Cheng C, Franck LS, Ye XY, et al. Evaluating the effect of Family Integrated Care on maternal stress and anxiety in neonatal intensive care units. J Reprod Infant Psychol 2021;39(2):166–79.
35. Dien R, Benzies KM, Zanoni P, et al. Alberta family integrated Care™ and standard care: a qualitative study of mothers' experiences of their journeying to home from the neonatal intensive care unit. Glob Qual Nurs Res 2022;9. 23333936221097113.
36. Mclean MA, Scoten OC, Yu W, et al. Lower maternal chronic physiological stress and better child behavior at 18 Months: follow-up of a cluster randomized trial of neonatal intensive care unit family integrated care. J Pediatr 2022;243:107–15.e4.
37. van Veenendaal NR, van der Schoor SRD, Broekman BFP, et al. Association of a family integrated care model with paternal mental health outcomes during neonatal hospitalization. JAMA Netw Open 2022;5(1):e2144720.
38. van Veenendaal NR, van Kempen AAMW, Broekman BFP, et al. Association of a zero-separation neonatal care model with stress in mothers of preterm infants. JAMA Netw Open 2022;5(3):e224514.
39. Banerjee J, Aloysius A, Mitchell K, et al. Improving infant outcomes through implementation of a family integrated care bundle including a parent supporting mobile application. Arch Dis Child Fetal Neonatal Ed 2020;105(2):172–7.
40. Moreno-Sanz B, Montes MT, Antón M, et al. Scaling up the family integrated care model in a level IIIC neonatal intensive care unit: a systematic approach to the methods and effort taken for implementation. Front Pediatr 2021;9:682097.
41. Zanoni P, Scime NV, Benzies K, et al. Alberta FICare in Level II NICU Study Team; Alberta FICare™ in Level II NICU Study Team. Facilitators and barriers to implementation of Alberta family integrated care (FICare) in level II neonatal intensive care units: a qualitative process evaluation substudy of a multicentre cluster-randomised controlled trial using the consolidated framework for implementation research. BMJ Open 2021;11(10):e054938.

42. Patel N, Ballantyne A, Bowker G, et al, Helping Us Grow Group (HUGG). Family Integrated Care: changing the culture in the neonatal unit. Arch Dis Child 2018; 103(5):415–9.
43. Toivonen M, Lehtonen L, Löyttyniemi E, et al. Close Collaboration with Parents intervention improves family-centered care in different neonatal unit contexts: a pre-post study. Pediatr Res 2020;88(3):421–8.
44. Axelin A, Ahlqvist-Björkroth S, Kauppila W, et al. Nurses' perspectives on the close collaboration with parents training program in the NICU. MCN Am J Matern/Child Nurs 2014;39(4):260–8.
45. Toivonen M, Lehtonen L, Ahlqvist-Björkroth S, et al. Effects of the close collaboration with parents intervention on the quality of family-centered care in NICUs [published online ahead of print, 2021 sep 30]. Adv Neonatal Care 2021. https://doi.org/10.1097/ANC.0000000000000953.
46. He FB, Axelin A, Ahlqvist-Björkroth S, et al. Effectiveness of the close collaboration with parents intervention on parent-infant closeness in NICU. BMC Pediatr 2021;21(1):28.
47. Itoshima R, Helenius K, Ahlqvist-Björkroth S, Axelin A, Lehtonen L. Effects of Close Collaboration with Parents intervention on length of stay and growth in preterm infants: a Finnish register study (under review).
48. Ahlqvist-Björkroth S, Axelin A, Korja R, et al. An educational intervention for NICU staff decreased maternal postpartum depression. Pediatr Res 2019;85(7):982–6.
49. Ahlqvist-Björkroth S, Axelin A, Setänen S, et al. Fewer maternal depression symptoms after the Close Collaboration with Parents intervention: two-year follow-up. Acta Paediatr 2022;111(6):1160–6.
50. Toivonen M, Lehtonen L, Ahlqvist-Björkroth S, et al. Key factors supporting implementation of A training program for neonatal family- centered care - a qualitative study. BMC Health Serv Res 2019;19(1):394.
51. Franck LS, Bisgaard R, Cormier DM, et al. Improving family-centered care for infants in neonatal intensive care units: recommendations from frontline healthcare professionals. Adv Neonatal Care 2022;22(1):79–86.
52. Family and infant neurodevelopmental education (FINE). Available at: https://www.finetraininguk.com. Accessed 29 October 2022.
53. Dharmarajah K, Seager E, Deierl A, et al. Mapping family integrated care practices in the neonatal units across the UK. Arch Dis Child Fetal Neonatal Ed 2020;105:F111–2.
54. Reid S, Bredemeyer S, Chiarella M. Perceptions of parents and healthcare professionals on family centred care in Australian neonatal units. J Neonatal Nurs 2022 (in press).
55. van Veenendaal NR, Labrie NHM, Mader S, et al. An international study on implementation and facilitators and barriers for parent-infant closeness in neonatal units. Pediatr Investig 2022;6(3):179–88.
56. van Veenendaal NR, Deierl A, Bacchini F, et al. International Steering Committee for Family Integrated Care. Supporting parents as essential care partners in neonatal units during the SARS-CoV-2 pandemic. Acta Paediatr 2021;110(7): 2008–22.
57. Kostenzer J, Zimmermann LJI, Mader S, EFCNI COVID-19 Zero Separation Collaborative Group. Zero separation: infant and family-centred developmental care in times of COVID-19. Lancet Child Adolesc Health 2022;6(1):7–8.
58. Raiskila S, Axelin A, Toome L, et al. Parents' presence and parent-infant closeness in 11 neonatal intensive care units in six European countries vary between and within the countries. Acta Paediatr 2017;106(6):878–88.

59. van Veenendaal NR, Heideman WH, Limpens J, et al. Hospitalising preterm infants in single family rooms versus open bay units: a systematic review and meta-analysis. Lancet Child Adolesc Health 2019;3(3):147–57.

60. van Veenendaal NR, van Kempen AAMW, Franck LS, et al. Hospitalising preterm infants in single family rooms versus open bay units: a systematic review and meta-analysis of impact on parents. EClinicalMedicine 2020;23:100388.

61. Axelin A, Feeley N, Campbell-Yeo M, et al. Symptoms of depression in parents after discharge from NICU associated with family-centred care. J Adv Nurs 2022;78(6):1676–87.

62. Lehtonen L, Lilliesköld S, De Coen K, et al. Parent-infant closeness after preterm birth and depressive symptoms: a longitudinal study. Front Psychol 2022;13:906531.

63. O'Brien K, Bracht M, Macdonell K, et al. A pilot cohort analytic study of Family Integrated Care in a Canadian neonatal intensive care unit. BMC Pregnancy Childbirth 2013;13(Suppl 1):S12.

64. Separation and Closeness Experiences in Neonatal Environment (SCENE) research group. Parent and nurse perceptions on the quality of family-centred care in 11 European NICUs [published correction appears in Aust Crit Care. 2017 Jan;30(1):53-54]. Aust Crit Care 2016;29(4):201–9.

65. Bloyd C, Murthy S, Song C, et al. National cross-sectional study of mental health screening practices for primary caregivers of NICU infants. Children 2022;9(6):793.

66. Profit J, Gould JB, Peña MM, et al. Improving the quality, safety, and equity of neonatal intensive care for infants and families. In Fannaroff A and Martin R Neonatal Perinatal Medicine, 12th (in press).

67. Centers for Disease Control and Prevention. Applying the knowledge to action (K2A) framework: questions to guide planning. Atlanta, GA: Centers for Disease Control and Prevention, US Dept of Health and Human Services; 2014.

68. Agency for Healthcare Quality. Evidence-based guidelines toolkit for QI partnership among patients, families, and health professionals. Available at: https://www.ahrq.gov/patient-safety/patients-families/engagingfamilies/index.html. Accessed 29 October 2022.

69. Donabedian A. The quality of care. How can it be assessed? JAMA 1988;260(12):1743–8.

70. McDonald KM, Sundaram V, Bravata DM, et al. Closing the quality gap: a critical analysis of quality improvement strategies, vol. 7. Rockville (MD): Agency for Healthcare Research and Quality (US); 2007. Care Coordination.

71. Braithwaite J, Herkes J, Ludlow K, et al. Association between organisational and workplace cultures, and patient outcomes: systematic review. BMJ Open 2017;7(11):e017708.

72. Institute for patient and family centered care. Better together: partnering with families in hospitals. Organizational self assessment. Available at: https://www.ipfcc.org/bestpractices/IPFCC_Better_Together_Self_Assessment_June_2021.pdf. Accessed 29 October 2022.

73. Kainiemi E, Flacking R, Lehtonen L, et al. Psychometric properties of an instrument to measure the quality of family-centered care in NICUs. J Obstet Gynecol Neonatal Nurs 2022;51(4):461–72.

74. Bruce B, Ritchie J. Nurses' practices and perceptions of family-centered care. J Pediatr Nurs 1997;12(4):214–22.

75. van Veenendaal NR, Auxier JN, van der Schoor SRD, et al. Development and psychometric evaluation of the CO-PARTNER tool for collaboration and parent participation in neonatal care. PLoS One 2021;16(6):e0252074.

76. Development of a COS for family interventions in the NICU. COMET Initiative. Available at: https://comet-initiative.org/Studies/Details/1925 [Accessed 29 October 2022.

77. Franck LS, Cormier DM, Hutchison J, et al. A multisite survey of NICU healthcare professionals' perceptions about family-centered care. Adv Neonatal Care 2021; 21(3):205–13.

78. Braithwaite J, Mannion R, Matsuyama Y, et al. Accomplishing reform: successful case studies drawn from the health systems of 60 countries. Int J Qual Health Care 2017;29(6):880–6.

79. Semaan A, Audet C, Huysmans E, et al. Voices from the frontline: findings from a thematic analysis of a rapid online global survey of maternal and newborn health professionals facing the COVID-19 pandemic. BMJ global health 2020;5(6): e002967.

80. Bainter J, Fry M, Miller B, et al. Family presence in the NICU: constraints and opportunities in the COVID-19 Era. Pediatr Nurs 2020;46:256.

The Electronic Health Record as a Quality Improvement Tool
Exceptional Potential with Special Considerations

Leah H. Carr, MD[a,b,c,d,*], Lori Christ, MD[a,b,c], Daria F. Ferro, MD[c,d,e]

KEYWORDS

- Electronic health record • Clinical informatics • Data analytics • Quality improvement

KEY POINTS

- The recent widespread adoption of electronic health records (EHRs) allows for new methods of discrete data capture and testing and implementation interventions within the EHR as part of quality improvement (QI) initiatives.
- Although there are many promising avenues for effective integration of the EHR within QI efforts, there are multiple special considerations needed for this type of work.
- Key factors that must be addressed when using the EHR as an improvement tool include, but are not limited to, inclusion of informatics-focused team members on improvement teams, attention to human factors during clinical decision support design, and recognition of the underlying data structure of the EHR.

INTRODUCTION

Electronic health records (EHRs) are software systems focused on comprehensive patient health. Unlike electronic medical records (EMRs), which represent a digitized version of prior patient charts, EHRs are intended to capture all aspects of clinical

[a] Division of Neonatology, Department of Pediatrics, Children's Hospital of Philadelphia, 3400 Civic Center Boulevard, Philadelphia, PA 19104, USA; [b] Division of Neonatology, Department of Pediatrics, Children's Hospital of Philadelphia Newborn Care at the Hospital of the University of Pennsylvania, 3400 Spruce Street, 8 Ravdin, Philadelphia, PA 19104, USA; [c] Department of Pediatrics, University of Pennsylvania Perelman School of Medicine, Philadelphia, PA, USA; [d] Department of Biomedical and Health Informatics, Children's Hospital of Philadelphia, 2716 South Street, Philadelphia, PA 19146, USA; [e] Division of General Pediatrics, Department of Pediatrics, Children's Hospital of Philadelphia, 3400 Civic Center Boulevard, Philadelphia, PA 19104, USA
* Corresponding author. Division of Neonatology, Children's Hospital of Philadelphia Main Hospital, 3400 Civic Center Boulevard, 2NW59, Philadelphia, PA 19104.
E-mail address: carrlh@chop.edu

Clin Perinatol 50 (2023) 473–488
https://doi.org/10.1016/j.clp.2023.01.008
perinatology.theclinics.com

care, offer support to providers while interacting with the system, and transcend singular patient practice.[1] The history of EHR development and adoption reflects recognition of these systems' promises to aid in improving patient care delivery at the individual and population levels.

Although the earliest versions of US-based EMRs and EHRs began in the 1960s, the immense growth was noted in the early 2000s, largely due to governmental efforts to encourage the broad implementation of EHRs through incentives and legislation.[2–4] Recently, passage of the twenty-first Century Cures Act in 2016 and the "Final Rule" interpreting this law in 2021 further legislated how information is shared in the EHR.[4,5] These governmental changes aligned with a marked rise in EHR adoption across clinical settings. As of 2019, 96% of nonfederal hospitals were noted to have a certified EHR.[6–9]

The EHR has the potential to serve as a strong quality improvement (QI) tool, acting as a vehicle to implement change ideas as well as for data creation, extraction, and presentation in support of measuring the impact of changes. However, usage of the EHR in QI comes with its own special considerations. In this review, the authors discuss how the EHR can be used to support QI through clinical decision support (CDS), data capture, and measurement. The authors also address potential unintended consequences of EHR usage in QI work. The authors provide context for the concepts discussed here with a clinical case example, to which the authors refer to reinforce select concepts (**Box 1**).

BUILDING THE NECESSARY TEAM

Beyond the clinical partners and support staff who may compose a typical QI team, if the QI initiative will include work involving the EHR, the team should be expanded beyond this core group. Although the titles and job descriptions may vary across institutions, there are a range of individuals with EHR-related expertise who are important to include in your QI team if you intend to test and implement EHR-based interventions and/or use EHR data to track project outcomes.

If planning to design and implement an EHR-based intervention, your team will need an individual capable of making this modification. This may mean bringing in an EHR analyst, typically a nonclinical, technical expert within a system's Information Services team or a provider builder, a clinician with the skills and permissions to modify your EHR. Analysts and builders are also knowledgeable about local governance processes required to ensure your project is meeting appropriate institutional standards for safety and maintenance purposes. For example, your institution may have a ticket queue for change requests and/or there may be a committee at your center where you need to present your proposed changes to obtain feedback or design recommendations before implementation.

Similarly, if planning to use automated data collection for you project, it is helpful to engage individuals with this expertise at the outset of the project to optimize the measurement plan. A data analyst is an individual who gathers data (ie, "queries") from EHR databases, transforms these data into useful visuals, and/or applies these skills to other digital data collection systems. A data analyst can also assist with the use of external databases and survey tools (eg, REDCap[11]) if needed. In working with a data analyst, you may choose to request data that is provided to you in a raw spreadsheet from which you can create run or control charts, or you might request this be handled by a data analyst. Data analysts may also be able to design dashboards where you can visualize and/or extract data at any time as opposed to waiting for intermittent or scheduled data delivery.

Box 1
Case example: introduction

A neonatology team notes that 50% of their very low birth weight (VLBW) infants admitted from the delivery room (DR) to the neonatal intensive care unit (NICU) have admission hypothermia.

Unit QI leaders propose a project to reduce the rate of admission hypothermia to <25% of all admitted VLBW infants within a year. The QI project lead assembles a team composed of NICU providers, staff, and nursing leaders.

The hospital has an EHR system that includes computerized order entry, digital provider documentation, and charting of vital signs, medication administration, and laboratory testing. Most of the EHR information is stored in a database that can be accessed by hospital personnel with the appropriate credentials. DR resuscitation information is recorded on paper.

The team identifies the following project measures.

- Outcome: Percent of infants with an admission temperature <36C

- Process:
  ○ Percent compliance with DR temperature regulation policies
  ○ Duration of DR resuscitation.

- Balancing: Percent of infants with hyperthermia defined as admission temperature >37.5C

The team evaluates current processes and observes several potential barriers to successful thermoregulation. They also recognize a missed opportunity to use the EHR for data collection and decision support.

The team begins implementing several initial interventions outside of the EHR through staged Plan-Do-Study-Act (PDSA) cycles.[10] They plan two PDSA cycles using the EHR to support reliable completion of all aspects of thermoregulation in the DR and to monitor performance with real-time feedback on outcomes, process, and balancing measures. These PDSA cycles include.

- PDSA ramp 1: Design of an electronic CDS tool that includes the key DR checklist items (eg, DR resuscitation duration, patient temperature leaving the DR, adherence to thermoregulation bundle elements).

- PDSA ramp 2: Creation of a project dashboard with automated extraction of related data.

To begin to work on these PDSA cycles, what are the team's next steps?

More broadly, it can be helpful to include staff with clinical informatics expertise to act as a bridge between clinical content experts and your technical support personnel (eg, EHR analyst, data analyst). Clinical informatics specialists have expertise in the creation, storage, retrieval, usage, and presentation of healthcare-related data. The American Board of Preventive Medicine, a group who oversees the certification of physician clinical informatics specialists, notes that those who practice in this area often "collaborate with other health care and information technology professionals to analyze, design, implement, and evaluate information and communication systems that enhance individual and population health outcomes."[12] In other words, those who work in clinical informatics often serve as a link between other clinical providers, QI teams, operational leaders, and the world of data and information technology. These specialists may at times serve multiple roles on a project team (eg, EHR analyst). If clinical informatics specialists are not available at your institution, these collaborative activities may be performed by an individual with some training in your specific EHR and may have a title such as EHR super user, EHR champion, and/or be the same person serving as your provider builder.

Last, if introduction of a significant EHR modification or additional task is under consideration for a project, particularly if it affects multiple clinical groups, you may also consider an executive informatics sponsor. In most health systems, this sponsor might be a chief medical information officer (CMIO) or a chief health informatics/information officer (CHIO). The CMIO/CHIO oversees the enterprise health informatics infrastructure at an executive level while traversing between clinical medicine and administration (**Box 2**).

INCORPORATING ELECTRONIC HEALTH RECORD-BASED INTERVENTIONS IN QUALITY IMPROVEMENT PROJECTS
General Principles for Electronic Health Record-Based Interventions

EHR-based interventions can be powerful tools to drive change. The "Fundamental Theorem" of bioinformatics states that, when designed and implemented properly, technology combined with human efforts can perform better than the human alone.[16] Designing a new EHR-based intervention requires consideration of concepts within a sector of clinical informatics called "cognitive informatics." This evolving field focuses on the convergence of behavioral sciences, including human factors engineering and healthcare-related information technology. Cognitive informatics aims to examine the interactions between humans, technology, and other aspects of the incredibly complex systems in which they are asked to perform their daily tasks.[17–19] Inclusion of cognitive informatics concepts when implementing an EHR-based QI intervention ensures that we are addressing multiple components of Deming's theory of "profound knowledge" which highlights psychology of change, theory of knowledge, and appreciation of a system[20] in optimizing the chances of an intervention's success. It is important to note that although EHR-based interventions are often considered by QI teams, low-technology efforts can often be as successful, especially in early stages, and may greatly inform ultimate EHR modifications.

Clinical Decision Support Interventions

Many proposed QI interventions involving the EHR will fall into the category of CDS. Broadly, CDS includes any tools that are intended to assist with decision-making by individuals working in health care and therefore may include noncomputer-based support systems such as paper checklists and digital non-EHR tools such as drug

---

Box 2
Case example: expanding the quality improvement team

Because the QI team working to reduce admission hypothermia intends to use the EHR to support reliable completion of thermoregulation care in the DR (via a digital checklist) and to monitor performance with real-time feedback of process, outcome, and balancing measures, they expand their team to include individuals with informatics and EHR-expertise.

They engage an EHR analyst and provider builder to help construct the digital DR checklist (PDSA 1) and involve a data analyst to assist with creating a project-specific dashboard to track key metrics (PDSA 2).

A clinical informaticist joins the team as a core member to assist in communicating with the builder and analysts and to ensure the team is going through the appropriate channels as they modify the system and work to obtain their data.

Finally, given the increased morbidity and mortality of cold stress on premature infants,[13–15] the CMIO is engaged to aid in removal of institutional barriers to prioritize the EHR-based modifications for the initiative.

The EHR analyst notes that once the digital checklist is created in the EHR, it will be difficult to modify often, so it should be in a finalized form before EHR design begins. How can the team ensure that the checklist will suit their needs before "going live?"

formulary guidance. CDS within the EHR might include groupings of orders (eg, order panels, order sets), documentation templates, information to guide a provider embedded within an order, and alerts. Like guidelines for medication administration safety, ideal CDS meets "Five Rights:" (1) delivering the right information (2) to the right people (3) through the right format (4) via the right channel (5) at the right time in the workflow.[21]

There have been several successful examples of CDS interventions leveraging the EHR within neonatal–perinatal QI initiatives. For example, in an initiative to decrease variability in time to discharge from last apnea of prematurity event using improved documentation, a QI team identified lack of complete documentation about apnea/bradycardia/desaturation events as a key driver of variability. They surveyed bedside NICU nurses and physicians regarding key elements needed for decision-making and drafted an updated EHR flow sheet based on this feedback. This improved flow sheet allowed for improved documentation with important clarifying information regarding the apnea/bradycardia/desaturation events added at point of entry. A team representative presented the updates to the health system EHR governance committee, which spans four hospitals with NICUs. All NICUs came to agreement on the updated flow sheet, and an EHR analyst made the changes within the EHR. Nursing and physician satisfaction with documentation increased and the team achieved their goal of decreasing variability in time to discharge for infants with apnea of prematurity.[22]

In another QI initiative designed to improve compliance with an NICU patient QI/safety checklist, the QI team started by developing and testing a paper version of novel checklist. Through the iterative cycles of learning and feedback, the team refined the paper checklist. Once use was sustained at a high level, they transitioned to an EHR-embedded checklist, with data that could then be captured in an automated manner.[23] Similarly, a newborn nursery QI team working to streamline clinical care and decrease time to discharge for low-risk term newborns and their birthing parents effectively used the EHR to facilitate their improvement work. Through partnership with an EHR analyst, low-risk criteria and aspects of discharge care were identified and displayed via an EHR-embedded dashboard, which was associated with a decrease in length of stay from 2.3 to 2 days.[24] In another instance, a level III NICU team sought to improve documentation for patients that may qualify for therapeutic hypothermia. Integration of an enhanced documentation template embedded with CDS correlated with an improvement in comprehensive documentation from 50% to 80%.[25]

Electronic Health Record-Based Interventions Require Culture Change

The implementation of new EHR-based interventions requires culture change. Even the introduction of relatively minor changes can be jarring for clinical staff. It is important to ensure that adequate timing is allocated for training and feedback as modifications are rolled out. In addition to initial planning, taking an agile approach with the ability for iterative change is especially helpful.[26] Flexibility in design will allow incorporation of this feedback from clinical users. It is also necessary to consider the varying needs of stakeholders. As Ash and colleagues highlight, there are "Special People" who often play a role in the successful roll out of EHR-based interventions and this concept extends to all stakeholder groups involved in QI efforts. They can include administrative leaders (ie, executive members), clinical leaders, and "bridgers," such as support staff and informaticists. Among the clinical leaders, it is essential to know who will champion your effort—"champions," who will have a valued, strong voice for or against the effort—"opinion leaders," and who will be vocal in skepticism, but may become the strongest supporters—"curmudgeons."[27] Buy-in from these roles is needed for implementation success and the value of "at-the-elbow" support cannot be diminished as you go through your roll-out (**Box 3**).

USING THE ELECTRONIC HEALTH RECORD FOR QUALITY IMPROVEMENT DATA CAPTURE AND MEASUREMENT

Data and measurement are fundamental to the Model for Improvement question, "How will I know that a change is an improvement?" Using EHR data in QI initiatives requires understanding EHR infrastructures to aptly define measures, assess data quality (output), access the needed data, and communicate effectively.

What Is Data?

Within health care, we commonly discuss the creation and interpretation of "data," and many QI projects involve the crafting of a "data request" for evaluation purposes. It is important to recognize that the term "data" may have different meanings to each team member. This can best be understood in the context of a frequently used model in information management, the data-information-knowledge-wisdom (DIKW) hierarchy (**Fig. 2**).

The DIKW pyramidal model displays data as comprising the largest amount of content in the rawest form, without context or meaning. Information sits immediately above data in the DIKW pyramid and is often what is desired when a team requests data. Information is a format that adds additional context. Knowledge sits above information in the DIKW pyramid. Knowledge applies some degree of evidence, interpretation, and further context to the information provided. At the very top of the pyramid, stands wisdom, the component of the hierarchy where further understanding can be used to convey judgment.[28,29] When the data are collected for use in a QI effort, collection in a raw form is often necessary. Context and judgment that are applied as the team progresses up the DIKW pyramid bring the data from raw to interpretable.

Box 3
Case example: developing an electronic health record-based checklist

As they embark on PDSA cycle 1 (digitization of their DR checklist), consideration of the Five Rights of CDS will be essential.

Fig. 1 demonstrates how the CDS Five Rights can be applied broadly in this QI project, and specifically regarding the design of CDS to support reliable implementation of the DR thermoregulation care practices.

Based on the Five Rights, opportunities for CDS could include easily accessible guidelines, a checklist specific to VBLW infants, and an embedded alert flag that indicates abnormal temperature values in a non-interruptive manner.

The team tests a paper checklist specific to VLBW infants and tests this paper checklist with known "champions" and "opinion leaders" to garner feedback through a series of PDSA cycles. With each successive version, feedback becomes more positive, and "champions" are asked to coach all clinicians to use the checklist in the DR.

Once consensus is reached by the team that the checklist is in a finalized state, it is presented to EHR governance and work begins to construct the checklist in the EHR. The EHR analyst checks back with the team frequently during the build to ensure that the checklist and associated CDS is functioning as expected.

Once the checklist is "live," the team wants to ensure that data can be queried to continue to inform their QI efforts. What else does the team need to know?

Clinical Decision Support Opportunity	CDS Five Rights				
	Right information	Right people	Right format	Right channel	Right time
VLBW Temperature Management	VLBW DR Management Policy	DR/NICU team	Reference, educational documentation	Health system intranet, link accessible from the EHR	Scheduled education session or "just in time" for anticipated VLBW deliveries
	VLBW DR Management Checklist	DR/NICU team	Brief statements with space for appropriate documentation of completion. If on paper – should be in a standard, easy-to-find location where the DR "recording" team member usually works. If in the EHR, access to the checklist should be highlighted for anticipated VLBW patients. Checklist should include a link to reference materials.	EHR	Pre-delivery DR huddle
	Abnormal temperature detected	NICU care team	Abnormal value flag (!) where vital signs are charted and in any reports that contain the value	EHR	Upon recording of and admission temperature that is outside the defined normative values

Fig. 1. Example of the application of the CDS Five Rights to a QI initiative to reduce admission hypothermia. An opportunity for CDS in this context may include easily accessible guidelines in the EHR or via hospital intranet, a checklist specific to VBLW infants accessed in the EHR in the predelivery huddle, or an embedded alert flag that indicates abnormal temperature values in a non-interruptive manner when the vital sign is charted in the EHR.

This is true for projects that leverage the EHR and those that do not. Understanding the EHR data structure helps to apply these data definition concepts when the EHR is being leveraged.

How Data Move into and Out of the Electronic Health Record

Health care data stored in the EHR are complex, partially because these are presented in many forms. Some data are stored discretely as a structured element that is more easily retrieved. Discrete data may include elements such as a patient's vital sign. This differs from unstructured health care data, which can include scanned documents, free text clinical notes, and imaging studies.[30] Additional complexity can be added when considering continuous data such as those from cardiorespiratory monitors. Metadata, defined as data regarding data, are also collected in the EHR.[31] The examples of metadata might include a timestamp of when a nurse enters and saves an admission temperature value.

Databases serve as repositories for all data. EHR data are often ultimately housed in "relational databases" which include multiple tables specific to different topics and

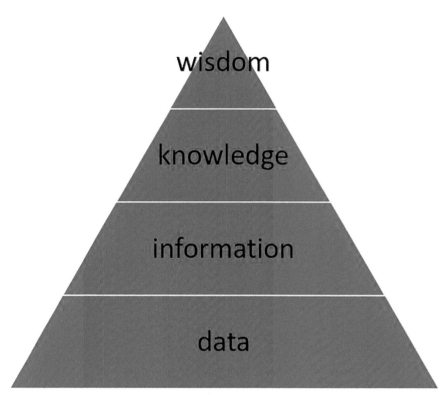

Fig. 2. Data-information-knowledge-wisdom (DIKW) hierarchy. Frequently used model of information management that represents relationships between data, information, knowledge, and wisdom. Each step reflects increasing amounts of value, interpretation, and context.

can be used for reporting purposes. Relational database tables can be joined together to make new tables and, ultimately, to create meaningful output for a clinical team. Commonly, databases used for EHR data go through a process called normalization where redundant values are filtered and information is stored in multiple tables which are updated and changed in an efficient manner.[32,33] To import data into a health system's database, an extract-transform-load (ETL) process is run on an established schedule (eg, daily at 0100). During ETL, data are extracted from the EHR interface used in clinical care or another database, transformed into a structure that is appropriate for the receiving database, and then loaded into the receiving database to be accessible for querying and reporting. This means that data pulled from these databases have a time lag where real-time information is not accessible. For example, if a hospital's ETL process runs daily at 0100 and an analyst pulls data from the database at 0059, the analyst's report will not include any information from the prior day. An overview of this workflow can be found in **Fig. 3**. Data can be obtained from tables of relational databases to support QI, research, or operational activities using a programming language, such as Structured Query Language (SQL).[34,35] Although further understanding of database structure and SQL programming is beyond the scope of this review, basic knowledge of this process and terminology can be helpful when working with your institution's data team and when submitting data requests related to projects. Data analysts hired by your individual group or

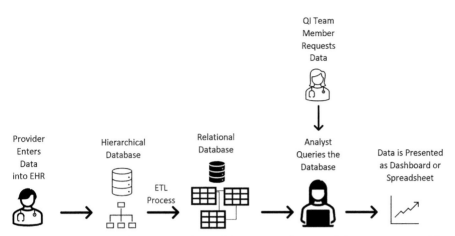

Fig. 3. Schematic of data flow into and out of the EHR. At the start of the process, a provider enters data into the EHR. This typically flows into a hierarchical database that stores a large amount of information (eg, all a patient's vitals in the last 24 hours, recent imaging studies, and recent clinical documentation), but can only display this information on a few individuals in real time. Hierarchical databases are often what providers interact with during clinical care. The information then undergoes an extract-transform-load (ETL) process that runs at a scheduled time and is moved into a relational database where it is stored in multiple tables. If a QI team requests information from the EHR, a data analyst will query the relational database and return this data in a form desired by the team.

centralized to the health system are typically responsible for directly accessing these databases.

Garbage In, Garbage Out

For all data types, interpretation is only as valuable as the quality of the values inputted into the system. The data quality mantra "garbage in—garbage out" reflects this fact.[36] A quick slip of the hand or misinterpretation of an input field could result in an erroneous value. Similarly, the lack of an appropriate charting technique may lead to incomplete data capture (eg, no defined location for charting temperature resulting in many unknown values). In addition, poor stakeholder buy-in can result in limited data collection. Adding in a field for data capture does not guarantee it will be used; providers must be willing participants in the project to ensure appropriate data entry. If data from the EHR are used to support process, outcome, and balancing measures, it can be useful to design tests of change with a focus on ensuring high data quality in ways that avoid disruption of existing, effective workflows, or encourage adoption of a new, desirable workflow.

Considerations for When to Use (or Avoid) Electronic Health Record Data for a Quality Improvement Effort

Automated data capture from the EHR can add efficiency, standardization, and ease to QI data processing. When using the EHR to capture data for QI, teams should aim for having accurate, valid, and complete data. To achieve this, they must build on the Five Rights (previously discussed) and consider existing workflows. Projects are set up for success when teams fit data capture into an already existing workflow, for example, pulling admission temperature values from the EHR database that are entered as a part of routine care. Alternatively, projects can be successful when data capture is included in improvements to existing workflows that are introduced as part of the QI process. For example, if a DR uses a checklist for all neonatal deliveries, then an intervention integrating it into the EHR may offer the opportunity to filter checklist items based on patient characteristics like gestational age.[37] Systems considerations may shape strategy depending on the type of user entering the data. For example, if a bedside nurse typically uses a specific portion of the EHR for vital sign documentation, any intervention regarding temperature recording should be done in the same location. However, an ordering provider may regularly document information regarding interpretation of vitals and management plans in a clinical note section of the EHR. Any intervention involving such a provider may then use embedded data capture in a note template as opposed to elsewhere in the chart. The best metrics to automatically extract from the EHR for the QI project are those in which the data elements are well-established, clearly defined, and routinely documented the EHR as standard practice. Metrics that are often good candidates for automated data extraction include medication orders in a system with standardized computer-based order entry, patient demographics, and vital signs.

Although there are many situations when automated data capture from the EHR can be effectively used in a QI project, it is not always an appropriate choice. New processes, metrics with operational definitions that may change, or data that is embedded in the EHR, but not consistently charted, cannot be reliably extracted in an automated fashion.

Using Electronic Health Record Data Aligns with Our Project, Now What?

If you plan to use EHR data in your QI project, early preparation is the key. First, investigate local processes for requesting data. Select QI leads may have programming know-how and training to request such access for themselves. If not, as stated earlier, generally, there is an analyst team that meets your health systems' specifications for credentialing and would be responsible for obtaining data from the EHR for QI efforts. Data extraction can take varying amounts of time depending on many things including the maturity of your health system's data structure, complexity and clarity of your request, and current workload of your analyst team. It is never too early to start planning your request!

Once you know who will be responsible for fulfilling your data request, you should explore methods by which you might file your request, which could include submission via an online portal, direct email with an analyst, or a survey platform. How you craft your data request depends on your institution's submission specifications, but the following suggestions can be universally helpful: (1) ensure your metrics are well-defined and (2) consider where the metrics may be collected from the EHR. Knowing the workflow behind data entry (eg, what role enters temperature measurement, where this is inputted in the EHR) as well as provision of several examples of specific data points (eg, Baby Bear's initial axillary temperature was 36.7 °C) can be very helpful for your analyst team as they validate their work. Including screenshots of where the data are entered in your EHR and what it looks like as an end-user can assist your analyst in knowing where to look when they query the EHR database. (3) If you intend to obtain a spreadsheet of outputted data, designing a draft result spreadsheet with defined values can be invaluable for your analyst team. For example, to obtain the data as shown in **Fig. 4**, the team would request a spreadsheet with one row per patient with the following columns: patient first name, last name, date of birth, time of birth, initial temperature value, initial temperature source, date and time of vital sign entry. Providing a spreadsheet with defined row granularity (eg, one row per patient,

```
with results as (
    select
        Last_name,
        First_name,
        Date_of_birth,
        Time_of_birth,
        Temp,
        Temp_source,
        Vitals_date,
        Vitals_time,
        row_number() over (partition by Patient.Patient_ID order by Vitals_date, Vitals_time) as vitals_row_num
    from
        Patient
        inner join Vitals
            on Patient.Patient_ID = Vitals.Patient_ID
    where
        Temp_source = 'axillary'
)|

select
    Last_name,
    First_name,
    Date_of_birth,
    Time_of_birth,
    Temp,
    Temp_source,
    Vitals_date,
    Vitals_time
from
    results
where
    vitals_row_num = 1
```

Last_name	First_name	Date_of_birth	Time_of_birth	Temp	Temp_source	Vitals_date	Vitals_time
Bear	Baby	3-21-2022	0015	36.7	axillary	3-21-2022	0045
Caterpillar	Hungry	3-21-2022	1920	36.2	axillary	3-21-2022	1740
Dumpty	Humpty	3-22-2022	0340	35.8	axillary	3-22-2022	0505

Fig. 4. Example of Structured Query Language (SQL) query and its results. Script from an SQL query based on data from the patient (see **Fig. 5**) and vitals (see **Fig. 6**) relational tables. This query will return the initial recorded temperatures for patients in the cohort if their initial temperature source was axillary with the following details: patient first name, last name, date of birth, time of birth, initial temperature value, initial temperature source, date and time of vital sign entry.

one row per patient visit, one row per medication administration) and defined column headers will ensure the data requesters' and analysts' expectations align (**Box 4**).

CONSIDERATION OF UNINTENDED CONSEQUENCES

There is immense potential in using the EHR in QI efforts. Although the preparation required for successful design and implementation can be overwhelming initially, the upfront work can result in great reward—improved patient outcomes, efficient data analytics, and novel technology-supported interventions. However, with this power comes substantial opportunity for unintended consequences.

If a QI team decided to test and implement EHR-based interventions like CDS, they must be aware of the potential pitfalls of these interventions. There is extensive literature on patterns of unintended consequences related to CDS. For example, commonly used tools such as interruptive alerts (ie, an indicator to someone using

> **Box 4**
> **Case example: extracting data from the EHR**
>
> The QI team responsible for reducing admission hypothermia knew up front wanted to prioritize EHR data to track project measures.
>
> Patient identifiers and admission temperature information are known to readily exist within this team's EHR. The presence of these widely established, clearly defined measures incorporated into the EHR as standard practice makes them ideal metrics for extraction.
>
> The data analyst on their team regularly queries the hospital relational databases to obtain the data needed to calculate the project's process, outcome, and balancing measures including: (1) percent of infants with an admission temperature <36 °C, (2) duration of DR resuscitation, and (3) percent of infants with hyperthermia defined as admission temperature >37.5 °C.
>
> The analyst runs an SQL query (see **Fig. 4**) to obtain the relevant pieces of data for this project from the hospital relational database. The examples of normalized tables that store data from the EHR related to our example of this QI project can be found in **Figs. 5** and **6**.
>
> The data from PDSA 1 (use of a digital checklist) may differ slightly. The team decides to leverage the knowledge that new processes in the EHR make take time to enculturate and includes "completion of digital checklist" to their process measures to track its usage over time as well as unintended consequences that occur once the checklist is "live" in the EHR. Once usage of the digital checklist becomes routine, the team may consider extracting specific elements of checklist completion for tracking purposes.

the EHR that impedes their ability to continue to interact with the system until they take a specific action) may result in unwanted workarounds such as dismissing the alert without fully acknowledging its content. The transition to computerized order entry has been noted to be associated with patient safety events.[38] In addition, the EHR has been connected in numerous studies to physician and provider burnout.[39–41] Furthermore, it is important to highlight that many of the disparities that exist in our health care system also exist in technological advances. CDS and other health information technology offer immense potential to improve inequities in care but may also worsen them. When taking part in intervention design and implementation, it is important for QI team members to ask themselves how different types of populations may be affected by the work based. Particularly with technology-based intervention, differences in access to technology and preferred language across the population may introduce inequities. Effort must be made to both recognize and mitigate this inequity while including end users of different background in the planning conversations.[42]

Patient_ ID	Last_ name	First_ name	Date_of_birth	Time_of_birth	Admit _NPI
1	Bear	Baby	3-21-2022	0015	1112223334
2	Pig	Little	3-22-2022	1330	2223334445
3	Caterpillar	Hungry	3-21-2022	1920	3334445556
4	Dumpty	Humpty	3-22-2022	0340	3334445556

Fig. 5. Example of a normalized EHR database table ("Patient"). Table devoted to patient-specific information including a patient's unique identifier, first and last name, date and time of birth, and the national provider identification (NPI) number specific to their admitting attending provider. Although this table shows one row per patient, there can be duplicate Admit_NPI numbers as the same admitting provider may admit multiple patients. Note that additional information regarding their attending provider would likely be featured in another table.

Patient_ID	Provider_ID	Vitals_date	Vitals_time	Temp	Temp_source	HR	BP	RR
1	15	3-21-2022	0045	36.7	axillary	156	64/40	38
1	21	3-21-2022	1230	37.0	axillary	168	78/36	36
1	15	3-22-2022	0052	37.2	axillary	144	66/46	34
1	16	3-22-2022	0819	36.3	axillary	138	68/28	44
2	10	3-22-2022	1400	37	rectal	142	78/28	48
3	13	3-21-2022	1740	36.2	axillary	146	92/46	42
3	8	3-22-2022	0145	36.6	axillary	130	70/44	40
3	13	3-22-2022	1254	36.4	axillary	144	72/38	32
4	22	3-22-2022	0505	35.8	axillary	120	64/40	40
4	16	3-22-2022	1349	36.5	rectal	133	74/42	38

Fig. 6. Example of a normalized EHR database table ("Vitals"). Table devoted to patient-level vital signs with one row per set of patient vital signs. Here, specific information regarding vital signs such as the unique provider identification number who recorded the vital signs, the time and date of vital sign charting, and the values of the vital signs are stored. There may be multiple rows per patient, as denoted by the outlined rows in this example.

In addition, the use of EHR data without consideration of its accuracy, completeness, and validity can hinder the success of a project or result in incorrect conclusions being drawn from the data. For example, if documentation in the EHR is unreliable or incomplete, the use of EHR data will underrepresent patients in the cohort because the population only includes patients who had EHR charting. Similarly, if a project relies on the EHR for a metric where the operational definition or "source of truth" in the EHR changes, this could also lead to incorrect conclusions. For example, if a team modifies its outcome metric to be defined as provider charting of a diagnosis code as opposed to the initial plan to use vital sign field, this may result in significantly different outcomes. If the provider documentation of diagnoses is unreliable or variable, there may be a significant undercount of patients with outcome of interest. A change in the middle of the project could give a false sense of improvement from special cause variation leading to improvement in patient outcomes when variation was secondary to a change in definition and data source. Constructing a well-rounded team that includes informatics expertise can increase likelihood that these unintended consequences are considered before they occur.

SUMMARY

The EHR is a widely adopted tool filled with immense promise for QI teams. From designing and implementing EHR-based interventions, collecting data, and analyzing outcomes, the EHRs potential uses in QI are manifold. However, EHR-integrated project success relies on an understanding and application of this tool's special considerations. Through an appreciation of EHR-based data structure, the complexities of building and incorporating high-technology interventions into the EHR, and recognition of potential unintended consequence, QI teams can position themselves for effective project design, application, and completion with the EHR as a core component of their success.

CLINICS CARE POINTS

- The EHR can be used in QI efforts for multiple purposes including as a venue for interventions and to aid in data collection.

• Successful integration of the EHR in a QI effort is dependent on appropriate team support, thoughtful design, and an understanding of how data is stored in the system.

DISCLOSURE

The authors have nothing to disclose.

REFERENCES

1. Seidman J, Garrett P. EMR vs EHR – what is the Difference? Health IT Buzz; 2011. Available at: https://www.healthit.gov/buzz-blog/electronic-health-and-medical-records/emr-vs-ehr-difference. Accessed July 1, 2022.
2. Simborg DW. Promoting electronic health record adoption. Is it the correct focus? J Am Med Inform Assoc 2008;15(2):127.
3. Atheron J. Development of the electronic health record. AMA J Ethics 2011;13(3):186–9.
4. Department of Health and Human Services. Department of health and human services fiscal year 2018 justification of estimates for appropriations committees message from the administrator. Available at: https://www.hhs.gov/sites/default/files/combined-onc.pdf. Published online 2017:16. Accessed June 30, 2022.
5. About ONC's Cures act final Rule. Available at: https://www.healthit.gov/curesrule/overview/about-oncs-cures-act-final-rule. Accessed July 15, 2022.
6. Gold M, McLaughlin C. Assessing HITECH implementation and lessons: 5 Years later. Milbank Q 2016;94(3):654.
7. Jha AK, DesRoches CM, Campbell EG, et al. Use of electronic health records in U.S. Hospitals. N Engl J Med 2009;360:1628–66.
8. National trends in hospital and physician adoption of electronic health records. healthit.gov. 2022. Available at: https://www.healthit.gov/data/quickstats/national-trends-hospital-and-physician-adoption-electronic-health-records. Accessed July 16, 2022.
9. Everson J, Rubin JC, Friedman CP. Reconsidering hospital EHR adoption at the dawn of HITECH: implications of the reported 9% adoption of a "basic" EHR. J Am Med Inform Assoc 2020;27(8):1198–205.
10. How to improve | IHI - institute for healthcare improvement. Available at: https://www.ihi.org/resources/Pages/HowtoImprove/default.aspx. Accessed July 22, 2022.
11. Harris PA, Taylor R, Minor BL, et al. The REDCap consortium: building an international community of software platform partners. J Biomed Inform 2019;95:103208.
12. Clinical informatics – American board of preventive medicine.
13. Laptook AR, Salhab W, Bhaskar B, et al. Admission temperature of low birth weight infants: predictors and associated morbidities. Pediatrics 2007;119(3):e643–9.
14. Yu YH, Wang L, Huang L, et al. Association between admission hypothermia and outcomes in very low birth weight infants in China: a multicentre prospective study. BMC Pediatr 2020;20(1):321.
15. Bhatt DR, White R, Martin G, et al. Transitional hypothermia in preterm newborns. J Perinatol 2007;27 Suppl(2):S45–7.
16. Friedman CP. A "fundamental Theorem" of biomedical informatics. J Am Med Inf Assoc 2009;16(2):169–70.

17. Patel VL, Kannampallil TG. Cognitive informatics in biomedicine and healthcare. J Biomed Inform 2015;53:3–14.

18. Dul J, Bruder R, Buckle P, et al. A strategy for human factors/ergonomics: developing the discipline and profession. Ergonomics 2012;55(4):377–95.

19. Dempsey PG, Wogalter MS, Hancock PA. What's in a name? Using terms from de® nitions to examine the fundamental foundation of human factors and ergonomics science. Theor Issues Ergon Sci 2000;1(1):3–10.

20. Mauro NJ. The Deming leadership method and profound knowledge: a global prescription. Cross Cult Manag: Int J 1999;6(3):13–24.

21. Osheroff J, Teich J, Levick D, et al. Improving outcomes with clinical decision support: an implementer's guide. Improving Outcomes with Clinical Decision Support: An Implementer's Guide 2012. Available at: https://scholarlyworks.lvhn.org/administration-leadership/54. Accessed June 19, 2022.

22. Coughlin K, Posencheg M, Orfe L, et al. Reducing variation in the management of apnea of prematurity in the intensive care nursery. Pediatrics 2020;145(2). https://doi.org/10.1542/PEDS.2019-0861/68275.

23. Carr LH, Padula M, Chuo J, et al. Improving compliance with a rounding checklist through low- and high-technology interventions: a quality improvement initiative. Pediatr Qual Saf 2021;6(4):e437.

24. Gartner C, Scalise L. Healing at home. In: Epic users group meeting 2020 - maternal safety webinar. 2020.

25. Peebles P, Carr LH, Presser L, et al. Improving the assessment of infants at-risk for hypoxic ischemic encephalopathy. In: 48th northeastern conference on perinatal research. 2022.

26. Beng Leau Y, Khong Loo W, Yip Tham W, et al. Software Development Life Cycle AGILE vs Traditional Approaches. Information and Network Technology; 2012.

27. Ash JS, Stavri PZ, Dykstra R, et al. Implementing computerized physician order entry: the importance of special people. Int J Med Inform 2003;69(2–3):235–50. https://doi.org/10.1016/S1386-5056(02)00107-7.

28. Rowley J. The wisdom hierarchy: representations of the DIKW hierarchy. J Inf Sci 2007;33(2):163–80. https://doi.org/10.1177/0165551506070706.

29. Dammann O. Data, information, evidence, and knowledge:: a proposal for health informatics and data science. Online J Public Health Inform 2018;10(3). https://doi.org/10.5210/OJPHI.V10I3.9631.

30. White SE. A review of big data in health care: challenges and opportunities. Published online 2014. https://doi.org/10.2147/OAB.S50519.

31. Rules for handling and maintaining metadata in the EHR. Available at: https://library.ahima.org/doc?oid=106378#.YtwxV3bMKUk. Accessed July 22, 2022.

32. Baxendale P, Codd EF. Information Retrieval A Relational Model of Data for Large Shared Data Banks.

33. Kent W. Parallel architectures for database systems. Commun ACM 1983;26(2):120–5.

34. Lee Xu, Souza D, Martin Z. Unlocking the potential of electronic health records for health research. International Journal of Population Data Science Journal Website 2020;5. https://doi.org/10.23889/ijpds.v5i1.1123. Available at: www.ijpds.org.

35. Dilling TJ. Artificial intelligence research: the utility and design of a relational database system. Advancesradonc 2020;5:1280–5.

36. Kilkenny MF, Biostats G/, Robinson KM. Data quality: "Garbage in-garbage out.". Health Inf Manag 2018;47(3):103–5.

37. Sittig DF, Wright A, Osheroff JA, et al. Grand challenges in clinical decision support v10. J Biomed Inform 2008;41(2):387–92.

38. Koppel R, Metlay JP, Cohen A, et al. Role of computerized physician order entry systems in facilitating medication errors. JAMA 2005;293(10):1197–203.
39. Gardner RL, Cooper E, Haskell J, et al. Physician stress and burnout: the impact of health information technology. J Am Med Inform Assoc 2019;26(2):106.
40. Linzer M, Poplau S, Babbott S, et al. Worklife and wellness in academic general internal medicine: results from a national survey. J Gen Intern Med 2016;31(9): 1004–10.
41. Shanafelt TD, Dyrbye LN, Sinsky C, et al. Relationship between clerical burden and characteristics of the electronic environment with physician burnout and professional satisfaction. Mayo Clin Proc 2016;91(7):836–48.
42. Craig S, McPeak KE, Madu C, et al. Health information technology and equity: applying history's lessons to tomorrow's innovations. Curr Probl Pediatr Adolesc Health Care 2022;52(1):101110.

Using Quality Improvement to Improve Value and Reduce Waste

Brian King, MD[a],*, Ravi M. Patel, MD, MSc[b]

KEYWORDS

- Value • Quality • Waste • Outcomes • Infant • Neonate

KEY POINTS

- Neonatologists should care about the value of care they provide.
- Improving the value of care should ideally focus on improving outcomes and reducing cost.
- There are several high-priority areas for improvement in value-based neonatal care that could be readily addressed by local quality improvement initiatives.

WHAT IS VALUE?

Value in health care has been best described by Michael Porter as "health outcomes achieved per dollar spent."[1] Value is often described as the output of an equation with health outcomes achieved in the numerator, and total costs of care in the denominator (Value = outcomes/cost). The emphasis on improving value in health care was emphasized in the Institute for Healthcare Improvement's "Triple Aim." This framework for optimizing health system performance focuses on the following: (1) improving the individual experience of care, (2) improving the health of populations, and (3) reducing the per capita costs of care for populations.[2] At its core, value is patient-centered and outcomes-focused. Importantly, it is not about the "amount" of health care provided but the actual outcomes achieved, and the cost needed to achieve those outcomes. Improving value is not simply cost reduction. Without concurrently measuring outcomes achieved, cost-reduction is "dangerous and self-defeating, leading to false savings and potentially limiting effective care."[1]

In neonatal medicine, Dukhovny and colleagues[3] argue that 3 key components of clinical practice should be combined to achieve value: (1) evidence-based medicine, (2) evidence-based economics, and (3) quality improvement (QI). One simple way to

Funding: None.
[a] Department of Pediatrics, University of Pittsburg School of Medicine; [b] Emory University School of Medicine and Children's Healthcare of Atlanta, 2015 Uppergate Drive, NE, Atlanta, GA 30322, USA
* Corresponding author. 3240 Craft Place, 2nd Floor, Suite 200, Pittsburgh, PA 15213.
E-mail address: kingbc2@upmc.edu

apply the concepts of evidence-based medicine and evidence-based economics is to consider the value of individual interventions across 2 axes on a "cost-effectiveness plane": outcomes and costs (**Fig. 1**). Evidence-based medicine helps to identify interventions that are most likely to improve outcomes (falling to the right of the y-axis). Evidence-based economics identifies which of those interventions are the "best bet for the money" (high value vs low value), often defined by some specific "cost-effectiveness" threshold.[4] Those interventions that have been shown to have worse (or no better outcomes) regardless of cost are considered nonvalue added care, or "waste." We can then use QI to ensure interventions that are cost-effective and most likely to improve outcomes (high-value care) reliably reach our patients, whereas lower value (and wasteful) interventions are minimized or eliminated. The provided visual aid is a simplification, and it is important to highlight that a single intervention may be in the high-value care category for a specific population or indication, whereas falling in the waste category in a different clinical scenario and/or indication (a theoretic example of overuse or misuse of an intervention).

One example would be the use of pasteurized donor human milk, which would be of relatively high value for use in very low-birth weight infants for the prevention of necrotizing enterocolitis (NEC) but of relatively lower value for in-hospital use in well newborns. In addition, although all interventions have an associated cost, some may lead to net cost savings overall, which could result in interventions plotting below the x-axis (with net benefits in terms of both outcomes and costs). For example, pasteurized donor human milk use could lead to a net cost-savings in units with high-NEC rates but might not be cost saving in populations with high mother's milk use.[5,6] The combination of evidence-based medicine, evidence-based economics and QI should consider the intervention along with the specific population and indication for use when determining the value of care being provided.

Although a significant focus in neonatal medicine has been on health outcomes, the numerator of the value equation, there has been less focus on costs, the denominator.

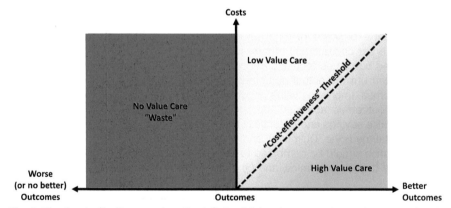

Fig. 1. The "cost-effectiveness plane"—defining high value care using outcomes and costs. A visual representation of value-based care. High-value care includes interventions that benefit patients (improve outcomes) and have costs less than a predetermined "cost-effectiveness" threshold. Low-value care includes interventions that benefit patients but have increased costs that place them above the threshold. Wasteful care does not benefit patients, regardless of costs. (*Adapted from* A Pandya, MPH, PhD. High and Low Value Care. Available at: https://vimeo.com/270682342. Accessed Oct 28 2022. Also refer: Pandya A. Adding Cost-effectiveness to Define Low-Value Care. JAMA. 2018;319(19):1977–1978. https://doi. org/10.1001/jama.2018.2856.

Both are important if we want to achieve the Triple Aim in neonatal medicine. A national survey of neonatologists found generally poor knowledge about the costs of commonly used tests, diagnostic studies, and hospitalization costs.[7] Understanding the structure of costs, because they relate to neonatal care, is an important first step when thinking about how to consider incorporating cost into efforts to improve the quality and value of neonatal care.

In this review, we summarize the successes of QI in improving the value of neonatal care. First, we make the case for why value is important for the neonatologist to consider. Next, we discuss how traditional QI focused on processes and outcomes has great potential to improve value but requires explicit cost accounting to demonstrate it. Then, we review important cost measures that can be incorporated into QI. Finally, we apply the concept of waste to examples of overuse of the neonatal intensive care unit, as well as categories of tests and treatments, while proposing additional QI opportunities to improve the value of neonatal care and reduce waste.

WHY SHOULD THE NEONATOLOGIST CARE ABOUT VALUE?

There are several reasons why neonatologists should care about value. Health-care spending in the United States continues to grow rapidly, and annual expenditures attributed to waste are estimated to account for more than US$900 billion dollars.[8,9] Lifetime excess costs related to prematurity are estimated to be more than US$25 billion dollars, a large contribution on health-care costs for a relatively small subset of the population.[10] Neonatal care also has long-term implications, being responsible for 4 of the top 25 leading causes of disability-adjusted life years (preterm birth, neonatal encephalopathy, neonatal sepsis, congenital anomalies).[11] Beyond the impact to society, the direct financial impact on families of infants requiring neonatal care, while understudied, is significant.[12] The American College of Physician's Manual of Ethics also argues that physicians have an ethical imperative to use health-care resources responsibly.[13] A focus on value can benefit our patients, by reducing spending while achieving better health, as well as providing greater efficiencies and patient satisfaction, and can benefit the health-care system and society as a whole by reducing long-term chronic morbidities.[14]

With the changing landscape of reimbursement, improving value through QI not only makes sense for our patients but also makes financial sense. Associated reductions of hospital costs from improvement efforts make a strong business case for investment in QI.[15] Health-care reimbursement is increasingly shifting toward methods that reward value instead of volume of care. Diagnostic-related groups-based and bundled payments, which set reimbursement rates based on a patient's condition rather than the amount of services delivered, incentivize efforts to reduce wasteful care.[16,17] Although these payment models do not specifically focus on value (outcomes and costs), value-based models have been expanding in adult medicine, and will likely also become more prevalent in pediatrics.[18,19]

INCORPORATING VALUE AND COST INTO TRADITIONAL QUALITY IMPROVEMENT

Although QI efforts are often focused on process or outcome measures, and not specifically cost, reduction in common neonatal morbidities have a great potential to reduce cost and improve value. Johnson and colleagues used a single institution sample of very-low birth weight infants infants to estimate the additional hospital costs related to bronchopulmonary dysplasia (BPD), NEC, brain injury and late-onset sepsis (LOS), after controlling for infant characteristics.[20] They estimated that those 4 morbidities added US$31,565, US$15,440, US$12,048, and US$10,055, respectively, to the inpatient costs related to the initial hospital stay. These are likely low estimates, as other studies have suggested higher costs, and they also do not include lifetime costs after discharge with long-term effects of these morbidities.[21–23] Common neonatal conditions such as hypoglycemia may also potentially have significant lifetime costs associated with them.[24] Given the costs (both immediate and across the child's lifetime) associated with these common morbidities, successful QI initiatives that reduce these outcomes can be presumed to also reduce cost.

Adverse events are also common targets for traditional QI in neonatology. These include reducing central-line associated bloodstream infections (CLABSIs) and unplanned extubation (UPE). Studies have estimated that the attributable cost and added length of stay related to these events in pediatric patients may surpass US$50,000, with 19 additional hospital days associated per CLABSI and 6.5 days for UPE.[25–27] A systematic review of economic evaluations related to QI interventions focused on reducing CLABSIs found substantial cost savings-related quality programs focused on reducing CLABSI events, with an estimated incremental net savings of US$1.85 million per hospital during 3 years.[28]

COST MEASURES IN QUALITY IMPROVEMENT

Although the potential for cost savings by reducing neonatal morbidities is clear, QI projects aiming to demonstrate value improvement need to include robust cost measures. At present, incorporating robust cost measures in traditional QI is relatively novel and underutilized. A systematic review of QI collaboratives found that few reported cost estimates or economic evaluations.[29] One of the earliest examples is from the work of Jeannette Rogowski and VON, where they showed significant sustainable cost savings because of collaborative QI efforts across neonatal intensive care units (NICUs).[30] Although treatment costs in control hospitals that did not participate in the QI collaboratives increased, they saw a decrease in treatment costs among infants with infection and chronic lung disease (the 2 areas of focus). After considering costs related to the QI collaboratives, the average savings per hospital in patient care costs were more than US$2 million in the year following interventions.

For those interested in incorporating robust cost measures in their QI efforts, hospital-billing data can be used to estimate total costs from the hospital perspective, using department-specific cost to charge ratios.[31] Thompson and colleagues provide an excellent review of cost structures because they relate to costing NICU care.[32] Cost measures should include fixed costs (eg, NICU bed-space) and variable costs (interventions eg, radiographs, laboratory tests, surfactant) involved in patient care. In a simplified way, separate departmental billing (room and board charges, laboratory charges, pharmacy charges, and so forth) can be combined with department-specific ratios of cost to charges to estimate the costs incurred within each department.

One approach that might be more practical for clinical teams without access to cost data would be to use published data on the costs of individual tests and treatments to estimate utilization. Cost data may not be hospital-specific but could estimate utilization and track changes over time. For example, a recent publication using cost estimates from cost-to-charge ratios averaged across US children's hospitals could allow estimation of per-day costs (eg, US$264 for parenteral nutrition, US$1593 for gas therapy such as nitric oxide, US$81 for blood chemistry) and allow calculation of potential cost reductions to decreases in per-day utilization.[33] Although this approach is imperfect, it might be a start for improvement teams that desire a general cost estimate for projects focused on the reduction of utilization without more intensive accounting efforts.

There are several alternative approaches that could also be considered to aid in cost measures for QI efforts. Ho and colleagues summarized simple examples of cost metrics that QI projects can measure in neonatology.[34] A modified version of their table is reproduced here (**Table 1**). Zupancic and colleagues developed a daily cost prediction model for NICU care and found that 8 tests and treatments predicted daily variable costs.[35] These resources were surfactant, chest radiographs, red blood cell transfusion, cranial ultrasound, abdominal radiograph, parenteral nutrition infusions, platelet transfusions, and echocardiograms. Individual projects can also utilize cost measures from the published literature that fit their needs, to combine with other types of cost data collection. For example, a QI effort focused on reducing CLABSI may be able to include published estimates of the incremental costs associated with CLABSI events in their assessment of changes in cost overtime. However, caution should be taken with this approach because it is important to measure both positive and negative cost measures (eg, cost-associated interventions introduced through QI such as added nursing time/staffing to adhere to central-line maintenance protocols) to fully estimate the influence on hospital costs.

Length of stay has also been used as a surrogate for cost measures. For example, Kaempf and colleagues examined value improvement in a subset of NICUs participating in a Vermont Oxford Network (VON) quality collaborative. They created a novel "value metric" where benefit (the numerator) was defined by risk-adjusted inverse rates of morbidities and cost (the denominator) was measured as mean total hospital length of stay in survivors. They found that value improved over time for NICUs involved in collaborative QI compared with other NICUs in VON, although the magnitude of value improvement was diminished by an increase in length of stay (cost) during the study period.[36] This highlights the importance of tracking not only benefit/outcomes but also cost to ensure a net gain in value.

Although methods of estimating costs based on a hospital or payer perspectives are most commonly used in neonatal QI, a societal approach to cost measures is

Table 1	
Cost categories for potential inclusion in quality improvement projects	
Cost Categories	**Examples**
Aggregate measures	Length of stay Ventilator days
Testing and treatment costs	Number of imaging studies (eg, radiographs, ultrasounds, echocardiograms) Number of laboratory studies Parenteral nutrition utilization (eg, parenteral nutrition days) Antibiotic days
Supply costs	Oxygen probes Near-infrared spectroscopy monitors Endotracheal tubes
Personnel costs	Nursing hours and ratios Physician hours and ratios Other support services (eg, respiratory therapy, nutrition, therapists)
Family costs	Lost productivity Travel costs (transportation, accommodation, meals) Equipment costs (eg, breast pump rentals)

Adapted from Ho T, Zupancic JAF, Pursley DWM, Dukhovny D. Improving Value in Neonatal Intensive Care. Clin Perinatol. 2017;44(3):617-625.

preferred. Expenses incurred by families that are related to interventions should be accounted.[37] These costs are understudied but are likely substantial and influence families.[12] In addition, potential cost savings from a reduction in morbidity must be weighed against changes in resource use (eg, new interventions introduced, or changes to staffing ratios) and labor costs associated with QI efforts themselves.[38]

OVERUSE/MISUSE OF NEONATAL INTENSIVE CARE

NICU care is costly and the use of the NICU itself can be considered a resource. Fixed room and bed costs are high, even before the addition of variable costs that inevitably occur following an intensive care admission. A recent study in children's hospitals estimated that more than 70% of total hospital costs were related to these fixed costs, with an average daily cost of US$2339.[10,33] There is a wide variability in NICU utilization, with some evidence that there is a growing use of NICUs for infants who may potentially not require intensive care (eg, infants who are not premature, do not have serious congenital anomalies and are not critically ill).[39,40] In a study of the VON database in 2018, there was wide variation in "short stay" (<3 days) NICU admissions for infants greater than 34 weeks (0%–100%), and only a small proportion of infants greater than 34 weeks were considered "high-acuity" admissions.[41] Evidence suggests that the use of the NICU for term infants of relatively low acuity has been increasing overtime.[42,43]

Safely reducing utilization by decreasing admissions of lower risk infants to the NICU can improve value. This idea was initially introduced by Pursley and Zupancic and has since been featured by VON in their "Using the NICU Wisely" campaign.[40,41] Enhancing resources available in newborn nurseries can safely reduce unnecessary NICU admissions with many other added benefits due to a reduction in maternal–infant separation. Interventions designed to allow for low-risk infants to be cared for in a well-newborn setting have included standardized, risk-based approaches to sepsis evaluations in asymptomatic infants, noninvasive approaches to the treatment of neonatal hypoglycemia, and changes to nonpharmacologic management for opioid-withdrawal syndrome. Many of these interventions also have the added benefit of reducing unnecessary testing and treatment, further reducing waste and improving value. Based on published evidence-based economics, the interventions below all have the potential to both improve patient outcomes while also producing net cost savings (falling below the x-axis on the cost-effectiveness plane in **Fig. 1**). We summarize the available evidence related to these interventions and their effectiveness at reducing potentially unnecessary NICU admissions below.

Well-Appearing Infants at Risk for Sepsis

Management of well-appearing term newborns with risk factors for sepsis has evolved during the recent decade, with national guidelines endorsing approaches including sepsis risk calculators and clinical surveillance that can be more easily performed in a well-newborn setting.[44] A cost–benefit analysis using a decision-tree model examined the impact of implementing a sepsis-risk calculator and demonstrated an incremental net benefit of US$3998 per infant in their base case analysis, in addition to a 67% reduction in antibiotic use.[45] Additionally, there was a net per-patient benefit of US$1930 in direct medical costs alone. Similar data from the implementation of the Kaiser calculator in affiliated NICUs showed a reduction in sepsis evaluations from 15% to 5% of newborns and an accompanying 50% reduction in antibiotic exposure.[46] Achten and colleagues demonstrated a significant reduction in hospital costs among term newborns, primarily driven by a decrease in length of stay, as well as decreases in antibiotic utilization. They found a relative 9% reduction in combined costs associated with early onset sepsis-related care per term newborn in their Dutch NICU.[47] In addition to demonstrating decreases in the overuse of sepsis laboratory evaluations and antibiotic treatment, several single-center studies have also shown significant reductions in NICU admissions, and reduced length of stay contributing to the value improvement seen with implementation of validated sepsis-risk calculators.[47–49]

Neonatal Hypoglycemia

Oral glucose gel has been studied as both a treatment of neonatal hypoglycemia and as prophylaxis in newborns at risk. When used to treat hypoglycemia, oral glucose gel can reduce NICU admissions and maternal–infant separation by allowing care to continue in a well-newborn setting. The Sugar Babies Trial,[50] a double-blind randomized trial in New Zealand that randomized infants who were hypoglycemic to receive 200 mg/kg 40% dextrose gel or placebo, observed a significant reduction in treatment failure (14% vs 24%, $P = .04$), as well as a reduction in NICU admissions for hypoglycemia (14% vs 25%, $P = .03$) and less formula feeding at 2 weeks of age (4% vs 13%, $P = .03$). Several studies reporting the experience of single centers implementing oral glucose gel for the treatment of hypoglycemia have shown reductions in NICU admissions, in addition to reductions in length of stay, costs, and improvements in exclusive breastfeeding.[51–53] A decision-tree analysis modeling costs related to oral glucose gel, based on data from The Sugar Babies Trial, found cost savings of US$1300 per infant, with cost savings persisting across a range of sensitivity analyses.[54] Although most of the published literature supports a positive cost–benefit assessment of oral glucose gel to treat hypoglycemia, the hPOD Trial of prophylactic glucose gel administration demonstrated reduced rates of hypoglycemia without a reduction in NICU admissions or maternal–infant separation.[55] Based on the available evidence, patient selection is important for QI efforts focused on glucose gel, if the goal is to reduce unnecessary NICU admissions.

Infants with Neonatal Abstinence Syndrome

The incidence of neonatal abstinence syndrome (NAS) or neonatal opioid withdrawal syndrome continues to increase in the United States. These infants are at increased risk of NICU admission, medication exposure, and prolonged lengths of stay, with significant associated economic burdens.[56,57] Efforts to improve care for this population, and specifically reduce NICU admission and decrease mother–infant separation, provide significant opportunities to improve the value of care. In 2017, Yale New Haven Children's Hospital published their QI initiative to improve care for infants with NAS, using an approach now referred to as "eat, sleep, console" (ESC). They significantly reduced NICU admissions (100% to 20%), length of hospital stay (22–6 days), and hospital costs (US$45,000–US$10,000 per patient), with no adverse events or increase in readmissions for NAS (**Fig. 2**).[58] In the last 5 years, many institutions have adopted ESC approaches and significantly reduced NICU admissions, length of stay and medication exposure for infants with NAS.[59–62] The Colorado Hospitals Substance Exposed Newborn Quality Improvement Collaborative employed ESC across 19 birthing hospitals in Colorado, and significantly reduced average LOS (14.8–5.9 days) and pharmacologic therapy (61%–23%). Admissions to Level III NICUs also decreased from a baseline mean of 16% to 12% (Unpublished data, courtesy of authors).[63] Even in a population of infants already admitted to a Level IV NICU with maternal–infant separation, the ESC method has reduced length of stay and medication exposure.[64]

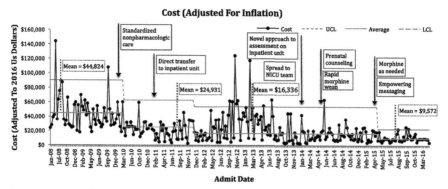

Fig. 2. Example of cost-based outcome measure: direct hospital costs per infant prenatally exposed to methadone. Figure shows hospital costs per-patient prenatally exposed to methadone in an initiative to improve care for infants with NAS using the ESC method. During the study period, average hospital costs decreased from US$44,824 to US$10,289, along with significant reductions in the use of pharmacologic therapy and the average length of stay. (Reproduced with permission from Pediatrics, 139(6):e20163360. © 2017 by AAP.)

OVERUSE OF POTENTIALLY UNNECESSARY TESTS AND TREATMENTS

Overuse and overtreatment is estimated to account for more than US$185 billion in wasteful spending per year and has been identified as the "next quality frontier" by Donald Berwick, former Administrator for the Centers for Medicare and Medicaid Services.[9,65] The challenge is distinguishing between appropriate use of tests and treatments, and inappropriate overuse. This is where efforts to improve value must combine QI methodologies with evidence-based medicine and evidence-based economics to identify the right tests and treatments in the right patients at the right time.[3] Some tests and treatments may be wasteful (or harmful) in specific populations, falling to the left of the y-axis on the cost-effectiveness plane (see **Fig. 1**), whereas others may provide only marginal benefits with added costs that make their "value for money" questionable.

There have been some efforts to set priorities for targeting high-yield areas of overuse in neonatology (**Table 2**). The "Choosing Wisely" campaign, an initiative that seeks to advance a national dialog on avoiding unnecessary tests and treatments, published their top 5 list in newborn care in 2015 using a national survey and modified Delphi approach to prioritizing topics.[66] Although this list offers an initial starting point based on expert consensus and an evidence-based review of the literature, one limitation is that it did not consider the prevalence of overuse among different test and treatment options commonly used in neonatology. Similarly, King and colleagues used billing data from freestanding children's hospitals to describe the cost of tests and treatments among preterm infants, and created a prioritization list by combining data on cost, hospital variation, and prevalence.[33,67] This data can also serve as a starting point for hospitals to identify and focus on areas for improvement that are large drivers of cost, based on high utilization and/or high costs for the specific test or treatment. Both of these approaches (Choosing Wisely and the King Prioritization Framework) offer reasonable starting points to identify high-yield areas of overuse. Here, we also propose and review a third "categorical" approach, that focuses on high-yield areas of overuse across key resource-type categories in neonatal care; laboratory use, imaging use, medication use, and feeding and nutrition.

Table 2
Potential targets to prioritize value-based efforts to reduce overuse and waste in the neonatal intensive care unit

Prioritization Tool	List
Choosing Wisely[66]	Avoid routine use of antireflux medications in preterm infants
	Avoid routine continuation of antibiotics beyond 48 h
	Avoid routine use of predischarge pneumograms for apnea in preterm infants
	Avoid routine use of daily chest radiographs
	Avoid routine screening term-equivalent MRI in preterm infants
Prioritization Framework[67]	Optimizing feeding advancement, use of TPN and reducing central line days
	Safely reducing commonly ordered routine laboratories (hematology, chemistry, blood gases)
	Safely reducing frequently ordered imaging studies (chest and abdominal radiographs, cranial ultrasounds)
Categorical Approach	Safely reducing laboratory utilization
	Safely reducing imaging utilization
	Safely reducing medication utilization
	Optimal use of parenteral nutrition and feeding advancement

Abbreviations: MRI, magnetic resonance imaging; TPN, total parenteral nutrition.

Reducing Laboratory Utilization

This area of focus is currently understudied in the NICU. In 2021 Yale New Haven Children's Hospital published their initiative to decrease laboratory utilization in the NICU (**Fig. 3**). In their baseline data, they found that 3 laboratory tests, glucose measurements, blood gases, and bilirubin levels, constituted more than two-thirds of all laboratory testing.[68] These findings are similar to a national study of inpatient billing within children's hospital NICU's.[69] During 2 years, interventions primarily targeting these 3 tests led to a 27% decrease in laboratory tests per 1000 patient days (51,000 tests), as well as a significant decrease in blood drawn and cost savings of more than US$250,000.[68] They also developed an online dashboard that allowed providers to review their own laboratory ordering practices and compare this to their peers. This is an effective way to make the system visible, and encourage discussion around utilization. More examples of successful QI projects focused on reducing laboratory utilization can be found in the Pediatric Hospital Medicine and Pediatric Cardiac ICU literature.[70–72]

In 2008, Intermountain Healthcare's Dixie Regional Medical Center in Utah launched a unique initiative called the POKE Program, which categorized all interventions on infants (painful and nonpainful) as "pokes" and sought to reduce unnecessary "pokes." They have reported improved care and outcomes from this program, including a reduction in more than 11,000 "pokes," a 28% reduction in operational costs, significant reductions in central-line associated blood stream infections, and a 21% reduction in length of stay.[73] This program has expanded to other NICUs across the country, although peer-reviewed publications are not yet available. These 2 QI efforts suggest that targeted reduction in laboratory utilization may provide both benefits in clinical outcomes, and reduced costs (Falling below the x-axis on the cost-effectiveness plane).

Reducing Unnecessary Imaging

Among the "Choosing Wisely" Top 5 list, 3 are types of diagnostic imaging (chest radiographs, brain MRI, and pneumograms). Wide variation in the use of radiographs,

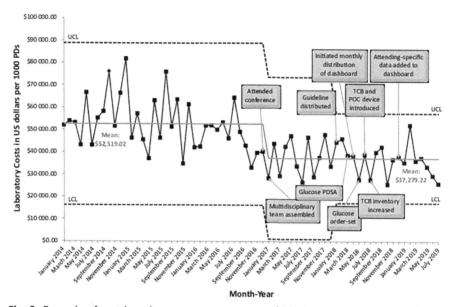

Fig. 3. Example of cost based outcome measure: monthly laboratory costs. Figure depicts monthly laboratory costs per 1000 NICU patient days during an initiative to reduce laboratory testing in the NICU. During a 30-month period, this initiative led to a savings of US$258,000, as well as a significant reduction in blood draws (approximately 8 L of blood). LCL, lower control limit; POC, point of care; PDSA, plan-do-study-act; TCB, transcutaneous bilirubin; UCL, upper control limit. (Reproduced with permission from Pediatrics. 148(1):e2020000570. © 2021 by AAP.)

brain MRI, and head ultrasounds have been described by Goodman and colleagues, across a variety of populations and payer types and largely unexplained by differences in illness severity.[74] In a Texas Medicaid population, they observed a greater than 7-fold variation in brain MRI, almost 3-fold variation in head ultrasounds, 4-fold variation abdominal radiographs, and 2-fold variation in chest radiographs, all after adjustment for illness severity.[75] When combining cost, prevalence, and hospital variation, King and colleagues's prioritization framework included both chest radiographs and head ultrasounds in their Top 10 list of overused tests and treatments.[67] Despite the wide variation in the use of brain MRI and high cost per test, it was not featured in the prioritization framework due to its relatively low overall prevalence and subsequently low total cost. This highlights costly procedures that are not commonly used may not be the most effective targets for value-based improvements. At the individual hospital level, NICUs with high brain MRI utilization rates could still consider this an excellent target for value-based improvement.

Single centers have reported on QI efforts aimed at reducing unnecessary radiographs. Motz and colleagues at Seattle Children's Hospital were able to reduce radiographs for peripherally inserted central catheter and endotracheal tube placement by more than 20% by instituting guidelines focused on optimal patient position, radiograph frequency, and endotracheal tube depth.[76] A QI initiative at Nationwide Children's aimed to primarily reduce UPE, also included a restrictive radiography policy in their interventions. They were able to decrease their UPE rate from 1.75 to 0.68 per 100 ventilator days while also cutting chest radiograph use in half.[77,78] Nathan and colleagues demonstrated an approximately 20% reduction in abdominal radiographs performed as part of a QI collaborative aimed at reducing the incidence of NEC.[79] These efforts highlight how QI initiatives aimed at more traditional quality outcomes can include resource utilization metrics to better demonstrate how their initiative changes resource use, and potentially improves value through a reduction in unnecessary imaging. Additional opportunities to potentially reduce the overuse of imaging studies could include reducing repetitive head ultrasounds to screen or follow intraventricular hemorrhage, periventricular leukomalacia, or posthemorrhagic hydrocephalus, and echocardiography to evaluate the patent ductus arteriosus or for pulmonary hypertension screening.

Reducing Unnecessary Treatments

Preterm neonates are exposed to a wide variety of medications and treatments, most of which are used off-label with limited safety or efficacy data.[80,81] For example, in infants with severe BPD admitted to US Children's Hospitals, Bamat and colleagues found a median of 30 medication exposures per patient, with significant variation in exposures across centers.[82] Although the lack of evidence should not completely preclude the use of certain medications in our population, routine use of medications without data to support its safety and efficacy is a questionable practice. Prioritizing potentially unnecessary treatments for targeted reduction should be based on the tenants of evidence-based medicine, by including the best available evidence with provider and patient values.[3] Particular attention should be made toward evidence for potential harm, particularly when high or moderate certainty of evidence for efficacy is lacking. Additional considerations could include evidence-based economics, when cost-effectiveness studies are available. By combining the best available evidence and economic data (when available), questionable interventions that are likely wasteful (fall to the left on the cost-effectiveness plane in **Fig. 1**) can be identified for targeted reduction.

The use of antireflux medications, one of the Top 5 in the "Choosing Wisely" list, is an example where QI initiatives have successfully reduced potentially unnecessary and harmful medication use. Wide variation in the diagnosis and treatment of gastroesophageal reflux among preterm infant have been reported, with up to 13-fold variation in diagnosis across children's hospitals, high rates of medication use, and significantly increased costs associated with diagnosis and treatment.[83,84] Following the "Choosing Wisely" initiative, multiple institutions have used relatively simple interventions, such as evidence-based guidelines and education, standardized documentation, and electronic medical record support, to successfully reduce the nonindicated use of antireflux medications in the NICU.[85–88] Although more recent population-level studies in the United States have not provided an overall estimate of the impact of QI efforts in reducing antireflux medication use, a recent national cohort study in England and Wales suggests continued frequent diagnosis and treatment of reflux in preterm infants, implying more efforts are needed.[89]

Although not included in the "Choosing Wisely" Top 5 list, inhaled nitric oxide (iNO) is a costly treatment with clear indications among term infants with hypoxic respiratory failure but has not been shown to improve outcomes among preterm infants.[90,91] Due to the lack of supporting data, there have been calls for reducing overutilization of iNO among preterm infants.[92] Wide variation in the use of iNO among preterm infants has been demonstrated in US centers, and a recent nationwide study in England that found increasing use.[93,94] As such, it is an ideal target for QI focused on maintaining use for the appropriate indications while limiting overuse. Although more evidence is needed to best identify appropriate indications among preterm infants, several "iNO stewardship" programs have successfully reduced utilization with no adverse effects.[95–97] Similar stewardship programs have also taken place in other critical care subspecialties, resulting in decreases in iNO utilization and expenditures.[98,99]

Optimizing Enteral Feeding and Reducing Unnecessary Parenteral Nutrition Use

The use of parenteral nutrition, intravenous fluids, and central venous access is associated with significant costs among preterm infants. King and colleagues found that parenteral nutrition accounted for the greatest proportion of total costs related to clinician-driven tests and treatments in preterm infants, and parenteral nutrition and intravenous-line related billing (eg, intravenous fluids, heparin-containing fluid infusions) featured prominently in their prioritization framework.[33,67] In addition, the harms and increased costs related to central line days and CLABSIs are well documented.[100,101] Therefore, optimizing enteral feeding regimens with subsequent reductions in central line days and parenteral nutrition use represents a significant opportunity to improve the value of care for neonates by reducing potentially unnecessary central line days involving parenteral nutrition. Additionally, increasing human milk feeding is a key target for value improvement. This has been reviewed in detail by Johnson and colleagues, and therefore, we refer readers to this detailed review.[102]

Similar to QI efforts previously highlighted, centers have used standardized protocols to decrease parenteral nutrition use in very-low birth weight infants. This has been achieved by earlier enteral feeding initiation and faster feeding advancement to shorten the time to full feeds, reduce central line days, decrease the use of parenteral nutrition, and reduce the length of stay while also improving growth outcomes.[103–105] For example, Chu and colleagues utilized a standardized feeding regimen among very preterm infants to shorten the time to full feeds (from 12.8 days to 7.7 days), reduce central line days by 35%, and reduce total parenteral nutrition (TPN)-related costs by approximately US$2500 per patient.[105] Beyond initial feeding advancement strategies, standardization of feeding advancement following medical and surgical NEC is another opportunity for improving value.[106,107] Patel and colleagues standardized feeding advancement after nonsurgical NEC and demonstrated a reduction in days to reach full feeds (24–15.7), central line days (16–11), and parenteral nutrition use.[107]

SUMMARY

Value-based care focuses on achieving the best health outcomes for patients for the lowest cost. QI plays an integral role in translating evidence-based medicine and evidence-based economics into clinical practice. Improving value through QI requires accounting for the costs of neonatal care to demonstrate cost savings from improvements in outcomes, as well as expenditures related to interventions. Opportunities to improve value through QI include interventions that focus on reducing unnecessary NICU admissions among term and late-preterm infants, as well as reducing potentially unnecessary care.

CLINICS CARE POINTS

- Incorporating cost metrics into QI can help provide a "business case" for quality improvement by demonstrating improvement in outcomes, while reducing costs.

- Reducing potential overuse of neonatal intensive care provides ample opportunities for value-based QI, with examples that include improvements in care for well-appearing infants at risk for sepsis, neonatal hypoglycemia and neonatal abstinence syndrome.

DECLARATION OF INTERESTS

R.M. Patel serves as a consultant for Noveome, Inc, receives honorarium from Mednax and serves on the data-safety monitoring committee for Infant Bacterial Therapeutics/Premier research.

REFERENCES

1. Porter ME. What is value in health care? N Engl J Med 2010;363(26):2477–81.
2. Berwick DM, Nolan TW, Whittington J. The triple aim: care, health, and cost. Health Aff 2008;27(3):759–69.
3. Dukhovny D, Pursley DM, Kirpalani HM, et al. Evidence, quality, and waste: solving the value equation in neonatology. Pediatrics 2016;137(3). https://doi.org/10.1542/PEDS.2015-0312/81392.
4. Bertram MY, Lauer JA, De Joncheere K, et al. Policy & practice Cost-effectiveness thresholds: pros and cons What are cost-effectiveness thresholds? Policy & practice. Bull World Health Organ 2016. https://doi.org/10.2471/BLT.15.164418.
5. Johnson TJ, Berenz A, Wicks J, et al. The economic impact of donor milk in the neonatal intensive care unit. J Pediatr 2020;224:57–65.e4.
6. Trang S, Zupancic JAF, Unger S, et al. Cost-ffectiveness of supplemental donor milk versus formula for very low birth weight infants. Pediatrics 2018;141(3). https://doi.org/10.1542/PEDS.2017-0737/37612.
7. Wei D, Osman C, Dukhovny D, et al. Cost consciousness among physicians in the neonatal intensive care unit. J Perinatol 2016;36(11):1014–20.
8. Moses H, Matheson DHM, Dorsey ER, et al. The anatomy of health care in the United States. JAMA 2013;310(18):1947–64.
9. Berwick DM, Hackbarth AD. Eliminating waste in US health care. JAMA 2012;307(14):1513–6.
10. Waitzman NJ, Jalali A, Grosse SD. Preterm birth lifetime costs in the United States in 2016: an update. Semin Perinatol 2021;45(3):151390.
11. Murray CJL, Lopez AD. Measuring the global burden of disease. N Engl J Med 2013;369(5):448–57.
12. King BC, Mowitz ME, Zupancic JAF. The financial burden on families of infants requiring neonatal intensive care. Semin Perinatol 2021;45(3). https://doi.org/10.1016/J.SEMPERI.2021.151394.
13. Snyder L. American College of physicians Ethics manual: sixth edition. Ann Intern Med 2012;156(1 Pt 2):73.
14. NEJM Catalyst. 2017. Available at: https://catalyst.nejm.org/doi/full/10.1056/CAT.17.0558. Accessed February 26th, 2023.
15. Fischer HR, Duncan SD. The business case for quality improvement. J Perinatol 2020;40(6):972–9.
16. What are bundled payments? NEJM catalyst. 2018. Available at: https://catalyst.nejm.org/doi/full/10.1056/CAT.18.0247. Accessed June 23, 2022.
17. Mihailovic N, Kocic S, Jakovljevic M. Review of diagnosis-related group-based financing of hospital care. Heal Serv Res Manag Epidemiol 2016;3. https://doi.org/10.1177/2333392816647892.
18. Liao JM, Navathe AS, Werner RM. The impact of medicare's alternative payment models on the value of care. Annu Rev Public Health 2020;41:551–65.
19. Wong CA, Perrin JM, Clellan M. Making the case for value-based payment reform in children's health care. JAMA Pediatr 2018;172(6):513–4.

20. Johnson TJ, Patel AL, Jegier BJ, et al. Cost of morbidities in very low birth weight infants. J Pediatr 2013;162(2). https://doi.org/10.1016/J.JPEDS.2012.07.013.

21. Lai KC, Lorch SA. Health care costs of major morbidities associated with prematurity in United States children's hospitals. J Pediatr 2022. https://doi.org/10.1016/J.JPEDS.2022.11.038.

22. Lapcharoensap W, Lee HC, Nyberg A, et al. Health care and societal costs of bronchopulmonary dysplasia. NeoReviews 2018;19(4):e211.

23. Ganapathy V, Hay JW, Kim JH. Costs of necrotizing enterocolitis and cost-effectiveness of exclusively human milk-based products in feeding extremely premature infants. Breastfeed Med 2012;7(1):29–37.

24. Glasgow MJ, Edlin R, Harding JE. Cost burden and net monetary benefit loss of neonatal hypoglycaemia. BMC Health Serv Res 2021;21(1):1–13.

25. Hatch LD, Hatch LD, Hatch LD, et al. Outcomes, resource use, and financial costs of unplanned extubations in preterm infants. Pediatrics 2020;145(6). https://doi.org/10.1542/PEDS.2019-2819.

26. Roddy DJ, Spaeder MC, Pastor W, et al. Unplanned extubations in children: impact on hospital cost and length of stay. Pediatr Crit Care Med 2015;16(6):572–5.

27. Goudie A, Dynan L, Brady PW, et al. Attributable cost and length of stay for central line–associated bloodstream infections. Pediatrics 2014;133(6):e1525–32.

28. Nuckols TK, Keeler E, Morton SC, et al. Economic evaluation of quality improvement interventions for bloodstream infections related to central catheters: a systematic review. JAMA Intern Med 2016;176(12):1843–54.

29. De La Perrelle L, Radisic G, Cations M, et al. Costs and economic evaluations of Quality Improvement Collaboratives in healthcare: a systematic review. BMC Health Serv Res 2020;20(1):1–10.

30. Rogowski JA, Horbar JD, Plsek PE, et al. Economic implications of neonatal intensive care unit collaborative quality improvement. Pediatrics 2001;107(1):23–9.

31. Shwartz M, Young DW, Siegrist R. The ratio of costs to chargees: how good a basis for estimating costs? Inquiry 1995;32(4):476–81.

32. Thompson C, Pulleyblank R, Parrott S, et al. The cost-effectiveness of quality improvement projects: a conceptual framework, checklist and online tool for considering the costs and consequences of implementation-based quality improvement. J Eval Clin Pract 2016;22(1):26–30.

33. King BC, Richardson T, Patel RM, et al. Cost of clinician-driven tests and treatments in very low birth weight and/or very preterm infants. J Perinatol 2020;41(2):295–304.

34. Ho T, Zupancic JAF, Pursley DWM, et al. Improving value in neonatal intensive care. Clin Perinatol 2017;44(3):617–25.

35. Zupancic JAF, Richardson DK, O'Brein BJ, et al. Daily cost prediction model in neonatal intensive care. Int J Technol Assess Health Care 2003;19(2):330–8.

36. Kaempf JW, Zupancic JAF, Wang L, et al. A risk-adjusted, composite outcomes score and resource utilization metrics for very low-birth-weight infants. JAMA Pediatr 2015;169(5):459–65.

37. Byford S, Raftery J. Economics notes: perspectives in economic evaluation. BMJ Br Med J (Clin Res Ed) 1998;316(7143):1529.

38. Schuster MA, Onorato SE, Meltzer DO. Measuring the cost of quality measurement: a missing link in quality strategy. JAMA 2017;318(13):1219–20.

39. Braun D, Edwards EM, Schulman J, et al. Choosing wisely for the other 80%: what we need to know about the more mature newborn and NICU care. Semin Perinatol 2021;45(3):151395.
40. Pursley DM, Zupancic JAF. Using neonatal intensive care units more wisely for at-risk newborns and their families. JAMA Netw Open 2020;3(6):e205693.
41. Edwards EM, Horbar JD. Variation in use by NICU types in the United States. Pediatrics 2018;142(5). https://doi.org/10.1542/PEDS.2018-0457/81654.
42. Braun D, Braun E, Chiu V, et al. Trends in neonatal intensive care unit utilization in a large integrated health care system. JAMA Netw Open 2020;3(6). https://doi.org/10.1001/JAMANETWORKOPEN.2020.5239.
43. Harrison W, Goodman D. Epidemiologic trends in neonatal intensive care, 2007-2012. JAMA Pediatr 2015;169(9):855–62.
44. Puopolo KM, Benitz WE, Zaoutis TE. Management of neonates born at ≥35 0/7 weeks' gestation with suspected or proven early-onset bacterial sepsis. Pediatrics 2018;142(6):20182894.
45. Gong CL, Dasgupta-Tsinikas S, Zangwill KM, et al. Early onset sepsis calculator-based management of newborns exposed to maternal intrapartum fever: a cost benefit analysis. J Perinatol 2019;39(4):571–80.
46. Kuzniewicz MW, Puopolo KM, Fischer A, et al. A quantitative, risk-based approach to the management of neonatal early-onset sepsis. JAMA Pediatr 2017;171(4):365–71.
47. Achten NB, Visser DH, Tromp E, et al. Early onset sepsis calculator implementation is associated with reduced healthcare utilization and financial costs in late preterm and term newborns. Eur J Pediatr 2020;179(5):727–34.
48. Bridges M, Pesek E, McRae M, et al. Use of an early onset-sepsis calculator to decrease unnecessary NICU admissions and increase exclusive breastfeeding. J Obstet Gynecol Neonatal Nurs 2019;48(3):372–82.
49. Gievers LL, Sedler J, Phillipi CA, et al. Implementation of the sepsis risk score for chorioamnionitis-exposed newborns. J Perinatol 2018;38(11):1581–7.
50. Harris DL, Weston PJ, Signal M, et al. Dextrose gel for neonatal hypoglycaemia (the Sugar Babies Study): a randomised, double-blind, placebo-controlled trial. Lancet 2013;382(9910):2077–83.
51. Makker K, Alissa R, Dudek C, et al. Glucose gel in infants at risk for transitional neonatal hypoglycemia. Am J Perinatol 2018;35(11):1050–6.
52. Rawat M, Chandrasekharan P, Turkovich S, et al. Oral dextrose gel reduces the need for intravenous dextrose therapy in neonatal hypoglycemia. Biomed Hub 2016;1(3):1–9.
53. Meneghin F, Manzalini M, Acunzo M, et al. Management of asymptomatic hypoglycemia with 40% oral dextrose gel in near term at-risk infants to reduce intensive care need and promote breastfeeding. Ital J Pediatr 2021;47(1):1–8.
54. Glasgow MJ, Harding JE, Edlin R, et al. Cost analysis of treating neonatal hypoglycemia with dextrose gel. J Pediatr 2018;198:151–5.e1.
55. Harding JE, Hegarty JE, Crowther CA, et al. Evaluation of oral dextrose gel for prevention of neonatal hypoglycemia (hPOD): a multicenter, double-blind randomized controlled trial. PLoS Med 2021;18(1):e1003411.
56. Patrick SW, Schumacher RE, Benneyworth BD, et al. Neonatal abstinence syndrome and associated health care expenditures: United States, 2000-2009. JAMA 2012;307(18):1934–40.
57. Patrick SW, Davis MM, Lehmann CU, et al. Increasing incidence and geographic distribution of neonatal abstinence syndrome: United States 2009-2012. J Perinatol 2015;35(8):650.

58. Grossman MR, Berkwitt AK, Osborn RR, et al. An initiative to improve the quality of care of infants with neonatal abstinence syndrome. Pediatrics 2017;139(6). https://doi.org/10.1542/PEDS.2016-3360.

59. Hein S, Clouser B, Tamim MM, et al. Eat, sleep, console and adjunctive buprenorphine improved outcomes in neonatal opioid withdrawal syndrome. Adv Neonatal Care 2021;21(1):41–8.

60. Achilles JS, Castaneda-Lovato J. A quality improvement initiative to improve the care of infants born exposed to opioids by implementing the eat, sleep, console assessment tool. Hosp Pediatr 2019;9(8):624–31.

61. Wachman EM, Grossman M, Schiff DM, et al. Quality improvement initiative to improve inpatient outcomes for Neonatal Abstinence Syndrome. J Perinatol 2018;38(8):1114–22.

62. Blount T, Painter A, Freeman E, et al. Reduction in length of stay and morphine use for NAS with the "eat, sleep, console" method. Hosp Pediatr 2019;9(8):615–23.

63. Hwang SS, Weikel B, Adams J, et al. The Colorado hospitals substance exposed newborn quality improvement collaborative: standardization of care for opioid-exposed newborns shortens length of stay and reduces number of infants requiring opiate therapy. Hosp Pediatr 2020;10(9):783.

64. Ponder KL, Egesdal C, Kuller J, et al. Project Console: a quality improvement initiative for neonatal abstinence syndrome in a children's hospital level IV neonatal intensive care unit. BMJ Open Qual 2021;10(2):e001079.

65. Berwick DM. Avoiding overuse-the next quality frontier. Lancet (London, England) 2017;390(10090):102–4.

66. Ho T, Dukhovny D, Zupancic JAF, et al. Choosing wisely in newborn medicine: five opportunities to increase value. Pediatrics 2015;136(2):e482–9.

67. King BC, Richardson T, Patel RM, et al. Prioritization framework for improving the value of care for very low birth weight and very preterm infants. J Perinatol 2021;41(10):2463–73.

68. Klunk CJ, Barrett RE, Peterec SM, et al. An initiative to decrease laboratory testing in a NICU. Pediatrics 2021;148(1). https://doi.org/10.1542/PEDS.2020-000570/179937.

69. King BC, Richardson T, Patel RM, et al. Cost of clinician-driven tests and treatments in very low birth weight and/or very preterm infants. J Perinatol 2020;41(2):295–304.

70. Tchou MJ, Girdwood ST, Wormser B, et al. Reducing electrolyte testing in hospitalized children by using quality improvement methods. Pediatrics 2018;141(5). e20173187-e20173187.

71. Johnson DP, Lind C, Parker SES, et al. Toward high-value care: a quality improvement initiative to reduce unnecessary repeat complete blood counts and basic metabolic panels on a pediatric hospitalist service. Hosp Pediatr 2016;6(1):1–8.

72. Algaze CA, Wood M, Pageler NM, et al. Use of a checklist and clinical decision support tool reduces laboratory use and improves cost. Pediatrics 2016;137(1). https://doi.org/10.1542/PEDS.2014-3019/52804.

73. Cheney C. How Intermountain reduced NICU infections, pain and blood loss. Health leaders media. 2019. Available at: https://www.healthleadersmedia.com/clinical-care/how-intermountain-reduced-nicu-infections-pain-blood-loss. Accessed June 20, 2022.

74. Goodman D, Little G, Harrison W, et al. The Dartmouth Atlas of Neonatal Intensive Care. The Dartmouth Institute for Health Policy and Clinical Practice; 2019.

75. Goodman DC, Ganduglia-Cazaban C, Franzini L, et al. Neonatal intensive care variation in medicaid-insured newborns: a population-based study. J Pediatr 2019;209:44–51.e2.

76. Motz P, Do J, Lam T, et al. Decreasing radiographs in neonates through targeted quality improvement interventions. J Perinatol 2019;40(2):330–6.

77. Galiote JP, Ridoré M, Carman J, et al. Reduction in unintended extubations in a level IV neonatal intensive care unit. Pediatrics 2019;143(5). https://doi.org/10.1542/PEDS.2018-0897/37162.

78. Ridore M, Carman J, Zell L, et al. Reducing unintended extubation rates in the children's national neonatal intensive care unit (NICU): a quality improvement project. Pediatrics 2018;142(1_MeetingAbstract):220. https://doi.org/10.1542/PEDS.142.1MA3.220.

79. Nathan AT, Ward L, Schibler K, et al. A quality improvement initiative to reduce necrotizing enterocolitis across hospital systems. J Perinatol 2018;38(6):742–50.

80. Laughon MM, Avant D, Tripathi N, et al. Drug labeling and exposure in neonates. JAMA Pediatr 2014;168(2):130.

81. De Lima Costa HTM, Costa TX, Martins RR, et al. Use of off-label and unlicensed medicines in neonatal intensive care. PLoS One 2018;13(9). https://doi.org/10.1371/JOURNAL.PONE.0204427.

82. Bamat NA, Kirpalani H, Feudtner C, et al. Medication use in infants with severe bronchopulmonary dysplasia admitted to United States children's hospitals. J Perinatol 2019;39(9):1291–9.

83. Jadcherla SR, Slaughter JL, Stenger MR, et al. Practice variance, prevalence, and economic burden of premature infants diagnosed with GERD. Hosp Pediatr 2013;3(4):335–41.

84. Slaughter JL, Stenger MR, Reagan PB, et al. Neonatal histamine-2 receptor antagonist and proton pump inhibitor treatment at United States children's hospitals. J Pediatr 2016;174:63–70.e3.

85. Shakeel FM, Crews J, Jensen P, et al. Decreasing inappropriate use of antireflux medications by standardizing gastroesophageal reflux disease management in NICU. Pediatr Qual Saf 2021;6(2):e394.

86. Angelidou A, Bell K, Gupta M, et al. Implementation of a guideline to decrease use of acid-suppressing medications in the NICU. Pediatrics 2017;140(6). https://doi.org/10.1542/PEDS.2017-1715/38226.

87. Reinhart RM, McClary JD, Zhang M, et al. Reducing antacid use in a level IV NICU: a QI project to reduce morbidity. Pediatr Qual Saf 2020;5(3):e303.

88. Thai JD, Rostas SE, Erdei C, et al. A quality improvement initiative to reduce acid-suppressing medication exposure in the NICU. J Perinatol 2021;1–8.

89. Binti Abdul Hamid H, Szatkowski L, Budge H, et al. Anti-reflux medication use in preterm infants. Pediatr Res 2021;1–6. https://doi.org/10.1038/s41390-021-01821-y.

90. Barrington KJ, Finer N, Pennaforte T. Inhaled nitric oxide for respiratory failure in preterm infants. Cochrane Database Syst Rev 2017;1(1):CD000509.

91. Barrington KJ, Finer N, Pennaforte T, et al. Nitric oxide for respiratory failure in infants born at or near term. Cochrane Database Syst Rev 2017;2017(1).

92. Soll RF. Inhaled nitric oxide for preterm infants: what can change our practice? Pediatrics 2018;141(3):e20174214.

93. Truog WE, Nelin LD, Das A, et al. Inhaled nitric oxide usage in preterm infants in the NICHD neonatal research network: inter-site variation and propensity evaluation. J Perinatol 2014;34(11):842–6.

94. Subhedar NV, Jawad S, Oughham K, et al. Increase in the use of inhaled nitric oxide in neonatal intensive care units in England: a retrospective population study. BMJ Paediatr Open 2021;5(1):e000897.

95. Ahearn J, Panda M, Carlisle H, et al. Impact of inhaled nitric oxide stewardship programme in a neonatal intensive care unit. J Paediatr Child Health 2020;56(2):265–71.

96. Elmekkawi A, More K, Shea J, et al. Impact of stewardship on inhaled nitric oxide utilization in a neonatal ICU. Hosp Pediatr 2016;6(10):607–15.

97. Hussain WA, Bondi DS, Shah P, et al. Implementation of an inhaled nitric oxide weaning protocol and stewardship in a level 4 NICU to decrease inappropriate use. J Pediatr Pharmacol Ther JPPT 2022;27(3):284.

98. Todd Tzanetos DR, Housley JJ, Barr FE, et al. Implementation of an inhaled nitric oxide protocol decreases direct cost associated with its use. Respir Care 2015;60(5):644–50.

99. Di Genova T, Sperling C, Gionfriddo A, et al. A stewardship program to optimize the use of inhaled nitric oxide in pediatric critical care. Qual Manag Health Care 2018;27(2):74–80.

100. Goudie A, Dynan L, Brady PW, et al. Attributable cost and length of stay for central line–associated bloodstream infections. Pediatrics 2014;133(6):e1525.

101. Karagiannidou S, Msce CT, Zaoutis TE, Papaevangelou V, Maniadakis Bsc N, Kourlaba G. Length of stay, cost, and mortality of healthcare-acquired bloodstream infections in children and neonates: A systematic review and meta-analysis. Published online 2020. doi:10.1017/ice.2019.353

102. Johnson TJ, Patel AL, Bigger HR, et al. Economic benefits and costs of human milk feedings: a strategy to reduce the risk of prematurity-related morbidities in very-low-birth-weight infants. Adv Nutr 2014;5(2):207–12.

103. Jadcherla SR, Dail J, Malkar MB, et al. Impact of process optimization and quality improvement measures on neonatal feeding outcomes at an all-referral neonatal intensive care unit. J Parenter Enteral Nutr 2016;40(5):646–55.

104. Culpepper C, Hendrickson K, Marshall S, et al. Implementation of feeding guidelines hastens the time to initiation of enteral feeds and improves growth velocity in very low birth-weight infants. Adv Neonatal Care 2017;17(2):139–45.

105. Chu S, Procaskey A, Tripp S, et al. Quality improvement initiative to decrease time to full feeds and central line utilization among infants born less than or equal to 32 0/7 weeks through compliance with standardized feeding guidelines. J Perinatol 2019;39(8):1140–8.

106. Jasani B, Patole S. Standardized feeding regimen for reducing necrotizing enterocolitis in preterm infants: an updated systematic review. J Perinatol 2017;37(7):827–33.

107. Patel EU, Head WT, Rohrer A, et al. A quality improvement initiative to standardize time to initiation of enteral feeds after non-surgical necrotizing enterocolitis using a consensus-based guideline. J Perinatol 2022;42(4):522–7.

Recent Progress in Neonatal Global Health Quality Improvement

Ashish KC, MBBS, MHCM, PhD[a,b], Rohit Ramaswamy, PhD, MPH[c],
Danielle Ehret, MD, MPH[d,e], Bogale Worku, MD[f,g],
Beena D. Kamath-Rayne, MD, MPH[h,*]

KEYWORDS

- Neonatal mortality • Global health • Quality improvement • Helping Babies Breathe
- Essential Newborn Care • Neonatal resuscitation

KEY POINTS

- Improvements in neonatal mortality have progressed at a slower pace than other age groups less than 5 years and now make up an overall greater proportion of less than 5-year mortality.
- Programs, such as Helping Babies Survive and Essential Newborn Care, provide training on important interventions to improve basic neonatal resuscitation practices and essential newborn care but must be coupled with quality improvement methodologies to support behavior change and health systems strengthening after a training event.
- Innovative approaches to support quality improvement after a training event include numerous online resources, in addition to both in-person and telementoring initiatives.
- Essential elements of successful learning health systems that support high-quality care include the provision of support for local leaders and champions; local systems for training, debriefing, and audits; a data collection system on a set of standardized indicators for basic processes of care and outcomes; and empowerment of health care professionals and community members to provide/demand high-quality care, respectively.

Continued

[a] Global Health, Institute of Medicine, Sahlgrenska Academy, School of Public Health and Community Medicine, Gothenburg University, Gothenburg, Sweden; [b] Department of Women's and Children Health, Uppsala University, Dag Hammarskjölds Väg 14B, Uppsala 751 85, Sweden; [c] Cincinnati Children's Medical Center Hospital, 3333 Burnet Avenue, Cincinnati, OH 45229, USA; [d] Global Health, University of Vermont Larner College of Medicine, 111 Colchester Avenue, Burlington, VT 05401, USA; [e] Vermont Oxford Network, 33 Kilburn Street, Burlington, VT 05401, USA; [f] Addis Ababa University, Addis Ababa, Ethiopia; [g] Ethiopian Pediatric Society, Addis Ababa Chapter Office, Family Building 5th Floor, Room 501, Addis Ababa, Ethiopia; [h] Global Newborn and Child Health, American Academy of Pediatrics, 345 Park Boulevard, Itasca, IL 60143, USA
* Corresponding author.
E-mail address: bkamathrayne@aap.org

Clin Perinatol 50 (2023) 507–529
https://doi.org/10.1016/j.clp.2023.02.003
0095-5108/23/© 2023 Elsevier Inc. All rights reserved.

perinatology.theclinics.com

Continued

- Because frameworks for quality improvement were developed in highly resourced settings, these may need to be adjusted to apply to lower-resourced settings through engaging with partners and collaborators in those settings and determining what their priorities are for improvement.

INTRODUCTION

Over the past 2 decades, substantial decreases have been achieved in global deaths of children less than 5 years of age, from 9.65 million in 2000 to 5.05 million in 2019.[1,2] Concurrently, reductions in neonatal mortality, defined as deaths in live-born babies within the first 28 days after birth, have been seen, from 4.0 million in 2000[3] to 2.42 million (48%) in 2019.[1] Although notable accelerations in reduction of global mortalities in children less than 5 years of age have been realized, the largest number of deaths, as well as the slowest progress, occurred in the early neonatal age group. In all income settings, declines in neonatal mortality have lagged behind mortality declines in other age groups.[2]

The 3 main reasons newborns die in the first month of life are prematurity, infection, and asphyxia-related complications.[4–6] Each year, approximately 10 million neonates do not cry or breathe at birth and require resuscitation to transition to extrauterine life.[7] Newborns who are born too soon or too small or who become sick are at the greatest risk of death and disability[8–10] and often need the most significant resuscitation at birth. As resuscitation and stabilization are occurring, all newly born infants also require assessment and intervention related to essential newborn care that must continue until the baby is ready for hospital discharge, and then beyond.[11]

Training programs, such as Helping Babies Breathe (HBB), led by the American Academy of Pediatrics (AAP) with other partners,[12,13] and the Essential Newborn Care (ENC) course of the World Health Organization (WHO)[14,15] have been successful at teaching cadres of more than 1 million health care professionals the skills of basic neonatal resuscitation and essential newborn care to address the most common causes of neonatal mortality. However, an important lesson learned from the undoubtable success of these programs is that training in these skills is only the start of a journey to high-quality care that must include behavior change and health systems strengthening.[16,17]

Indeed, high-quality care requires an integrated, resilient health system, multidisciplinary teams, and innovation.[18] High-quality care requires investment in quality improvement (QI) systems with enough health care providers with the skills to care for small or sick newborns, working in partnership with parents and families.[19] High-quality care also involves facilities that use evidence-based practices; are well-organized, accessible, and adequately resourced; are safe, efficient, equitable, timely, and people-centered; and ensure optimal clinical, developmental, and social outcomes for small and sick newborns.[20] Most importantly, it is important to acknowledge that most of the theories, models, and frameworks used in QI and implementation science have been developed in higher-resourced settings, that may not be universally applicable to heterogeneous global contexts.[21] It is and will continue to be critical to apply the lens of decolonization to the partnerships, collaborations, and frameworks through which this work is undertaken.

In this article, the authors further describe some of these lessons learned in disseminating educational programs related to basic neonatal resuscitation and essential newborn care globally, as well as complementing those programs with QI and health systems strengthening initiatives that must follow training, with the overall goal of improving neonatal outcomes and decreasing neonatal mortality worldwide.

LESSONS LEARNED FROM HELPING BABIES BREATHE

In 2010, the AAP, in conjunction with other collaborators in a public/private Global Development Alliance, introduced the HBB program.[13] Emphasizing skills-based practice and adult learning techniques, HBB was developed to aid health care professionals in resource-limited settings to learn the critical skills of basic newborn resuscitation.[12] Two companion curricula, Essential Care for Every Baby[22] and Essential Care for Small Babies,[23] were developed to address essential newborn care and specialized care for low-birth-weight and preterm infants, respectively. Together with HBB, these curricula are known as the Helping Babies Survive (HBS) suite of programs and address the 3 most common causes of preventable newborn mortality: prematurity, infection, and perinatal asphyxia.

HBS training programs have been formally adopted into national health systems in many low- and middle-income countries (LMICs).[24] A wide body of literature now exists supporting that training with the HBS programs does decrease early neonatal mortality as well as stillbirth rates.[25–28] However, in the decade since its initial release, much has been learned regarding best practices for effective trainings, overcoming challenges to implementation, and sustaining impactful HBS interventions around the world.[29] One of the most important lessons from 10 years of HBB training and implementation is that a 1-day workshop by itself is insufficient to change neonatal outcomes.[30] Although training on the best-evidence-based practices is an important first step to improving outcomes, ongoing practice and local implementation are other key aspects to improving care.[31] Acquisition and maintenance of new complex skills for health care workers are not single events.[31,32] It requires a number of activities for knowledge acquisition, skills practice for acquisition and retention,[33–35] follow-on mentorship,[36] behavior change,[37] systems improvement, and monitoring of new skills in clinical application. The model of training health care workers in hotel conference rooms away from their health facilities for multiple days has become obsolete. HBB training has been encouraged within the health care facility itself, so that workers in their own workplace can contextualize the training approach, identify gaps in care, and problem solve as a team.[38] In addition to clinical training, this requires staff to be trained and oriented in basic QI methods to approach implementation challenges systematically.[39]

Helping Babies Breathe, 2nd Edition[40] attempted to provide some resources to start the QI journey that must occur after training, including directing learners to ask questions to identify gaps in care at the end of the workshop.[41] These questions included: "What are you going to do differently?" "What will you no longer do?" and finally, "How are you going to make these changes happen?" Under the heading "Commit to making a difference," the Action Plan (**Fig. 1**), which serves as the backbone of the essential life-saving steps to be performed, was used as a directive toward investigating gaps in care, with each step of the algorithm pointing to a process or outcome indicator that could serve as the basis of a QI project. These resources encouraged the learners to begin to consider gaps in care that could be remediated through QI processes.

Indeed, several teams have demonstrated that using QI methodologies after HBB training was essential for further acquiring and maintaining skills learned in the course through the establishment of "newborn corners" to perform low-dose/high-frequency

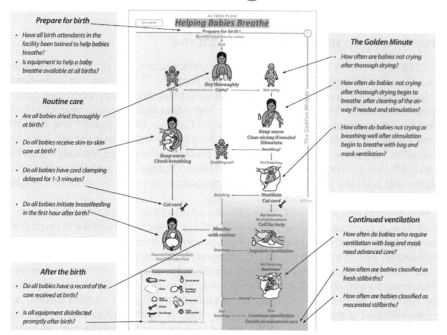

Fig. 1. Helping Babies Breathe, 2nd Edition, action plan linking key outcome and process indicators to the steps of basic neonatal resuscitation. The * is internal to the image of the Action Plan itself and its corresponding * is the equipment list pictured in the box at the bottom left of the image. HMS, helping mother survive. (*From* Niermeyer S, Kamath-Rayne B, Keenan W, Little G, Singhal N, Visick M, eds.; for Helping Babies Survive. *Helping Babies Breathe: Facilitator Flip Chart* [log-in required]. 2nd ed. American Academy of Pediatrics, Laerdal Global Health; 2016. http://internationalresources.aap.org/Resource/ShowFile?documentName=HBB_Flipbook_Second_Edition_20-00371_Rev_E.pdf. Accessed Jan 2 2022.)

practice,[42] the establishment of data collection systems to acquire, follow, and show data to health care professionals and hospital leadership to promote change,[43] and the establishment of audit teams that debriefed difficult delivery room resuscitations and reviewed cases of neonatal mortality to determine how to improve care.[17]

ESSENTIAL NEWBORN CARE NOW!

Because of the success of HBB dissemination and impact, the WHO chose to update their ENC course using HBB imagery and teaching methodologies[44] to teach neonatal resuscitation and essential newborn care.[44] This partnership between AAP and the WHO was forged to encourage greater adoption by Ministries of Health or other national health care leaders of the learning methodologies proven so successful by HBB, thereby allowing for a wider reach of the program. Essential newborn care involves immediate care at birth (delayed cord clamping, thorough drying, assessment of breathing, skin-to-skin contact, and early initiation of breastfeeding), thermal care, resuscitation when needed, support for breast milk feeding, nurturing care, infection prevention, assessment of health problems, recognition and response to danger signs, and timeline and safe referral when needed. These topics are fundamental in the HBS curricula. Using HBS programs as the foundation, the WHO, after partnership with AAP and others, updated the content in accordance with their own guidance and released the interim version of their ENC course, 2nd Edition, in April 2022. The goal is for this new ENC course to be the most updated educational program to train health care professionals in essential newborn care and basic neonatal resuscitation, serving as the next generation of HBB. It builds upon the in-person training modeled by HBB with the addition of online modules that cover certain topics with additional detail and that can be performed asynchronously. The face-to-face version of the course was field tested in Tanzania in 2019, and the goal is to release the final version in Spring 2023.

However, restrictions during the COVID-19 pandemic and beyond have required that capacity building of health care providers be reorganized to ensure continuity of services. Restrictions in gathering of groups and travel have prohibited health care workers to meet for training, much less leave frontline positions in clinical care for consolidated blocks for training.[45] AAP, in conjunction with Laerdal Global Health, launched ENC Now! The goal of ENC Now! was to allow for the most updated version of the WHO ENC content to be immediately available and accessible for training. Rather than printing paper flip charts and other teaching materials, the WHO ENC digital flip chart is available through an online digital platform available at hmbs.org [46] that can be used to teach the WHO ENC course remotely, led by an online facilitator who could be located anywhere in the world and who was supported by an onsite facilitator who could focus on the hands-on skills practice so engrained in HBB.[47]

The ENC Now! program has been field tested in Bangladesh, Nepal, Nigeria, South Africa, and Ethiopia, with initial positive feedback and improvement in educational outcomes.[48–50] The blended learning methodology allows for learners to view the materials before the course, adhering to a flipped classroom model, and greater flexibility exists to do distributed learning (short chunks divided over several sessions), rather than consolidated learning, as had been historically popular with HBB workshops.

ENC Now! provides a vehicle for a new way of thinking about delivery of high-quality care, thereby increasing adherence to protocols and reducing mortality. When paired with a culture of empowerment and innovation, health care workers can track their progress in implementing their new skills, measuring frequency, effectiveness, patient outcomes, and more. QI teams who look at data together from their own facilities gain insight into what is actually happening versus what they believe is happening. A case study done in Nepal (**Fig. 2**) indicates how ongoing QI efforts implemented after an ENC Now! training workshop can continue to improve clinical outcomes, parallel to what was seen when QI methods were implemented after HBB training.

METRICS FOR EVALUATING ESSENTIAL NEWBORN CARE

Implementation of HBS programs has shown that health institutions that used quality metrics to routinely track care and outcomes had improved readiness for care, performance, and survival.[12,24] Therefore, the development of a standard set of metrics to monitor and evaluate essential newborn care was desirable for comparability across settings. Gaps in care are highly individualized to patient populations, hospital facilities, and geographic locations, and thus, QI efforts must be adapted to local environments based on needs assessment. Indicators should be selected based on infrastructure, clinical context, QI goals, and resources.

The Every Newborn Action Plan (ENAP) was published in 2014 to provide a roadmap of strategic actions that the global community could be taking to reduce neonatal

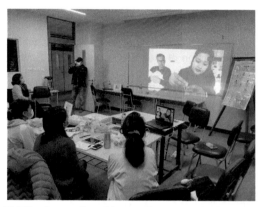

Fig. 2. Case study: ENC Now! was piloted in Nepal to assess the feasibility, acceptability, and adherence to online teaching. The ENC Now! training for a batch of health care professionals (HCPs) was done in 3-hour sessions for 3 consecutive days after their clinical services. A set of essential newborn care indicators were measured and monitored over the period before ENC Now! was introduced. The HCPs reviewed the indicators together during the ENC Now! training and based on the new learnings developed a QI plan using a PDSA process.[16,81] After the ENC Now!, clinical performance data were reviewed every 2 weeks. A daily skill drill was also introduced in the labor and delivery room so that HCPs could practice during their free time. During the pilot phase of 12 weeks, 1887 mothers were admitted in the labor room; 1836 (97%) were enrolled in the project, and 1795 (98%) mothers delivered their babies in the delivery room, the delivery events of which were observed by an independent research officer. Forty-one (2%) mothers were transferred to the operation theater for emergency cesarean section. HCPs' practice of greeting mothers before delivery significantly increased from 15.7% in baseline period to 33.3% during the intervention ($P<.001$). Likewise, during the baseline period, preparation of resuscitation equipment before delivery was done in 9.6% deliveries, whereas during the intervention period it increased to 43.7% ($P<.001$). The fetal heart rate was monitored as per national protocol in 83.7% of the mothers during the baseline period, which increased to 91.3% during the intervention period ($P = .002$). As compared with the baseline period, health workers practicing immediate and essential quality newborn care demonstrated improvements in handwashing before conducting every delivery (16.9% vs 36.6%; $P<.001$), continued skin-to-skin contact for at least 1 hour after birth (0.8% vs 22.9%; $P<.001$), initiation of breastfeeding within 1 hour after birth inside delivery room (58.9% vs 76.2%; $P<.001$). Although none of the noncrying/nonbreathing babies received ventilation within the Golden Minute after birth during the baseline period, this increased to 22% during the intervention period ($P = .86$). The median time of ventilation decreased from 141 seconds in the baseline period to 90 seconds in the intervention period. The research team is continuing to follow up clinical outcomes. (*Courtesy of* O Basnet, M.Sc, Lalitpur, Nepal.)

deaths and stillbirths.[51] These strategic actions included investing in care during labor/birth and the first week of life, improving the quality of maternal and newborn care, reaching every woman and newborn to reduce inequities, harnessing the power of parents, families, and communities, and counting every newborn through measurement, program tracking, and accessibility.[52] Using these strategic actions, the goal was to reduce each country's national neonatal mortality rate to 10 per 1000 live births or less, resulting in a global average of 7 per 1000 live births or less by 2035.[52]

To measure the progress of ENAP, a set of indicators were recommended for use by the WHO in 2015 (**Table 1**).[53,54] However, several challenges are notable around these measures. First, the indicators desired by the global community to follow

Table 1
Every Newborn Action Plan metrics

Level of Indicator	ENAP Indicators	Numerator	Denominator
Impact (expected effect of maternal and neonatal interventions)	Maternal mortality ratio[b]	Number of maternal deaths per year during pregnancy and childbirth or within 42 d of termination of pregnancy, irrespective of the duration and site of the pregnancy	100,000 live births
	Stillbirth rate[b]	Number of infants per year born with no sign of life and weighing ≤1000 g or after 28 wk' gestation	1000 total live and stillborn births
	Neonatal mortality rate[b]	Number of live-born infants per year who die before 28 completed days of age	1000 live births
	Intrapartum stillbirth rate[a]	Number of stillbirths per year born occurring during labor	1000 total live and stillborn births
	Low-birth-weight rate[a]	Number of live-born infants per year with birth weight <2500 g	1000 live births
	Preterm birth rate[a]	Number of live-born infants per year born with gestational age <37 wk	1000 live births
	Small for gestational age[a]	Number of live-born infants with weight <10 centile as per the gestational age	1000 live births
	Neonatal morbidity rates[a]	Number of sick infants before 28 completed days of age	1000 live births
	Disability after neonatal conditions[a]	Number of infants with disability	1000 live births

(continued on next page)

Table 1
(continued)

Level of Indicator	ENAP Indicators	Numerator	Denominator
Coverage: Care for All Mothers and Newborns	Skilled attendant at birth[b]	Number of women aged 15–49 y who received a health check within 2 d after delivery	Number of women aged 15–49 y with a live birth
	Early postnatal care for mothers[b]	Number of live births assisted by a skilled provider (doctor, nurse midwife auxiliary nurse/midwife)	Number of women aged 15–49 y with a live birth
	Early postnatal care for babies[b]	Number of last live births with a postnatal health check in the first 2 day after birth	Total number of live births
	Essential newborn care with early initiation of breastfeeding as tracer indicator[b]	Number of live-born infants (in the 2 y before the survey) who are breastfed within 1 h of birth	Total number of live-born infants
	Antenatal care[a]	Number of women aged 15–49 y who had 4 antenatal checkups	Total number of live births
	Exclusive breastfeeding up to 6 mo[a]	Number of infants aged 0–5 mo who are exclusively breastfed	Total number of live-born infants
Coverage: Complications and Extra Care	Antenatal corticosteroid use[b]	All women who give birth in facility at <34 completed weeks and received 1 dose of antenatal corticosteroids for risk of preterm birth	Total births in the facility
	Neonatal resuscitation[b]	Number of newborns who received any positive pressure ventilation using any device (most commonly via bag and mask)	Total births in the facility (including stillbirths)
	Kangaroo mother care[b]	Number of admitted newborns with a birthweight <2500 g who were initiated on kangaroo mother care	Number of admitted newborns with a birth <2500 g anywhere in the facility

		Numerator	Denominator
	Treatment of serious neonatal infections[b]	(placed in the kangaroo position) anywhere in the facility Number of infants within 28 d who received at least 1 injection of antibiotic for possible serious bacterial infection in the facility	Total number of live-born infants
	Cesarean section rate[a]	Number of women aged 15–49 y with a live birth delivered by cesarean section	Women aged 15–49 y with a live birth
	Chlorhexidine cord cleansing[a]	Number of newborns who received at least 1 dose of chlorhexidine (7.1%) to the cord within 24 h of birth	Total number of live-born infants
Input: Service Delivery Packages for Quality of Care	Emergency obstetric care[a]	Number of facilities in area providing basic or comprehensive emergency obstetric care	Population of area by 500,000
Input: Counting	Birth registration[b]	Number of births registered in the local government office	
	Death registration, cause of death[a]	Number of deaths registered in the local government office with cause of death	

[a] Core indicator.
[b] Additional indicators.

Data from World Health Organization and UNICEF. Every Newborn Action Plan 2015-2030. Geneva 2014. and Lawn JE, Blencowe H, Oza S, et al. Every Newborn: progress, priorities, and potential beyond survival. Lancet 2014;384(9938):189-205.

improvements made in neonatal health coverage may not be feasible to collect at national and subnational levels in countries facing the greatest challenges with neonatal mortality. Second, it is widely recognized that delving deeper into a country's data reveals health inequities at the subnational level, which are important to acknowledge and work toward lessening in order for countries to meet ENAP targets. Finally, in trying to focus on a set of core indicators, a tension exists between an indicator for coverage versus an indicator for quality; for example, having 8 antenatal care visits is an indicator for coverage, but recording number of antenatal visits by itself reveals nothing about the quality of those visits.

To evaluate the accuracy of reporting of ENC indicators (neonatal resuscitation, immediate breastfeeding, immediate skin-to-skin contact, delayed cord clamping, and antibiotic treatment of infection) in routine registers and maternal recall survey, a multicountry validation of the indicators was done between 2017 and 2019.[55] Performance of certain ENC indicators was measured through review of hospital registers and via exit surveys of postpartum women at the time of hospital discharge, compared with the gold standard of independent observation. Exit surveys had 100% agreement with observations for skin-to-skin contact, but underestimated neonatal resuscitation with bag-mask ventilation (0.8% vs 4.4% observed) and antibiotic treatment of neonatal infection (74.7% vs 96.4% observed) and overestimated early breastfeeding coverage (53.2% vs 10.9% observed). Register data underestimated neonatal resuscitation with bag-mask ventilation (4.3% vs 5.1% observed), kangaroo mother care (KMC) (92.9% vs 100% observed), and overestimated early breastfeeding (85.9% vs 12.5% observed). The investigators noted the interhospital heterogeneity to be higher for register-recorded coverage than for the exit survey report. Hospital register design and completeness are less standardized than surveys, resulting in variable data quality, however with good validity for the best performing sites.

Challenges also exist regarding the unifying definition of various indicators. For example, "neonatal resuscitation" or "resuscitation with a bag and mask" requires further definition—was the baby in the 5% to 10% who require bag and mask ventilation at all after drying and stimulation were performed? Or, did the baby have properly performed bag and mask ventilation after it was determined that it was needed? These are subtle but important differences. As a step forward in capturing data around neonatal resuscitation, a working group of the International Liaison Committee on Resuscitation Neonatal Task Force produced an Utstein-style report of core and supplemental indicators for neonatal resuscitation.[56] In 1990, the first standard reporting guidelines for out-of-hospital cardiac arrest were published after a meeting at the Utstein Abbey in Norway; since that time, more than 30 Utstein-style reports have been generated using similar procedures and for varying patient populations.[57] The Neonatal report was produced following the same process. Core and supplemental indicators across 7 domains (setting, patient, antepartum, birth/preresuscitation, resuscitation process, postresuscitation process, and outcomes) were represented.[56] In addition to demographic variables, core indicators included antenatal corticosteroid exposure, umbilical cord clamping timing and cord milking, Apgar scores, use of supplemental oxygen, positive pressure ventilation, and other delivery room resuscitation interventions, initial temperature, and outcomes, such as mortality, duration of hospital stay, hypoxic-ischemic encephalopathy, and prematurity outcomes, such as bronchopulmonary dysplasia, retinopathy of prematurity, necrotizing enterocolitis, intraventricular hemorrhage, and periventricular leukomalacia. Supplemental indicators included complete antenatal corticosteroid course, umbilical cord pH, number of times cord milked, timing of delivery room resuscitation interventions, number of providers in delivery room, transfer to higher level of care, glucose measurements, and neurodevelopmental impairment at 18 to 24 months corrected age.

Currently, in light of these challenges, the ENAP leadership group, in conjunction with its partner group Ending Preventable Maternal Mortality, is working toward streamlining the core indicators further, providing more direction with definitions of indicators (numerator and denominator), and determining how to improve capacity in data collection and analysis at the local level. Furthermore, linkages of various data dashboards that capture core data, as well as digitalization of data, are innovations being considered.

Several upcoming global maternal/neonatal health meetings in 2023 are expected to provide further guidance and improvements in data metrics to empower the global community toward meeting ENAP targets.

QUALITY IMPROVEMENT RESOURCES

Lessons learned from HBB demonstrated that a package of education in QI combined with mentorship or coaching on a focused QI initiative is valued by health care teams charged with changing the culture of their units, and improving quality of care. To that end, several open access resources are available to health care workers, teams, and coaches, providing a framework and complement of foundational QI education (Table 2).

As more people are aware of these resources, they are being used to support QI activities after initial training workshops. For example, the AAP worked with partners to create the *Improving Care of Mothers and Babies* Quality Improvement Workbook to take learners through some simple steps of the QI process, including setting goals for improving care, problem identification, development of a plan to overcome the problem, and a continual process of reviewing the progress.[58] Several studies evaluating the use of the QI workbook demonstrated greater effectiveness when learners had the support of a mentor through the process, rather than self-directed learning.[59,60]

By understanding the need for innovation to change the trajectory of improvement in neonatal mortality, several strategies for QI education, coaching, and remote mentorship have been trialed in Ethiopia. Using the guide *Improving Care of Mothers and Babies* QI Workbook,[58] it was feasible for midwifery teams without experience in QI to implement a large-scale change in their labor and delivery units when this curriculum was paired with QI coaching.[61] Emphasizing the importance of mentorship when first applying QI methodology to an identified quality gap in the clinical setting, investigators found that QI teams supported by in-person mentorship generally made more progress toward their QI aim than teams supported by remote QI mentorship. Although not specifically trained in data science, QI mentors provide guidance on the need for available, accurate, and actionable data for the purpose of QI. Although clinical data review at the bedside is within the purview of an on-site mentor, data quality is important for all teams regardless of the mentorship structure.

The importance of mentorship after HBB/ENC training to support ongoing implementation cannot be understated. The AAP has also developed CRISP, a Customized mentorRship, and Implementation Support Package, to develop a cadre of global mentors who are trained to provide supplemental mentorship and deliver resources on topics to support implementation, knowledge, and skills transfer and an approach to health systems strengthening. These topics include the following: monitoring and evaluation, QI, facilitator strengthening, systems for ongoing skills practice, and simulation/debriefing, among others. The facilitators who go through CRISP mentorship

Table 2
Open-access resources to support quality improvement in health care facilities in low-resource settings

Resource	Authoring Organization(s)	Brief Description	Target Audience	Link
Improving Care of Mothers and Babies	AAP and University Research Company	QI guide that outlines 6 steps for implementing QI	Facility-based QI team leaders and members	https://internationalresources.aap.org/
Quality of care toolkit	World Health Organization	Framework containing 8 domains of quality care for the time around childbirth	Health facility leaders, planners, managers, and providers	Quality Toolkits Home Page (who.int)
Standards for Improving Quality of Maternal and Newborn Care in Health Facilities	World Health Organization	Framework containing 8 standards of care and 31 quality statements for maternal and newborn health	Health facility leaders, planners, managers, and providers	https://cdn.who.int/media/docs/default-source/mca-documents/qoc/quality-of-care/standards-for-improving-quality-of-maternal-and-newborn-care-in-health-facilities.pdf
Coaching for QI	Healthqual and UCSF Institute for Global Health Sciences	Guide to implementation of coaching strategies and spread of QI knowledge in low-resource settings	QI coaches	https://healthqual.ucsf.edu/sites/g/files/tkssra931/f/coachingtoolkit-complete_printable_updated%20%282%29.pdf
Point-of-care QI training model	World Health Organization Regional Office for Southeast Asia, World Health Organization Collaborating Center for Training and Research in Newborn Care, AIIMS New Delhi, and ASSIST Project	Multiple resources, including: Coaching for QI, Improving the Quality of Care for Mothers and Newborns in Health Facilities (Learner's and Facilitator's Manuals), Setting Up and Managing a QI Program at District Level, and POCQI Virtual Workbook	QI teams, coaches, and leadership supporting QI teams	http://www.pocqi.org

| Institute for Healthcare Improvement Open School | Institute for Healthcare Improvement | An international and interprofessional community of learners with access to online courses, local chapters, and project-based learning through virtual training programs | Individuals with passion for improvement of patient care | Resources | IHI - Institute for Healthcare Improvement |

Abbreviations: AIIMS, All India Institute of Medical Sciences; ASSIST, applying science to strengthen and improve systems; POCQI, point-of-care quality improvement; UCSF, University of California San Francisco.

Adapted from Ehret DEY, Patterson JK, Kc A, Worku B, Kamath-Rayne BD, Bose CL. Helping Babies Survive Programs as an Impetus for Quality Improvement. Pediatrics. 2020 Oct;146(Suppl 2):S183-S193.

are equipped to support the roll-out of ENC to health care workers providing care to mothers and newborns.

TELEMENTORING INITIATIVES

Although access to care, including delivery in a health facility, remains a challenge in many LMIC settings, "access to care" is no longer viewed as a competing priority with "quality of care" by those implementing newborn health programs globally.[62–64] Simultaneously improving access and quality, however, requires innovation. With the intent of guiding redesign of health care systems with a focus on quality and transitions to population health, the "Triple Aim" was developed as a framework for high-value care with 3 overarching goals: improving the individual experience of care; improving the health of populations; and reducing the per capita cost of health care.[65] Recently, this has been broadened into the "Quadruple Aim," adding the goal of improving the health care team's experience of providing care.[63,66] During the COVID-19 pandemic and in humanitarian or fragile settings, a focus on the Quadruple Aim has highlighted the opportunity for telementoring to support health care teams when on-site local support is not possible. One strategy has been to use remote mentorship, or telementoring, on QI.

The AAP has had experience with telementoring through identifying gaps in care after needs assessments and developing educational curricula to address those gaps in care,[67] as well as health systems strengthening through Extending Community Healthcare Outcomes (ECHO) programs.[68,69] The ECHO program was originally developed as a hub-and-spoke model for dispersion of medical subspecialist expertise combined with supporting providers to deliver care in remote sites to meet the needs of patients, families, and communities.[70] As a pediatric superhub that has the ability to train other organizations to be ECHO hubs, the AAP has leveraged the ECHO model to rapidly disseminate the "all teach, all learn" model not only to communities of learners in domestic settings but also in global health settings. Through use of the ECHO model, the AAP has partnered with local professional associations to provide mentorship using case-based learning to cover content on topics as diverse as developmental surveillance and screening in the era of Zika, COVID-19, and maternal/neonatal health.

Several LMICs have incorporated QI capability building into their national plans to improve newborn survival. Ethiopia serves as an example, whereby innovation in QI for the LMIC setting is ongoing, and collaboration with international and nongovernmental organization partners has contributed to global learning in this space.[71,72] QI mentors may also serve a dual role as clinical mentors when the appropriate cadre is selected, necessary and requested training is provided, and the responsibility of advising colleagues is matched with a leadership platform to share collective experiences, advocating for resources necessary to implement and fully use QI education and clinical investments to realize improvement opportunities. The Ethiopian Pediatrics Society (EPS), in collaboration with UNICEF, the Ethiopian Federal Ministry of Health, and regional health bureaus, implemented in-person mentorship, with a focus on clinical support in addition to quality of care for 2 leading causes of mortality, intrapartum-related events/birth asphyxia, and infections/sepsis.[72] Mentors received education on HBS, QI, and low-dose/high-frequency training to combat known knowledge and skill retention issues following initial HBB training as well as an algorithm for identification and management of neonates with sepsis. Mentors facilitated establishment of QI teams at each of the participating facilities, 6 hospitals and 26 health centers, in low-performing woredas, or zones, across 5 different Ethiopian regional states.

The implementation of QI teams improved communication between the neonatal intensive care unit (NICU) and delivery ward staff, and early identification and treatment of infection as an improvement goal have been associated with a reduction in newborn morbidity and mortality.[73]

The national endorsement of QI in the Ethiopian context facilitated a pivot to trial QI telementoring and continued innovations and adaptations to support improvement in neonatal care. To that end, the ECHO model was implemented in Ethiopia through a collaboration between AAP and EPS, with EPS serving as the hub. The 8-community hospital "spokes," led by midwifery QI coaches, were linked with AAP members with expertise in QI. Ethiopian teams used the LIVEBORN application to collect real-time data on timing of cord clamping in observed deliveries.[74] Monthly interactive virtual sessions reviewed content from *Improving Care of Mothers and Babies* and directly applied this knowledge to team-based QI projects aiming to improve rates of delayed cord clamping. In addition to success in improving rates of delayed cord clamping at all participating sites, the virtual platform and pairing of AAP QI advisors with each Ethiopian coach allowed for cross-cultural collaboration over the 12-month project period, which would not have been feasible in person.[75]

Successful telementoring in 1 environment, however, does not necessarily translate to success in another. Important aspects to consider are the QI coach's experience leading a successful project, the foundation of QI in the health care system, and the complexity of the quality gap of focus. The Ethiopian Neonatal Network (ENN), a joint collaboration between EPS and Vermont Oxford Network and supported by the Ethiopian Federal Ministry of Health, embarked on a telementoring QI collaborative aiming to improve the quality of continuous positive airway pressure (CPAP) delivered to preterm infants with respiratory distress syndrome (RDS) in the participating ENN NICUs in an effort to continue momentum during the COVID-19 pandemic.[76] The ENN had fostered a robust community through 3 years of applying QI education and methodology to the review of standardized inpatient data and in-person meetings to share lessons learned, forming a community voice and a platform for advocacy. Despite the strengths of this community, Ethiopian mentors and teams unanimously advocated for a hybrid approach to mentorship, including at least 1 in-person session per year, when possible and safe, as the identified quality gap (inability to provide quality CPAP) reflected a complex and new skillset for most team members, utilization of new medical equipment, and comprised an important element of critical care. The hybrid model with an on-site visit of national nursing and physician CPAP champions combined with telementoring allowed for implementation feedback, and assessment of skills that are challenging and often not permissible via phone or video (use of CPAP in the NICU setting), while contributing to relationship and community building.[77]

TRANSCENDING QUALITY IMPROVEMENT TO IMPLEMENTATION SCIENCE IN PERINATAL HEALTH

As mentioned previously, clinical training alone is not adequate to ensure successful implementation in clinical settings. The field of implementation science, which is the study of techniques to get evidence-based interventions and proven best practices into everyday clinical care, has identified 4 activities needed to facilitate implementation. They are as follows: training, technical assistance (ie, supervision and coaching), tools (eg, job aids and documented protocols), and quality assurance and improvement (monitoring for compliance, and improvement of operational processes).[78]

Although the first 3 ingredients are directly related to the intervention or clinical practice, and therefore are primarily targeted at the clinicians providing perinatal care, developing an infrastructure for improvement is a foundational skill for the entire facility. It requires engagement and ownership at multiple levels of the facility, and at the health system level, and building effective QI capability requires targeted training and support at each level. On the front lines, staff who are motivated and trusted need to be engaged as change agents and trained in routine monitoring of implementation indicators (eg, adherence or fidelity) as well as in the use of Plan-Do-Study-Act (PDSA) cycles to develop and test solutions to improve performance of these indicators. At the facility level, ward in-charges and others in midlevel leadership positions need to be trained in more formal QI methods (eg, the Model for Improvement) to identify and prioritize system problems (eg, related to equipment or human resources) and to create and coach improvement teams to address them. At the facility leadership level, the leadership team needs to be trained in accountability processes that involve setting improvement priorities, monitoring of progress of QI projects, facilitating the availability of resources to engage in QI, and to build enthusiasm for improvement through appropriate reward and recognition activities. At the cross-facility level and health system levels, there needs to be planned opportunities for sharing implementation challenges and solutions, and regular communications with systems leaders about any policy changes that need to be made to support scale up and sustainment (eg, hiring or transfer policies that ensure that resources to support and maintain implementation are always available in facilities).

Knowledge and training are important, but there are several other key ingredients for a successful QI program. There needs to be an intentional effort to keep staff engaged and motivated in QI motivation, through incentive systems and recognition. In government systems, monetary incentives may not be feasible and may even be detrimental to collaboration, but nonmonetary incentives are available and should be used and communicated. Some examples of these are public recognition ceremonies with certificates, opportunity for conference travel and presentations, small gifts such as mobile phone airtime cards, names and accomplishments on bulletin boards, competition across sites to be the best, team awards, and so forth. Evidence on the relative effectiveness of monetary and nonmonetary incentives is mixed and is context dependent,[79] but in global health settings, there is anecdotal and research evidence of the motivating effect of nonmonetary incentives.[80]

In addition, QI programs are dependent on data, and a key ingredient for success is the ability to routinely collect and analyze process data. Although data on outcomes (eg, mortality) or on key clinical indicators may be available in registers, or in reports, data on adherence or implementation barriers need to be manually collected and analyzed in a way that does not unnecessarily burden the clinical staff or adversely affect clinical operations. Tests of improvement ideas using PDSAs require small amounts of data to be collected at specific points in time and need careful decision making on what data should be collected and when.[81] Getting leadership support for the need for data and building institutional capacity for local manual data collection analysis (eg, using data officers, developing easily customizable templates, training on spreadsheet, and simple statistical software tools) are more critical components for the successful use of QI to support implementation of perinatal interventions.

Finally, it is important to recognize that each of these key ingredients (leadership support and a culture of improvement, capability in the science of QI, incentives to motivate staff, and the availability of data) is not an independent factor but needs to exist together as part of an integrated "Learning Health System" (LHS). An LHS is defined as "a conceptual approach wherein science, informatics, incentives, and culture are aligned to support continuous improvement, innovation, and equity, and seamlessly embed knowledge and best practices into care delivery." The WHO has

---

Box 1
Key activities to create a learning health system to improve perinatal care

1. Adapt learning materials and training curricula to local contexts

2. Provide equipment and supplies simultaneously with training

3. Create a local leadership team and establish an accountability plan for leadership support

4. Identify front-line staff to be local champions and change agent

5. Train champions to conduct frequent, brief refresher training, debriefing, and audits

6. Create and support the function of facility-level perinatal quality-improvement teams

7. Develop a system to collect and report local data on a standardized set of indicators of basic processes of care and patient outcomes

8. Institute a process for reporting and feedback to/from all levels of the health system and the front line

9. Engage and empower health care providers, families, and the broader community in the initiative

---

recently produced guidelines on developing such systems to scale up and sustain maternal/newborn/child health interventions. These guidelines should inform the creation of QI programs to improve quality of perinatal care and include the elements noted in **Box 1**.[82,83]

An example of an LHS approach into perinatal care is the currently on-going MEBCI 2.0 (Making Every Baby Count Initiative) in Ghana. This version of the initiative is focused on improving the quality of advanced newborn care in 4 tertiary hospitals in Ghana. The initial version of this program (MEBCI 1.0) focused on improving the ability of staff in district-level facilities in 4 regions in Ghana to provide newborn care at the time of birth.[84] Staff were trained in 3 evidence-based interventions for newborn care: Helping Babies Breathe; Essential Care for Every Baby; and Infection Prevention. Knowledge and skills were tested using the programs' Knowledge checklist and Objective Structured Clinical Examinations tools.

Evaluation of MEBCI 1.0 revealed that although the program was effective in enhancing the knowledge and skills of staff, the interventions were not enough to care for the sickest babies, many of whom were treated at tertiary hospitals. Moreover, care of the sickest newborns not only required advanced knowledge of clinical care but also necessitated the development of operational processes for rapid transfer of babies, stabilization during transfer, maintenance of equipment, and so forth. MEBCI 2.0 has been designed for implementation in tertiary hospitals as an initiative that supplements advanced clinical training with capacity building in systems strengthening. In each of the 4 facilities, an interdisciplinary team of staff is chosen to serve as implementation coaches and champions, supported by a leadership team. Coaches and champions are trained in the use of data to identify gaps in key operational and clinical processes and in creating and facilitating teams to launch projects to close these gaps. Results from these projects are fed back to the leadership team that is ultimately accountable for achieving results for facilitation and support. Overall, using a mixture of leadership, QI, and implementation science methods, MEBCI 2.0 is designed to create a system of learning and improvement that incentivizes finding solutions to systems' barriers in implementation. Regular learning sessions where teams from each facility meet to share good practices facilitate the dissemination of learning across hospitals.

Finally, as we work to build successful LHSs with our global colleagues, we must do so using the lens of decolonization to assure that historical, systemic power imbalances are mitigated. Importantly, the frameworks for QI and implementation science were developed in highly resourced settings, thereby requiring adaptation for application in heterogenous global contexts.[21] A recent Global Conference for Implementation Science held in Dhaka, Bangladesh in 2019 had more than 250 delegates from 30 countries, with 80% of participants from lower-resourced countries. When the participants were asked to generate ideas regarding the 1 priority action to promote LMIC leadership in implementation science and 1 priority action to develop implementation research in LMIC settings, the themes that emerged included the following: (1) policymakers in LMICs do not set research agendas or fund implementation research; (2) implementation science theories, models, and frameworks are developed in high-income countries; (3) high-income countries monopolize opportunities for knowledge sharing; and finally, (4) equity and community participation are not currently emphasized in the implementation research agenda.[21]

To correct these asymmetries that have characterized global health partnerships, the conference participants envisioned the following to create transformation in implementation science through a decolonized lens: (1) decentralized knowledge creation; (2) equitable access and opportunity for learning and knowledge sharing; (3) research driven by local policymakers trained in implementation science; and finally, (4) implementation research centered on the voices of the vulnerable.[21]

SUMMARY

To achieve improved outcomes in neonatal mortality globally, educational training must be coupled with QI methodologies and implementation science to improve health care systems and create lasting behavior change. Ongoing mentorship is often needed beyond an initial training event to continue to support local leaders and champions; following, interpreting, and developing strategies to address gaps in care through data collection systems and audits; and empowering health care professionals to provide and demand high-quality care. The development of successful LHSs with these characteristics can support achievement of high-quality care for mothers and newborns. Finally, as we continue to move beyond training programs to incorporate QI methodologies into building high-quality health care systems, we must take a much broader approach in including our global health partners embedded with the local contexts themselves in the process from beginning to end, so that the systems continue to address the needs of the communities involved and have the highest chance for sustainability.

CLINICS CARE POINTS

- Training in neonatal resuscitation and essential newborn care must be followed by QI initiatives to strengthen health systems and improve neonatal outcomes.
- The support of QI initiatives after training can utilize innovative techniques, such as in-person and telementoring methods, in addition to numerous online resources.
- Frameworks for quality improvement should include engagement with partners and collaborators in the settings affected and incorporate their priorities for improvement.

DISCLOSURES

Dr B. Kamath-Rayne is currently an employee of the American Academy of Pediatrics. Before her employment, she was the Associate Editor of Helping Babies Breathe, 2nd Edition. Dr A. KC and Dr D. Ehret serve on the American Academy of Pediatrics Helping Babies Survive Planning Group, which has been responsible for developing and disseminating the Helping Babies Survive Curricula. Dr D. Ehret receives salary support in the form of protected nonclinical time at the University of Vermont for her leadership role at Vermont Oxford Network. Dr A. KC has received funding from the Laerdal Foundation for Acute Medicine for evaluation of Helping Babies Breathe.

REFERENCES

1. GDB Collaborators Under-5-Mortality. Global, regional, and national progress towards Sustainable Development Goal 3.2 for neonatal and child health: all-cause and cause-specific mortality findings from the Global Burden of Disease Study 2019. Lancet 2021;398(10303):870–905.
2. UNICEF WHO, World Bank Group and United Nations. Levels and trends in child mortality: report 2021. NewYork: UN Inter-agency Group for Child Mortality Estimation (IGME); 2021.
3. Lawn JE, Cousens S, Zupan J, et al. 4 million neonatal deaths: when? Where? Why? Lancet 2005;365(9462):891–900.
4. Bhutta ZA, Boerma T, Black MM, et al. Optimising child and adolescent health and development in the post-pandemic world. Lancet 2022;399(10337):1759–61.
5. Vaivada T, Lassi ZS, Irfan O, et al. What can work and how? An overview of evidence-based interventions and delivery strategies to support health and human development from before conception to 20 years. Lancet 2022;399(10337):1810–29.
6. World Health Organization and UNICEF. Every Newborn Action Plan Progress Report 2018. Geneva2019.
7. Lee AC, Cousens S, Wall SN, et al. Neonatal resuscitation and immediate newborn assessment and stimulation for the prevention of neonatal deaths: a systematic review, meta-analysis and Delphi estimation of mortality effect. BMC Publ Health 2011;11(Suppl 3):S12.
8. Chawanpaiboon S, Vogel JP, Moller AB, et al. Global, regional, and national estimates of levels of preterm birth in 2014: a systematic review and modelling analysis. Lancet Glob Health 2019;7(1):e37–46.
9. March of Dimes P. Save the children, World Health Organization. Born too soon. Geneva: The global action report on preterm birth; 2014.
10. Lawn JE, Kinney MV, Belizan JM, et al. Born too soon: accelerating actions for prevention and care of 15 million newborns born too soon. Reprod Health 2013;10(Suppl 1):S6.
11. Aziz K, Lee HC, Escobedo MB, et al. Part 5: neonatal resuscitation: 2020 American Heart Association guidelines for cardiopulmonary resuscitation and emergency cardiovascular care. Circulation 2020;142(16_suppl_2):S524–50.
12. Singhal N, McMillan DD, Savich R, et al. Development and impact of helping babies breathe educational methodology. Pediatrics 2020;146(Suppl 2):S123–33.
13. Niermeyer S, Keenan W, Little G, et al. For helping babies survive. Helping babies breathe: action plan. American Academy of Pediatrics. Laerdal Global Health; 2010.
14. Carlo WA, Goudar SS, Jehan I, et al. Newborn-care training and perinatal mortality in developing countries. N Engl J Med 2010;362(7):614–23.

15. Chomba E, Carlo WA, Goudar SS, et al. Effects of essential newborn care training on fresh stillbirths and early neonatal deaths by maternal education. Neonatology 2017;111(1):61–7.

16. Ehret DEY, Patterson JK, KC A, et al. Helping babies survive programs as an impetus for quality improvement. Pediatrics 2020;146(Suppl 2):S183–93.

17. KC A, Wrammert J, Clark RB, et al. Reducing perinatal mortality in Nepal using helping babies breathe. Pediatrics 2016;137(6).

18. Kruk ME, Gage AD, Arsenault C, et al. High-quality health systems in the Sustainable Development Goals era: time for a revolution. Lancet Glob Health 2018; 6(11):e1196–252.

19. Moxon SG, Guenther T, Gabrysch S, et al. Service readiness for inpatient care of small and sick newborns: what do we need and what can we measure now? J Glob Health 2018;8(1):10702.

20. Zaka N, Alexander EC, Manikam L, et al. Quality improvement initiatives for hospitalised small and sick newborns in low- and middle-income countries: a systematic review. Implement Sci 2018;13(1):20.

21. Bartels SM, Haider S, Williams CR, et al. Diversifying implementation science: a global perspective. Glob Health Sci Pract 2022;10(4).

22. Singhal N, Berkelhamer S. For helping babies survive. Essential care for small babies: action plan. American Academy of Pediatrics. Laerdal Global Health; 2015.

23. Bose C, Singhal N. For helping babies survive. Essential care for every baby: action plan. American Academy of Pediatrics. Laerdal Global Health; 2014.

24. Perlman JM, Velaphi S, Massawe A, et al. Achieving country-wide scale for helping babies breathe and helping babies survive. Pediatrics 2020;146(Suppl 2): S194–207.

25. Msemo G, Massawe A, Mmbando D, et al. Newborn mortality and fresh stillbirth rates in Tanzania after helping babies breathe training. Pediatrics 2013;131(2): e353–60.

26. Bellad RM, Bang A, Carlo WA, et al. A pre-post study of a multi-country scale up of resuscitation training of facility birth attendants: does Helping Babies Breathe training save lives? BMC Pregnancy Childbirth 2016;16(1):222.

27. Goudar SS, Somannavar MS, Clark R, et al. Stillbirth and newborn mortality in India after helping babies breathe training. Pediatrics 2013;131(2):e344–52.

28. Versantvoort JMD, Kleinhout MY, Ockhuijsen HDL, et al. Helping Babies Breathe and its effects on intrapartum-related stillbirths and neonatal mortality in low-resource settings: a systematic review. Arch Dis Child 2020;105(2):127–33.

29. Patterson J, Niermeyer S, Lowman C, et al. Neonatal resuscitation training and systems strengthening to reach the sustainable development goals. Pediatrics 2020;146(Suppl 2):S226–9.

30. Merali HS, Visick MK, Amick E, et al. Helping babies survive: lessons learned from global trainers. Pediatrics 2020;146(Suppl 2):S134–44.

31. KC A, Wrammert J, Nelin V, et al. Evaluation of Helping Babies Breathe Quality Improvement Cycle (HBB-QIC) on retention of neonatal resuscitation skills six months after training in Nepal. BMC Pediatr 2017;17(1):103.

32. Ersdal HL, Vossius C, Bayo E, et al. A one-day "Helping Babies Breathe" course improves simulated performance but not clinical management of neonates. Resuscitation 2013;84(10):1422–7.

33. Gurung R, Gurung A, Sunny AK, et al. Effect of skill drills on neonatal ventilation performance in a simulated setting- observation study in Nepal. BMC Pediatr 2019;19(1):387.

34. Tabangin ME, Josyula S, Taylor KK, et al. Resuscitation skills after Helping Babies Breathe training: a comparison of varying practice frequency and impact on retention of skills in different types of providers. Int Health 2018;10(3):163–71.

35. Rule ARL, Tabangin M, Cheruiyot D, et al. The Call and the challenge of pediatric resuscitation and simulation research in low-resource settings. Simul Healthc 2017;12(6):402–6.

36. Wrammert J, Sapkota S, Baral K, et al. Teamwork among midwives during neonatal resuscitation at a maternity hospital in Nepal. Women Birth 2017; 30(3):262–9.

37. KC A. Neonatal Resuscitation: understanding challenges and identifying a strategy for implementation in Nepal. Uppsala: Department of Women's and Children's Health, Uppsala University; 2016.

38. Enweronu-Laryea C, Dickson KE, Moxon SG, et al. Basic newborn care and neonatal resuscitation: a multi-country analysis of health system bottlenecks and potential solutions. BMC Pregnancy Childbirth 2015;15(Suppl 2):S4.

39. West F, Bokosi M. Helping babies survive and empowering midwives and nurses to provide quality newborn care. Pediatrics 2020;146(Suppl 2):S223–5.

40. Niermeyer S, Kamath-Rayne B, Keenan W. American Academy of Pediatrics, Laerdal Global Health 2016.

41. Kamath-Rayne BD, Thukral A, Visick MK, et al. Helping Babies Breathe, second edition: a model for strengthening educational programs to increase global newborn survival. Glob Health Sci Pract 2018;6(3):538–51.

42. Mduma E, Ersdal H, Svensen E, et al. Frequent brief on-site simulation training and reduction in 24-h neonatal mortality–an educational intervention study. Resuscitation 2015;93:1–7.

43. Rule ARL, Maina E, Cheruiyot D, et al. Using quality improvement to decrease birth asphyxia rates after 'Helping Babies Breathe' training in Kenya. Acta Paediatr 2017;106(10):1666–73.

44. World Health Organization, American Academy of Pediatrics, Laerdal Global Health. Essential Newborn Care Course, 2nd edition. Geneva2022.

45. KC A, Peterson SS, Gurung R, et al. The perfect storm: disruptions to institutional delivery care arising from the COVID-19 pandemic in Nepal. J Glob Health 2021; 11:5010.

46. Laerdal Global Health. Helping Mothers and Babies Survive, hmbs.org. Norway2021.

47. American Academy of Pediatrics and Laerdal Global Health. Essential Newborn Care Now! United States2021.

48. Savich RDNS, Meseret Y, Tabansi PN, et al. Covid 19: mitigating impact on neonatal mortality through remote training and support in Nigeria. Denver: Colorado Pediatric Academic Societies; 2022.

49. Molla MAM HL, Hattar N, Alex-Adeomi M, et al. Mitigating Impact on Neonatal Mortality utilising digital tools to enhance Neonatal Resuscitation knowledge & skills among skilled birth attendants in Rohingya Refugee camps of Cox's Bazar, Bangladesh. Annual Scientific Conference. Belfast, Ireland: Royal College of Emergency Medicine; 2022.

50. Tessema M, Tesfay S, Grønbæk A, et al. Essential newborn care (ENC) Digital Training: a feasibility study of teaching methods and practice frequency. Consortium of Universities in Global Health; 2021.

51. Every newborn action plan 2015-2030. Geneva: World Health Organization and UNICEF; 2014.

52. WHO technical consultation on newborn health indicators: every newborn action plan metrics. Geneva: World Health Organization; 2015.

53. Lawn JE, Blencowe H, Oza S, et al. Every Newborn: progress, priorities, and potential beyond survival. Lancet 2014;384(9938):189–205.

54. Mason E, McDougall L, Lawn JE, et al. From evidence to action to deliver a healthy start for the next generation. Lancet 2014;384(9941):455–67.

55. Day LT, Sadeq-Ur Rahman Q, Ehsanur Rahman A, et al. Assessment of the validity of the measurement of newborn and maternal health-care coverage in hospitals (EN-BIRTH): an observational study. Lancet Glob Health 2021;9(3): e267–79.

56. Foglia EE, Davis PG, Guinsburg R, et al. Recommended guideline for uniform reporting of neonatal resuscitation: the neonatal Utstein style. Pediatrics 2023; 151(2). e2022059631.

57. Otto Q, Nolan JP, Chamberlain DA, et al. Utstein Style for emergency care - the first 30 years. Resuscitation 2021;163:16–25.

58. Bose C, Hermida J, For Survive & Thrive Global Development Alliance. Improving care of mothers and babies: a guide for improvement teams. American Academy of Pediatrics, University Research Co LLC; 2016.

59. Weinberg S, Jones D, Worku B, et al. Helping babies survive training programs: evaluating a teaching Cascade in Ethiopia. Ethiop J Health Sci 2019;29(6): 669–76.

60. Perez K, Patterson J, Hinshaw J, et al. Essential Care for Every Baby: improving compliance with newborn care practices in rural Nicaragua. BMC Pregnancy Childbirth 2018;18(1):371.

61. Patterson J, Worku B, Jones D, et al. Ethiopian Pediatric Society Quality Improvement Initiative: a pragmatic approach to facility-based quality improvement in low-resource settings. BMJ Open Qual 2021;10(1).

62. Fink G, Ross R, Hill K. Institutional deliveries weakly associated with improved neonatal survival in developing countries: evidence from 192 Demographic and Health Surveys. Int J Epidemiol 2015;44(6):1879–88.

63. Tura G, Fantahun M, Worku A. The effect of health facility delivery on neonatal mortality: systematic review and meta-analysis. BMC Pregnancy Childbirth 2013;13:18.

64. Chaka EE, Mekurie M, Abdurahman AA, et al. Association between place of delivery for pregnant mothers and neonatal mortality: a systematic review and meta-analysis. Eur J Public Health 2020;30(4):743–8.

65. Berwick DM, Nolan TW, Whittington J. The triple aim: care, health, and cost. Health Aff 2008;27(3):759–69.

66. Sikka R, Morath JM, Leape L. The Quadruple Aim: care, health, cost and meaning in work. BMJ Qual Saf 2015;24(10):608–10.

67. Merali HS, Hemed M, Fernando AM, et al. Telementoring initiative for newborn care providers in Kenya, Pakistan and Tanzania. Trop Med Int Health 2022; 27(4):426–37.

68. Bernstein HH, Calabrese T, Corcoran P, et al. The power of Connections: AAP COVID-19 ECHO accelerates responses during a public health emergency. J Public Health Manag Pract 2022;28(1):E1–8.

69. Joshi S, Gali K, Radecki L, et al. Integrating quality improvement into the ECHO model to improve care for children and youth with epilepsy. Epilepsia 2020;61(9): 1999–2009.

70. Arora S, Thornton K, Murata G, et al. Outcomes of treatment for hepatitis C virus infection by primary care providers. N Engl J Med 2011;364(23):2199–207.

71. Health sector transformation plan II (HSTP II) 2020/21 - 2024/25. Ethopia: Ethopia MoH; 2021.
72. National healthcare quality and safety bulletin. Integrated people-centered health services: the pathways for better clinical outcomes and confidence in the system. Ethopia: UNICEF & MoH Ethopia; 2021.
73. Worku B. The 6th Ethiopian annual health care quality and safety summit proceeding people-centered and integrated health services: the pathways for better clinical outcomes and confidence in the system. Ethopia: Ethopia MoH-; 2020. p. 6–7.
74. Bucher SL, Cardellichio P, Muinga N, et al. Digital health innovations, tools, and resources to support helping babies survive programs. Pediatrics 2020;146(Suppl 2):S165–82.
75. Rent SJA, Johnson J. Improving delayed cord clamping in Addis Ababa, Ethiopia: a virtual partnership experience between the American Academy of Pediatrics and the Ethiopian Pediatrics Society. US: Convention AAoPN; 2022.
76. Stevenson AG, Tooke L, Edwards EM, et al. The use of data in resource limited settings to improve quality of care. Semin Fetal Neonatal Med 2021;26(1):101204.
77. Ehret DEY AM, Worku B, Musyoka E, et al. The development of an objective structured clinical examination (OSCE) for respiratory distress syndrome (RDS) in Ethiopia: a learning and assessment tool for neonatal continuous positive airway pressure (CPAP). Brussels: Grand Challenges Exposition; 2022.
78. Wandersman A, Chien VH, Katz J. Toward an evidence-based system for innovation support for implementing innovations with quality: tools, training, technical assistance, and quality assurance/quality improvement. Am J Community Psychol 2012;50(3–4):445–59.
79. Hanna M, Sittenthaler AM. Cash, non-cash, or mix? Gender matters! The impact of monetary, non-monetary, and mixed incentives on performance. J Bus Econ 2020;90.
80. Carmichael SL, Mehta K, Raheel H, et al. Effects of team-based goals and non-monetary incentives on front-line health worker performance and maternal health behaviours: a cluster randomised controlled trial in Bihar, India. BMJ Glob Health 2019;4(4):e001146.
81. Bhattarai P, Gurung R, Basnet O, et al. Implementing quality improvement intervention to improve intrapartum fetal heart rate monitoring during COVID-19 pandemic- observational study. PLoS One 2022;17(10):e0275801.
82. Institute of Medicine (US). In: Olsen L, Aisner D, McGinnis JM, editors. Roundtable on evidence-based medicine. The learning healthcare system: workshop summary. Washington (DC): National Academies Press (US); 2007.
83. Ersdal HL, Singhal N, Msemo G, et al. Successful implementation of helping babies survive and helping mothers survive programs-an Utstein formula for newborn and maternal survival. PLoS One 2017;12(6):e0178073.
84. Chinbuah MA, Taylor M, Serpa M, et al. Scaling up Ghana's national newborn care initiative: integrating 'helping babies breathe' (HBB), 'essential care for every baby' (ECEB), and newborn 'infection prevention' (IP) trainings. BMC Health Serv Res 2020;20(1):739.

Measuring Equity for Quality Improvement

Nina Menda, MD, MHQS[a],*, Erika Edwards, PhD, MPH[b,c,d]

KEYWORDS

- NICU • Quality improvement • Equity • Disparities • Measurement

KEY POINTS

- Health disparities are pervasive in the United States, including in perinatal care.
- The first step in addressing equity is acknowledging that disparities exist, which requires measurement.
- Measuring equity in support of quality improvement is possible and should be done to ensure that disparities are being addressed, not magnified.

BACKGROUND

The landmark report "Crossing the Quality Chasm,"[1] published by the Institute of Medicine in 2001, promoted equity as one of 6 fundamental pillars of quality health care. Equity is defined as providing care that does not vary in quality because of personal characteristics such as gender, ethnicity, race, geographic location, and socioeconomic status. Despite the call to action in "Crossing the Quality Chasm," disparities in health-care delivery continue to be rampant within the United States (US). A devastating example of racial/ethnic health disparity is infant mortality. In 2020, the US had an infant mortality rate (IMR) of 5.4 deaths per 1000 live births, much higher than comparable countries across the world; however, in 2019, the IMR of Black infants was more than double that of White infants (10.6 vs 4.5 deaths per 1000 live births).[2] The preterm delivery rate is nearly 50% higher for Black compared with White birthing parents.[3] Black infants are 4 times more likely to die due to younger gestational ages and low birth weights, contributing to the high Black IMR.[4]

Every 10 years, the US Department of Health and Human Services and Office of Disease Prevention and Health Promotion release data-driven national objectives to improve health and well-being during the next decade; the most recent is Healthy

[a] Department of Pediatrics, University of Wisconsin, 202 South Park Street, McConnell Hall, 4th Floor, Madison, WI 53715, USA; [b] Vermont Oxford Network, Burlington, VT 05401, USA; [c] Department of Pediatrics, Robert Larner, MD, College of Medicine, University of Vermont, Burlington, VT 05405, USA; [d] Department of Mathematics and Statistics, College of Engineering and Mathematical Sciences, University of Vermont, Burlington, VT 05405, USA
* Corresponding author.
E-mail address: menda@wisc.edu

Clin Perinatol 50 (2023) 531–543
https://doi.org/10.1016/j.clp.2023.01.010
perinatology.theclinics.com
0095-5108/23/© 2023 Elsevier Inc. All rights reserved.

People 2030.[5] An overarching goal of Healthy People 2030 aims to "eliminate health disparities, achieve health equity, and attain health literacy to improve the health and well-being of all." Healthy People 2030 defines health equity as "the attainment of the highest level of health for all people." A key strategic component to promote health equity includes utilization of data to track health disparities to inform program and policy development.

Unfortunately, health disparities cross the perinatal spectrum and extend into the neonatal intensive care unit (NICU). A 2019 systematic review revealed complex racial/and or ethnic disparities in common structure, process, and outcome measures in NICU populations, including intraventricular hemorrhage, necrotizing enterocolitis, and retinopathy of prematurity.[6] Racial/ethnic disparities have also been noted in antenatal corticosteroid administration and human breast milk feeding at discharge between Black and White infants.[7,8] A recent study of very low birth weight (VLBW) infants across the Vermont Oxford Network (VON) from 2015 to 2019 revealed minority infants scored higher on outcome measures but lower on process measures, potentially reflecting organizational and institutional biases.[9] Studies have demonstrated that Black and Hispanic babies are more likely to receive care in NICUs with lower quality ratings, with segregation being a contributing factor.[10–12] Infants of color are more likely to be born at NICUs that score lower on process and structural measures, predisposing them to receiving a lower quality of health care. Factors such as primary language[13,14] and household income[15] also influence the care infants may receive in the NICU.

In 2011, Profit and colleagues developed a framework to assess NICU quality of care using the Baby-MONITOR composite quality metric.[16,17] Composite measures combine "two or more individual measures into a single measure that results in a single score" as defined by the National Quality Forum.[18] Because composite measures are multidimensional, they provide an overview of the quality of care delivered within an NICU. An examination of the Baby-MONITOR metric across California demonstrated significant racial and ethnic variation in the quality of care *within* NICUs.[19] In 2021, the Baby-MONITOR composite measure was used to identify differences in the quality of care, by race and ethnicity across and within 737 NICUs in the US. This study confirmed that the alarming patterns observed in California were similar on a national scale.[9]

Quality of care is a crucial and potentially modifiable factor that contributes to disparities affecting outcomes of very preterm infants.[20] Accurate and meaningful data is critical to efforts to improve health equity. In this review, we will demonstrate the value of measuring health equity, delineate potential data sources, describe data analysis methods, and subsequently explain how to move from data to action to address health disparities.

Value of Measurement

Health-care inequities are pervasive in the US and result in worse outcomes for Black, Indigenous, and people of color.[21,22] The first step in addressing equity is acknowledging that disparities exist, which requires measurement. Disparity and equity expand beyond race and ethnicity and reflect differences between the most advantaged group versus the least advantaged group in a particular category,[23] including geography, language, payor status, education, religion, gender, sexual orientation, and socioeconomic status.

Measuring inequities can help identify whether an intervention will improve outcomes evenly and equally across the population or will have a greater impact in an advantaged or disadvantaged group. Improving outcomes evenly across the population can perpetuate disparities, whereas improving outcomes in an advantaged population can widen a disparity gap and improving outcomes in a disadvantaged population can narrow a gap.[24] (**Fig. 1**) Applying an equity lens to quality improvement (QI) by collecting, reviewing, and using data that are stratified by potential inequities can address these issues.

Data Sources for Stratifying Measures by Potential Inequities

Electronic medical records (EMRs) are one source of data on health inequities that can be used by individual NICUs. Although the scope of social determinants of health data included in the EMR is limited, the EMR does typically include data on race and insurance status, which can be used to examine inequities in care. However, accessing that data can be challenging. Chart review is commonly used but is extremely time and labor intensive. Recently, data exploration tools, such as Epic's Slicer/Dicer, have been incorporated into the EMR to facilitate data queries. Additionally, institutional healthcare informatics departments can assist in building data reports that examine quality measures stratified by potential inequities.

Other data sources may have information on race and ethnicity that is more easily accessible. Registry data from state-based perinatal quality collaboratives or international databases such as the VON database, can be used to examine inequities in key neonatal process and outcomes. VON members abstract standardized data from chart review. Participating NICUs have access to comprehensive real-time reports to serve as the foundation for local QI projects and improvement opportunities and can stratify all measures by race and ethnicity (**Fig. 2**).[25,26] Similarly, California (**Fig. 3**), Massachusetts, and Illinois are reporting data by race, ethnicity, and other social determinants of health,[27] which help teams benchmark disparities within and between NICUs.

Claims-based databases including Vizient Clinical Data Base/Resource Manager, Premier Healthcare Database, Pediatric Health Information System (PHIS), or the National Perinatal Information Center's (NPIC) Perinatal Center Database (PCDB) can also be used to examine quality of care stratified by potential inequities.[28] Vizient

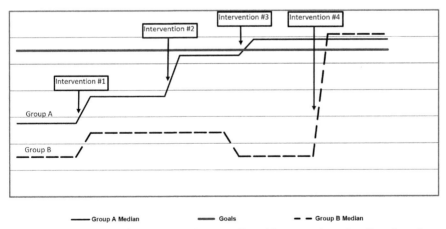

Fig. 1. Possible impact of QI interventions on disparities over time. Baseline data shows Group A performing better than Group B but both groups are well below the goal. After Intervention #1, Groups A and B benefitted equally. After Intervention #2, Group A continued to demonstrate improvement but Group B remained unchanged, widening disparities. After Intervention #3, Group A continued to improve performance, while Group B had decreased performance, further amplifying existing disparities. After Intervention #4, the gap between Group A and B began to narrow and both groups achieved the goal.

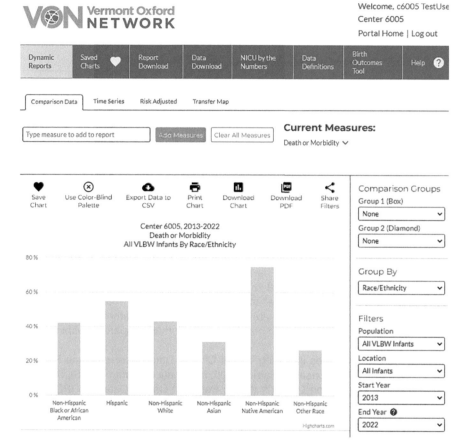

Fig. 2. Screenshot of VON's Nightingale Internet Reporting System with death or morbidity for all very-low-birth-weight infants stratified by race and ethnicity.

contains patient-level and hospitalization level data from more than 95% of academic medical centers and affiliated hospitals across the country. Vizient provides benchmarking data to guide health-care resource utilization.[29] Premier Healthcare Database is one of the largest US inpatient billing and discharging databases, capturing one-seventh of all US inpatient hospitalizations including demographic and billing information.[30] The PHIS offers comparative clinical and resource utilization data for inpatient, ambulatory surgery, emergency department, and observation unit encounters from more than 45 children's hospitals and can be used to examine inequities. NPIC's PCDB focuses on obstetric and newborn care.[31] Variables include hospital identifier, admission and discharge date, age, race, payor, zip code, birth weight, diagnosis, procedure codes, and charges. Each measure can be compared against individual hospital performance, subgroup performance, 5-year trends, NPIC database trends, and other national benchmarks.[28] NPIC also uses case-mix adjustment. Performance feedback utilizing claims data is frequently suggested to promote data-driven QI. Specific measures include NICU admissions, length of stay, and readmissions, all of which have limitations as quality measures. Although claims data may be helpful in examining trends over extended periods (quarterly or annually), it is severely limited by timely feedback for real-time continuous QI.

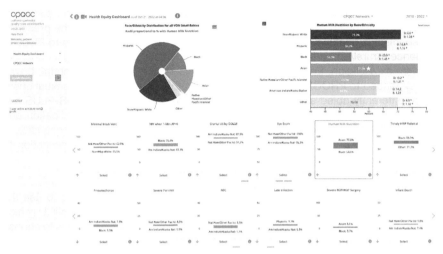

Fig. 3. Screenshot of California Perinatal Quality Collaborative's Health Equity Dashboard stratified by race and ethnicity for Human Milk Nutrition.

One measurement strategy that can be used to bolster data on equity issues is to map external data sources to patients' addresses using geocoding. Tools such as the Child Opportunity Index have been used to examine acute care utilization for children with medical complexity[32] and high-risk infant follow-up program participation.[33] Neighborhood geospatial data have been used to understand neonatal morbidity and mortality[34] and provision of breast milk at discharge among very-low birth weight infants.[35] The California Perinatal Quality Care Collaborative created extensive neighborhood-level databases describing population, socioeconomic status, built environment, businesses, retail food and restaurant environments, and traffic, and added these neighborhood-level measures to a dashboard for its members.[36]

Although not every NICU has access to such extensive data, in the US, nonprofit hospitals must do community health needs assessments every 3 years that represent the broad interests of the community served by the hospital.[37] The results of every hospital's needs assessment will be different but demographic data, which are reported routinely in these assessments, describe the population using the hospital including the NICU. Community health needs assessments are often found on hospital websites; see UnityPoint Health Meriter Hospital (https://www.unitypoint.org/madison/community-health-needs-assessment.aspx [38]) as one example. Community health needs assessments are multifactorial, and frequently include community survey data, provider survey data, key stakeholder interviews, community input sessions, evaluation of health outcomes, community resources, and access to care. Identifying and working with the team conducting the needs analysis and applying the data collected in these needs assessments to stratify unit level metrics using social determinants of health measures can help inform QI efforts.

Challenges with Equity Data

Available measures do not capture the full spectrum of factors contributing to inequity

As previously described, there is a range of data sources that can be used to examine quality of care for potential inequities; however, these data sources typically include data on a limited range of factors that can result in disparities. Several frameworks have been developed delineating factors that contribute to variations in health outcomes. The acronym PROGRESS was developed in 2003 to highlight the presence of disparities in health outcomes beyond income.[39,40] PROGRESS refers to Place of residence (rural/urban/inner city), Race/ethnicity/culture/language, Occupation, Gender/sex, Religion, Education, Socio-economic status, and Social capital. It was later expanded to PROGRESS-PLUS, to include other features such as sexual orientation, differently abled status, age, and immigration status. PROGRESS-PLUS has been used in systematic reviews as a framework to support data stratification and examine health outcomes for disparities. To be able to fully measure inequities in care delivery and outcomes, existing databases need to expand data collection to include more of these attributes.

Defining the metric for comparing groups

There are different methods to choosing a comparison group.[41] One is to use the context-specific majority population, such as the majority population in a NICU (which may be different from the majority population in another context). Another is to choose the "best off" group, or the group with the lowest rates. That will likely mean having a different comparison group for each measure, which is not ideal. A third option is to choose a fixed or target rate, such as from published literature, or the population average. A fourth option is to use a rate from an earlier time point in the same group. Ultimately, the choice of a comparison group should be based on the question that the QI initiative is trying to address and will require careful team discussion of the pros and cons of each option.

Reliability and validity of equity-related data

Establishing the validity and reliability of equity-related data can be challenging. Self-reported data, such as items collected with social determinants of health screening tool, may have response bias. Further, data on social determinants of health, aside from race and insurance status, are rarely stored in electronic health records, and social determinants of health data that are stored often suffer from accuracy and misclassification.[42] Combining sources, such as EMR data and birth certificates, can improve misclassification[43] and help impute missing data. Neonatal databases such as the VON database, and partners that use its definition, specify that race and ethnicity information is to be obtained "by personal interview with the mother or review of the birth certificate or medical record, in that order of preference."[44] Such specificity could improve reliability if site abstractors consistently follow the definition.

Analysis Methods

Understanding between group variation

Whether using data from data aggregators, community health needs assessments, or chart review, every NICU can and should evaluate process and outcome measures stratified by race and ethnicity. However, to identify disparities, NICUs need to understand between group variation. One method is to use absolute or relative differences. The absolute difference is excess risk in one group compared with another group. For example, the excess risk in preterm birth between African American women (12.2%) and White women (7.4%) in 2020 was 4.8%. The relative difference is a measure of the probability of an event occurring in one group compared with another group. The relative difference in preterm birth rates was 12.2% divided by 7.4% or 1.65; African American women were 1.65 times more likely to experience preterm birth than White women. Relative risk summarizes 2 numbers into one but conceals the absolute risks in each group; absolute risk may be easier to interpret for that reason. Major NICU databases provide infant-level data stratified by race and ethnicity that can be used to calculate absolute or relative risk. Small sample sizes overall and within groups will be a challenge for most NICUs but can be addressed by aggregating data over multiple years.

Stratifying run and control charts in quality improvement efforts

Stratifying run charts or statistical process control charts by groups can help evaluate the effects of QI interventions and identify if the intervention is perpetuating, reducing, or amplifying disparities (**Fig. 4**). Another advantage of stratification is not having to choose a comparison group (see **Fig. 4**A, B). Again, teams should interpret results with caution if sample sizes are small, or aggregate time points to create bigger groups. Some QI interventions may require collecting race, ethnicity, language, socioeconomic status, or other data as part of the project to evaluate disparities.

Monitoring of disparities on a local equity dashboard

One mechanism to highlight racial and ethnic inequalities in preterm birth includes the creation of a NICU health equity dashboard. As more emphasis is placed on addressing disparities in health care, the value of using health equity dashboards has increasingly become apparent. Dashboards influence behavioral change to drive QI, help prioritize specific projects, and assist with data visualization; they act as powerful communication tools for clinical staff and hospital administration. Most importantly, dashboards facilitate regular monitoring of data critical for effective decision-making.[45] Dashboards provide real-time feedback, which is necessary to drive improvement. Measurements displayed on dashboards can also promote accountability within organizations and highlight strategic goals. **Fig. 5** shows an example of an NICU equity dashboard developed by UnityPoint Health Meriter to track areas with the potential for disparities. It is updated and reviewed quarterly to provide feedback to clinical teams and hospital administration to monitor and drive change. Children's Minnesota has developed a similar Pediatric Health Equity Dashboard to promote equitable, disparities-targeted QI interventions and drive organizational transparency on health inequities.[46] Health equity dashboards have demonstrated success in driving improvements.[47]

Moving from Data to Action to Reduce Inequities

Once measurement has occurred and gaps identified, then QI methodology can be used to address and potentially eliminate modifiable disparities. QI efforts affect

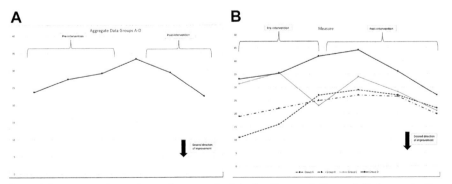

Fig. 4. (A) Annotated run chart of aggregate data for Groups A through D demonstrating improvement after an intervention. (B) Annotated run chart in which data was stratified by groups, demonstrating disparities, particularly between Groups A and D. The intervention resulted in improvement for all groups and demonstrated a decrease in disparity gaps.

NICU (A) Clinical Quality & Operations Dashboard FY 21						
Clinical Quality						
	Q1	Q2	Q3	Q4	FY 21 Target (VON 2020 Median)	NICU (A) FY 20 Scores
Measure	NICU (A)	NICU (A)	NICU (A)	NICU (A)		
Readmissions within 7 days of discharge from NICU ("n")	0%	0%	0%	1.1% (n=2)	0	0
% Black infants discharged home from NICU on any human milk (admitted < 7 days; discharged before 120 days - expanded VON database)	62.7%	61%	70%	50%	>/=80%	70.0%
% Black VLBW infants discharged home from NICU on any human milk (admitted <7days; discharged before 120 days)	50.0%	38%	50%	55%	>/=70%	50.0%
% Black infants admitted to the NICU	18%	12%	17%	15%	14%	16.80%

Fig. 5. Example of NICU Equity Dashboard used by an individual NICU. The first column lists the measure of interest with the percent meeting the measure represented on a quarterly basis. Measures of interest include key outcomes for the most disadvantaged group. The sixth column shows the prior fiscal year's (FY) VON Median and the last column shows the prior fiscal year (FY) performance.

different populations differently and a uniform approach can unintentionally widen disparity gaps. In theory, when health-care quality improves across the board, disadvantaged groups that suffer from lower quality care have the most to gain. Despite best intentions, such outcomes are not guaranteed. Thus, initiatives to improve quality and reduce disparities should be carefully integrated to ensure success of reducing disparities.[48] Interventions may need to be tailored to specific characteristics of vulnerable groups, or they may need to address social determinants of health. An "intervention-generated inequality" can occur when an intervention disproportionately benefits an advantaged group due to improved accessibility, adoption, adherence, or efficacy.[24,49] QI models need to establish equity as a cross-dimensional theme of every component of quality.[50] Because quality and equity are codependent, true QI cannot be achieved without addressing disparities. Equity must be an explicit goal of every QI initiative. Teams can also move to developing SMARTIE goals that include Inclusive and Equitable with the traditional Specific, Measurable, Achievable, Relevant, Time-bound (SMART) framework. The inclusive goal ensures that marginalized people will be included in processes, activities, and decision-making in a way that shares power while the equitable goal seeks to address systemic injustice or inequity by including an element of fairness. SMARTIE goals specify how the project will advance equity in tactics, benchmarks, or metrics while ensuring that the project will not create or perpetuate disparities.

There are several examples in the literature that support the role of QI methodology in reducing disparities.[51–53] In 2015, Dereddy and colleagues utilized a multipronged approach to improving breast milk feeding rates from 22% to 88% in VLBW infants in a largely Black population. Interventions included increased training for staff and mothers, electric pump distribution to mothers, and increased lactation consultant support.[54] Woods and colleagues targeted low-income children with asthma, decreasing emergency department visits, hospitalizations, and hospital costs, along with days of limited physical activity, missed school, and missed work.[55] A QI collaborative reduced the relative risk in severe maternal morbidity from hemorrhage between Black and White mothers from 1.33 (1.16–1.52) to 0.99 (0.76–1.29); the collaborative did not have a stated goal of reducing the difference but because severe maternal morbidity from hemorrhage was higher in Black women, the collaborative had a larger impact in that group.[56]

QI is only truly effective by involving key stakeholders, including families of color and community organizations. Engaging community organizations strengthens the effectiveness of interventions and assist in rebuilding trust with health-care systems.

When jointly developed, interventions are more likely to meet the needs of the community, as in the case of childhood asthma and immunization rates.[57]

In 2012, Chin and colleagues described a 6-step roadmap to reduce disparities.[58] The first step of this process is directly related to measurement, which is to recognize disparities and commit to reducing them by stratifying performance data by race, ethnicity, and language. The second step recommends implementation of a basic QI methodology by creating a multidisciplinary team to address identified disparities. The third step highlights the importance of making equity an integral component of QI efforts by recognizing equity as a cross-dimension of quality. The fourth step relates to designing the intervention to account for root causes and contextual contributions to disparities. A key component of designing interventions includes input from families of marginalized groups and nonhealth-care partners. The fifth and sixth steps include implementation, evaluation, and adjustment of the intervention and, if effective, sustainment of the intervention. The National Quality Forum convened a multidisciplinary group to develop a similar roadmap to address health equity with a 4-pronged approach: identify and prioritize areas to reduce health disparities, implement evidence-based interventions to reduce disparities, invest in the development and utilization of health equity performance measures, and incentivize the reduction of health disparities and achievement of health equity.[59] Using these frameworks, individual NICUs can identify opportunities to improve equity and the quality of care.

BEST PRACTICES

We recommend individual NICUs evaluate their own outcome data through the lens of racial equity and search for gaps using national, state, or local data. Teams should try to understand the reliability and validity of the race and ethnicity data they use and should be aware of the sample sizes in each group, aggregating over multiple time points as needed. Teams should discuss the choice of a comparison group and how to measure between-group variation. Once disparities are identified, QI methodology can be applied to decrease variation and improve the quality of care for all infants. Stratifying run charts by race and ethnicity will help teams understand if they are ameliorating or aggravating disparities. We must continue to address health-care inequities with QI because every baby deserves the opportunity to achieve the best outcome possible.

CLINICS CARE POINTS

- Individual NICUs should evaluate their own outcome data through the lens of racial equity.
- It is critical to understand the validity of race and ethnicity data, with particular awareness of sample size and the need to aggregate multiple points to search for equity gaps.
- When designing interventions to improve quality, consider if those interventions may exacerbate existing disparities.

DECLARATION OF INTERESTS

E. Edwards receives salary support from Vermont Oxford Network.

ACKNOWLEDGMENTS

The authors acknowledge Dr Jochen Profit for sharing the California Perinatal Quality Collaborative's Health Equity Dashboard for inclusion in this article. The authors also acknowledge Dr Gabrielle Hester for giving us permission to include Children's Minnesota Pediatric Health Equity Dashboard.

REFERENCES

1. Baker A. Crossing the quality chasm: a new health system for the 21st century. Washington, DC: The National Academies Press; 2001.
2. Infant mortality. Division of reproductive health, national center for chronic Disease prevention and health promotion. Available at: https://www.cdc.gov/reproductivehealth/maternalinfanthealth/infantmortality.htm#mortality. Published 2022. Accessed 7/13, 2022.
3. Osterman MJ, Hamilton BE, Martin JA, et al., Births: final data for 2020. 2022 March of Dimes Report Card. Available at: www.marchofdimes.org/sites/default/files/2022-11/March-of-Dimes-2022-Full-Report-Card.pdf. Accessed February 27, 2023.
4. Riddell CA, Harper S, Kaufman JS. Trends in differences in US mortality rates between black and white infants. JAMA Pediatr 2017;171(9):911–3.
5. Healthy people 2030 framework. U.S. Department of Health and Human Services; 2022. Available at: https://health.gov/healthypeople/priority-areas/health-equity-healthy-people-2030. Accessed 07/13, 2022.
6. Sigurdson K, Mitchell B, Liu J, et al. Racial/ethnic disparities in neonatal intensive care: a systematic review. Pediatrics 2019;144(2).
7. Lee HC, Lyndon A, Blumenfeld YJ, et al. Antenatal steroid administration for premature infants in California. Obstet Gynecol 2011;117(3):603.
8. Lee HC, Gould JB. Factors influencing breast milk versus formula feeding at discharge for very low birth weight infants in California. J Pediatr 2009;155(5):657–62. e652.
9. Edwards EM, Greenberg LT, Profit J, et al. Quality of care in US NICUs by race and ethnicity. Pediatrics 2021;148(2). e2020037622.
10. Morales LS, Staiger D, Horbar JD, et al. Mortality among very low-birthweight infants in hospitals serving minority populations. Am J Publ Health 2005;95(12):2206–12.
11. Howell EA, Hebert P, Chatterjee S, et al. Black/white differences in very low birth weight neonatal mortality rates among New York City hospitals. Pediatrics 2008;121(3):e407–15.
12. Horbar JD, Edwards EM, Greenberg LT, et al. Racial segregation and inequality in the neonatal intensive care unit for very low-birth-weight and very preterm infants. JAMA Pediatr 2019;173(5):455–61.
13. Brignoni-Pérez E, Scala M, Feldman HM, et al. Disparities in kangaroo care for premature infants in the neonatal intensive care unit. J Dev Behav Pediatr 2022;43(5):e304–11.
14. Palau MA, Meier MR, Brinton JT, et al. The impact of parental primary language on communication in the neonatal intensive care unit. J Perinatol 2019;39(2):307–13.
15. Bourque SL, Weikel BW, Palau MA, et al. The association of social factors and time spent in the NICU for mothers of very preterm infants. Hosp Pediatr 2021;11(9):988–96.
16. Profit J, Gould J, Zupancic J, et al. Formal selection of measures for a composite index of NICU quality of care: baby-MONITOR. J Perinatol 2011;31(11):702–10.

17. Profit J, Zupancic JA, Gould JB, et al. Correlation of neonatal intensive care unit performance across multiple measures of quality of care. JAMA Pediatr 2013; 167(1):47–54.
18. National Quality Forum. Composite measure evaluation framework and national voluntary consensus standards for mortality and safety—composite measures: a consensus report. Washington, DC: NQF; 2009.
19. Profit J, Gould JB, Bennett M, et al. Racial/ethnic disparity in NICU quality of care delivery. Pediatrics 2017;140(3):e20170918.
20. Beck AF, Edwards EM, Horbar JD, et al. The color of health: how racism, segregation, and inequality affect the health and well-being of preterm infants and their families. Pediatr Res 2020;87(2):227–34.
21. Matthew DB. Just medicine: a cure for racial inequality in American health care. New York, NY: NYU Press; 2018.
22. Gee GC, Ford CL. Structural racism and health inequities: old issues, New Directions1. Du Bois Rev 2011;8(1):115–32.
23. Braveman P. Health disparities and health equity: concepts and measurement. Annu Rev Public Health 2006;27:167–94.
24. Reichman V, Brachio SS, Madu CR, et al. Using rising tides to lift all boats: Equity-focused quality improvement as a tool to reduce neonatal health disparities. Semin Fetal Neonatal Med 2021;26(1):101198.
25. Horbar JD. The Vermont Oxford Network: evidence-based quality improvement for neonatology. Pediatrics 1999;103(Supplement_E1):350–9.
26. Edwards EM, Ehret DE, Soll RF, et al. Vermont Oxford Network: a worldwide learning community. Transl Pediatr 2019;8(3):182.
27. Mason CL, Collier CH, Penny SC. Perinatal quality collaboratives and birth equity. Curr Opin Anaesthesiol 2022;35(3):299–305.
28. Rochin E, Reed K, Rosa A, et al. Perinatal quality and equity—indicators that address disparities. J Perinat Neonatal Nurs 2021;35(3):E20–9.
29. Mahendra M, Steurer-Muller M, Hohmann SF, et al. Predicting NICU admissions in near-term and term infants with low illness acuity. J Perinatol 2021;41(3):478–85.
30. Hardy JR, Pimenta JM, Pokras S, et al. Risk of hospitalization for common neonatal morbidities in preterm and term infants: assessing the impact of one or more major congenital anomalies. J Perinatol 2019;39(12):1602–10.
31. Wright LL, Papile LA. US neonatal databases: methods and uses. Seminars in Neonatology 1997;2(3):159–69.
32. Fritz CQ, Hall M, Bettenhausen JL, et al. Child Opportunity Index 2.0 and acute care utilization among children with medical complexity. J Hosp Med 2022; 17(4):243–51.
33. Fraiman YS, Stewart JE, Litt JS. Race, language, and neighborhood predict high-risk preterm Infant Follow up Program participation. J Perinatol 2022;42(2): 217–22.
34. Janevic T, Zeitlin J, Egorova NN, et al. Racial and economic neighborhood segregation, site of delivery, and morbidity and mortality in neonates born very preterm. J Pediatr 2021;235:116–23.
35. Romaine A, Clark RH, Davis BR, et al. Predictors of prolonged breast milk provision to very low birth weight infants. J Pediatr 2018;202:23–30. e21.
36. Padula AM, Shariff-Marco S, Yang J, et al. Multilevel social factors and NICU quality of care in California. J Perinatol 2021;41(3):404–12.
37. Lopez L, Dhodapkar M, Gross CP. US nonprofit hospitals' community health needs assessments and implementation strategies in the era of the patient protection and affordable care act. JAMA Netw Open 2021;4(8):e2122237.

38. UnityPoint Health Meriter Community Needs Assessment. Available at: https://www.unitypoint.org/madison/community-health-needs-assessment.aspx. Accessed October 29, 2022.

39. O'Neill J, Tabish H, Welch V, et al. Applying an equity lens to interventions: using PROGRESS ensures consideration of socially stratifying factors to illuminate inequities in health. J Clin Epidemiol 2014;67(1):56–64.

40. Evans T, Brown H. Road traffic crashes: operationalizing equity in the context of health sector reform. Inj Control Saf Promot 2003;10(2):11–2.

41. Harper S, Lynch J. Methods for Measuring Cancer Disparities: Using Data Relevant to Healthy People 2010 Cancer-Related Objectives. In: NCI Cancer Surveillance Monograph Series, Number 6. Bethesda, MD: National Cancer Institute; 2005.

42. Cook LA, Sachs J, Weiskopf NG. The quality of social determinants data in the electronic health record: a systematic review. J Am Med Inf Assoc 2022;29(1):187–96.

43. Smith N, Iyer RL, Langer-Gould A, et al. Health plan administrative records versus birth certificate records: quality of race and ethnicity information in children. BMC Health Serv Res 2010;10(1):1–7.

44. Vermont Oxford Network Manual of Operations: Part 2. Data definitions and infant data booklet, 2021, Burlington, VT.

45. Randell R, Alvarado N, McVey L, et al. Requirements for a quality dashboard: Lessons from National Clinical Audits. AMIA Annu Symp Proc 2020;2019:735–44.

46. Hester G, Nickel AJ, Griffin KH. Accountability through measurement: using a dashboard to address pediatric health disparities. Pediatrics 2020;146(6). e2020024448.

47. Blagev DP, Barton N, Grissom CK, et al. On the journey toward health equity: data, culture change, and the first step. NEJM Catal Innov Care Deliv 2021; 2(7):1–17.

48. Weinick RM, Hasnain-Wynia R. Quality improvement efforts under health reform: how to ensure that they help reduce disparities—not increase them. Health affairs 2011;30(10):1837–43.

49. Veinot TC, Mitchell H, Ancker JS. Good intentions are not enough: how informatics interventions can worsen inequality. J Am Med Inf Assoc 2018;25(8):1080–8.

50. Cook SC, Goddu AP, Clarke AR, et al. Lessons for reducing disparities in regional quality improvement efforts. Am J Manag Care 2012;18(6 0):s102.

51. Fox P, Porter PG, Lob SH, et al. Improving asthma-related health outcomes among low-income, multiethnic, school-aged children: results of a demonstration project that combined continuous quality improvement and community health worker strategies. Pediatrics 2007;120(4):e902–11.

52. Mangione-Smith R, Schonlau M, Chan KS, et al. Measuring the effectiveness of a collaborative for quality improvement in pediatric asthma care: does implementing the chronic care model improve processes and outcomes of care? Ambul Pediatr 2005;5(2):75–82.

53. Szilagyi PG, Schaffer S, Shone L, et al. Reducing geographic, racial, and ethnic disparities in childhood immunization rates by using reminder/recall interventions in urban primary care practices. Pediatrics 2002;110(5):e58.

54. Dereddy NR, Talati AJ, Smith A, et al. A multipronged approach is associated with improved breast milk feeding rates in very low birth weight infants of an inner-city hospital. J Hum Lactation 2015;31(1):43–6.

55. Woods ER, Bhaumik U, Sommer SJ, et al. Community asthma initiative: evaluation of a quality improvement program for comprehensive asthma care. Pediatrics 2012;129(3):465–72.
56. Main EK, Chang S-C, Dhurjati R, et al. Reduction in racial disparities in severe maternal morbidity from hemorrhage in a large-scale quality improvement collaborative. Am J Obstet Gynecol 2020;223(1):123. e121–e123. e114.
57. Chin MH, Alexander-Young M, Burnet DL. Health care quality-improvement approaches to reducing child health disparities. Pediatrics 2009;124(Supplement_3): S224–36.
58. Chin MH, Clarke AR, Nocon RS, et al. A roadmap and best practices for organizations to reduce racial and ethnic disparities in health care. J Gen Intern Med 2012;27(8):992–1000.
59. National Quality Forum. A roadmap for promoting health equity and eliminating disparities: the four I's for health equity. Available at: https://www.qualityforum.org/Publications/2017/09/A_Roadmap_for_Promoting_Health_Equity_and_Eliminating_Disparities__The_Four_I_s_for_Health_Equity.aspx. Accessed February 27, 2023.

Moving?

Make sure your subscription moves with you!

To notify us of your new address, find your **Clinics Account Number** (located on your mailing label above your name), and contact customer service at:

Email: journalscustomerservice-usa@elsevier.com

800-654-2452 (subscribers in the U.S. & Canada)
314-447-8871 (subscribers outside of the U.S. & Canada)

Fax number: 314-447-8029

Elsevier Health Sciences Division
Subscription Customer Service
3251 Riverport Lane
Maryland Heights, MO 63043

*To ensure uninterrupted delivery of your subscription, please notify us at least 4 weeks in advance of move.